THE NATIONAL HEALTH SERVICE IN SCOTLAND

THE NATIONAL HEALTH SERVICE IN SCOTLAND

ORIGINS AND IDEALS, 1900–1950

Morrice McCrae

TUCKWELL PRESS

First published in Great Britain in 2003 by
Tuckwell Press Ltd
The Mill House
Phantassie
East Linton
East Lothian, Scotland

ISBN 1 86232 216 3

The publishers acknowledges the generous support of
the Scotland Inheritance Fund
in the publication of this volume

A catalogue record for this book is available
on request from the British Library

Typeset by Hewer Text Ltd, Edinburgh
Printed and bound by Cromwell Press, Trowbridge, Wiltshire

Contents

List of Illustrations

List of Tables and Figures

Abbreviations

BHA   British Hospitals Association
BMA   British Medical Association
BMJ   British Medical Journal
CAB   Cabinet
DC   University of Glasgow Archive
HC   House of Commons
EHS   Emergency Hospital Scheme
EMS   Emergency Medical Service
HIMS   Highlands and Islands Medical Service
IMR   Infant Mortality Rate
LCC   London County Council
LHB   Lothian Health Board Archive
MMR   Maternity Mortality Rate
MOH   Medical Officer of Health
NAS   National Archives of Scotland
NHI   National Health Insurance
NHS   National Health Service
PEP   Political and Economic Planning
PRO   Public Record Office
RCPE   Royal College of Physicians of Edinburgh
SCEC   Scottish Central Emergency Committee

Introduction and Acknowledgements

In 1948, two National Health Services were created in Britain. The National Health Service Act, 1946 that set up the National Health Service in England and Wales did not apply to Scotland. The National Health Service was established separately by the National Health Service (Scotland) Act, 1947. On introducing the Bill in the House of Commons in December 1946, the Secretary of State for Scotland stressed that it was a Scottish Bill and that its revision and approval would be for the Scottish Grand Committee.

That there should be two separate Acts was accepted at the time almost without comment, and over the years commentators on the National Health Service have paid little or no attention to the separate existence of two services operating in parallel yet retaining quite distinctive characteristics. No published history has yet explained how services in the two countries came to be so different or how the histories of the creation of the two services relate to each other. In one of the most authoritative histories, John Pater wrote that 'in Scotland the National Health Service has a history peculiar to itself.'[1] As he acknowledged, as a senior member of the Ministry of Health in the 1940s, he was not witness to the making of the National Health Service in Scotland.

In the official history of the National Health Service, Charles Webster dismisses the separate legislation for Scotland as no more than a late modification of the National Health Service Bill for England and Wales, made in March 1946, to 'permit [its] adaptation to the characteristic administrative and geographical conditions of Scotland.' Since no other historian has yet offered an alternative, Webster's assessment has come to be widely accepted.

My experience of the National Health Service, on both sides of the border, began as a medical student within months of the Appointed Day in July 1948. Over more than fifty years I have found the differences between the two services, in ethos and in practice, to be too fundamental to allow the dismissive official history of their separation to stand. The purpose of this book is to offer an account of the origins of the National Health Service as was seen in Scotland.

As Richard Titmuss has observed, 'when we study welfare systems we see

1 J. E. Pater, *The Making of the National Health Service* (London, 1981).

that they reflect the dominant cultural and political characteristics of their societies.'[2] In the 1920s and 1930s, the cultural and political circumstances of Scotland were not those of England. Scotland was then a proletarian society with an established culture of poverty. Scotland had its own long-established medical services and institutions and a quite different medical tradition. It also had a deep sense of nationalism and a separate health bureaucracy. In the depths of the Depression, the Department of Health for Scotland openly acknowledged that the existing medical services were inadequate and must be reformed. In 1936, the Department published, in the Cathcart Report, a plan for the introduction of a comprehensive state health service. That plan represented a consensus in Scotland and, by the early years of the Second World War, much of it had already been implemented.

Between the wars, the Ministry of Health failed to recognise the extent of the deficiencies in health care in England and Wales and no effective co-operation had been established among the medical services in England and Wales. When, in 1942, the Government's acceptance of the Beveridge Report suddenly committed it to the creation of a state health service, the Ministry of Health had no plan of its own. A scheme for England and Wales had to be put together in some haste. Agreement was difficult to reach, and as its official historian has observed, in the path towards the NHS for England and Wales there was 'a notable lack of consensus.'[3]

This book discusses the social conditions, political actions and medical traditions that put Scotland at the forefront of the development of the National Health Service on both sides of the border. The structure of the book was suggested by the speech made by the Secretary of State for Scotland when he introduced the National Health Services (Scotland) Bill for its Second Reading in the House of Commons on 10 December 1946. He informed the House that the comprehensive state health service success-fully operated by the Highlands and Islands (Medical Service) since 1913 had provided 'the necessary pointers' towards a comprehensive service for the whole country.[4] He also made it clear that it was the Cathcart Report[5] that had provided the basis for the Scottish Bill presented in 1946.

The Highlands and Islands Medical Service (HIMS) is discussed as the forerunner of – as a potential pilot study for – the National Health Service,

2 B. Abel-Smith and R. Titmuss, *The Philosophy of Welfare* (London, 1987).
3 C. Webster, *The National Health Service: A Political History* (Oxford, 1998), p. 3.
   Webster first commented that there had 'been little sign of consensus', in Webster, 1988, *op. cit.*, p. 28. In a hostile review, D. M. Fox, in 'Anti-intellectual History?', *Social History of Medicine*, iii, 1990, pp. 101–105, claimed that the assertion had been made with insufficient evidence. In the same issue of the journal Webster reasserted the judgement quoted here.
4 *Hansard*, xlxxxi, HC 10 December 1946, col. 998.
5 Report of the Committee on Scottish Health Services, 1939, Cmd. 5204.

not only for Scotland, but for England and Wales. The Archive of the Royal College of Physicians of Edinburgh has provided important material relating to the medical services in the Highlands and Islands in the nineteenth century and on the formation of the HIMS. The records of the Highland parishes were studied in the archives of the Highland Council in Inverness.

The greater part of the book takes the Cathcart Report as the framework for a discussion of the development of Scotland's devolved health bureaucracy, its response to the unique health and social problems of Scotland and the influence of traditions of the medical profession in Scotland – the essential elements in the separate development of health services in Scotland.

The papers relating to the formation and the deliberations of the Cathcart Committee were destroyed as a fire precaution at St. Andrew's House early in the Second World War. However, there are many published reports of the Scottish Board of Health, the Department of Health for Scotland and the Registrar General for Scotland that have not previously been used in this context. With a few referenced exceptions, the statistics quoted are all taken from these sources.

Invaluable material has been found in the archives of the University of Edinburgh, the University of Glasgow, the Scottish Record Office (now the National Archives of Scotland), the Public Record Office, the Royal College of Physicians of Edinburgh, the Royal College of Surgeons of Edinburgh, and the Royal College of Physicians and Surgeons of Glasgow. In London, the archives of the Royal College of Physicians of London, the British Medical Association, the General Medical Council and the Royal Medical Society have also proved very helpful. I am most grateful for the generous efforts made on my behalf by the archivists and staff of all these bodies.

I am indebted to those civil servants, administrators, nurses and doctors who had taken part in the planning and establishment of the NHS in the 1940s and who agreed to be interviewed. Their evidence, recorded on tape,[6] has been invaluable in assessing the attitudes, circumstances and events in Scotland before and during the Second World War and at the introduction of the new service in 1948. I am particularly indebted to those former senior civil servants who carried major responsibilities for the creation of the structure of the NHS in Scotland.

Ekkeharde von Kuenssberg, a general practitioner in Edinburgh and the first President of the Royal College of General Practitioners, has allowed me to read his unpublished autobiography. The papers of Sir Douglas Haddow, private secretary to the Secretary of State for Scotland during the

---

6 The tapes are now in the Archive of the Royal College of Physicians of Edinburgh.

Second World War, were kindly lent by his son. Professor James Williamson has contributed a number of valuable papers relating to the control of tuberculosis.

In setting the context for the new material presented in this book it has been necessary to consult and refer to a large number of secondary sources and these have been acknowledged and listed in the bibliography.

In carrying out the research and in the preparation of this book, I have enjoyed the guidance and encouragement of John Brown of the Department of History, University of Edinburgh who has shown great kindness and understanding to a neophyte converting to a new discipline. Michael Barfoot, Steve Sturdy, Malcolm Nicolson and Roger Davidson have been sound and ready sources of advice. I am also deeply grateful to Ian Milne, Librarian of the Royal College of Physicians of Edinburgh and his staff, for their constant and willing help. I have also had the expert assistance of Emily Naish, Archivist of the BMA, James Beaton, Librarian of the Royal College of Physicians and Surgeons of Glasgow, Professor Michael Moss, Archivist of the University of Glasgow, Margaret Gladden of the Department of Physiology, University of Glasgow and Robert Steward, Archivist of the Highland Council.

Over many months, I have been sustained by the interest and encouragement of the Senior Fellows of the Royal College of Physicians of Edinburgh. The opinions and conclusion are mine but they have been tested and influenced by many conversations with friends and former colleagues.

I

The Highlands and Islands Medical Service

On 12 July 1913 Parliament voted £42,000 to fund Britain's first comprehensive state medical service. Within a few years the Highland and Islands Medical Service (HIMS) had earned a 'high reputation internationally and locally'[1] as a well organised and administered medical service giving 'medical care of high quality to the people.'[2] In 1946, when presenting the National Health Service (Scotland) Bill to the House of Commons, the Secretary of State for Scotland acknowledged the part played by the HIMS in 'carrying us forward to the health services of today' and in providing 'the necessary pointers towards . . . a full and comprehensive service in Scotland.'[3]

This groundbreaking service has gone almost unnoticed by historians of the National Health Service (NHS). However, in her *History of Scotland*, Rosalind Mitchison briefly noticed the Highlands and Islands Medical Service as 'a forerunner of the National Health Service.'[4] But in what sense was it a forerunner? For over forty years, the HIMS was seen as relevant only to its own time and place. Only after the Second World War was it recognised that the HIMS offered 'pointers toward a full and comprehensive health service'[5] and that closer attention to its organisation and development might have corrected some of the unrealistic assumptions made in the planning of the National Health Service.

Early in the twentieth century the Highlands and Islands had 'become something of a laboratory for administrative and legislative experiments' in Britain since 'it is in these remote districts that experimental remedies may, with comparative impunity, be tried.'[6] In 1913, the people of the Highlands and Islands provided an ideal population for a great social experiment – the introduction of a comprehensive state medical service.

However, the HIMS was not set up as a social experiment. It was created as an expedient to overcome difficulties in implementing the National Insurance Act in the crofting community of the Highlands and Islands. The

1 *The Lancet*, i, 1950, p. 580.
2 *Ibid.*
3 *Hansard*, xlxxxi, HC 10 December 1946, col. 996.
4 R. Mitchison, *A History of Scotland* (London, 1982), p. 415.
5 *Hansard*, 10 December 1946, *op. cit.*
6 J. Day, *Public Administration in the Highlands and Islands of Scotland* (London, 1918), p. 6.

object of Lloyd George's Act was to give much needed protection to the industrial workforce from the extremes of poverty during periods of cyclical unemployment. As presented in 1911, the National Insurance Bill provided for the compulsory contributory insurance of all manual workers – both men and women – between the ages of sixteen and seventy, who were employed under a contract of service. It also provided for the insurance, on a voluntary basis, of anyone who was wholly or mainly dependent for his livelihood on some regular occupation and whose annual income did not exceed £160.[7] Together the employee and the employer were to pay 7d a week (6d for women); the state added a contribution of 2d. Voluntary contributors were required to pay both the employee's and the employer's contributions. For each contributor to the scheme the financial benefits were to be operated by the Approved Society (Friendly Society, Trade Union or Industrial Insurance Company) of which he or she was a member. Those who were not members of an Approved Society – generally assumed to be 'the very poorest of the poor'[8] – were to be insured as Deposit Contributors in an arrangement administered by the Post Office. Although Lloyd George's Insurance scheme was principally intended to protect against poverty, contributors also became entitled to a medical benefit. This was to take the form of such medical attendance, treatment and medicines as would normally be provided by a general practitioner together with Maternity Benefit (as a sum of money) and an ill-defined right to treatment for tuberculosis.

Those responsible for drawing up the Bill 'realised from the beginning that there were various categories of employed people, for whom by reason of their occupation, the general conditions of the scheme would need modification.'[9] The population of the Highlands and Islands of Scotland made up one such category.

The Crofting Community as a Special Case

The Highlands and Islands made up a unique part of Britain. Remote and almost untouched by industrialisation, it was populated very largely by crofters and landless cottars. In 1884, an inquiry into the condition of the people[10] had led in 1886 to the Crofters Holdings Act which established a Crofters Commission to administer the distribution and settlement of the land on which too many crofters were struggling to find space to provide for

---

7 This provision was intended to protect 'white collar' workers on low incomes.
8 *Hansard*, xxxi, HC 21 November 1911, col. 921.
9 W. J. Braithwaite, quoted by Sir Leslie Mackenzie, *Lancet*, ii, 1928, p. 105.
10 *Report of the Inquiry into the Condition of the Crofters and Cottars of the Highlands and Islands of Scotland*, 1884, Cd. 3980 (Napier Report).

their families. The Crofting Counties, the area designated for this special administrative provision, comprised Shetland, Orkney, Caithness, Sutherland, Ross and Cromarty, Inverness and Argyll. For the purposes of the Act a crofter was defined as a 'small farmer with or without a lease, who finds in the cultivation of his holding a material portion of his occupation, earnings and sustenance and who pays rent to the proprietor.' This definition of 'crofter' was further defined as tenants paying £30 or less per annum in rent, although in practice few crofters had holdings carrying rents of over £6.[11]

In 1851, Sir John McNeil, the Chairman of the Board of Supervision in Scotland, had estimated that, to provide a living for a family, a croft ought to have at least 10 acres with access to grazing.[12] But he had to accept that there was not enough arable land available to the crofting population for this to be possible. In 1886 the Crofters Holdings Act set the minimum size of a croft at six acres. On plots of this size crofters could barely maintain their families unless supported by cash income from other seasonal work or from contributions from the wages of family members who had found employment away from the croft. Since crofters, with their peculiar form of rural economy, made up the bulk of the population, the idea of the Highlands and Islands as a special case deserving special treatment was already established in the minds of British policy makers well before the introduction of the National Insurance Bill in 1911.

Almost by definition crofters were poor. In 1911 a weekly contribution of even a few pennies to the National Insurance Scheme represented an unaffordable proportion of a very low cash income. It was almost unknown for crofters to be members of Friendly Societies or subscribers to industrial insurance companies. Medical Associations – in which a small membership fee had entitled the member and his family to the services of a general practitioner – had been introduced in the Highlands and Islands in the nineteenth century and in the most prosperous areas a few had survived, at least for a time. But in most cases Associations had been formed, the initial fees paid and doctors engaged, but had then failed as members found it impossible to keep up the required cash payments. In 1911 the proposed compulsory weekly contribution to the state insurance scheme promised to be equally impossible.

This was not the only problem. Since neither crofters nor cottars were generally members of an Approved Friendly Society or contributors to an Approved Industrial Insurance Company, it was only open to them to join the National Insurance scheme as Deposit Contributors. As Deposit Con-

---

11 J. Hunter, *The Making of the Crofting Community* (Edinburgh, 1976).
12 F. Gillanders, 'The West Highland Economy,' *The Transactions of the Gaelic Society of Inverness*, 1962, p. 257.

tributors they were at a great disadvantage. While the Approved Societies operated by collecting contributions from a very large number of contributors to create a fund from which each contributor could draw at times of need, in the Post Office scheme there was no such accumulation of a common fund. The scheme for Deposit Contributors operated on a 'dividing out' basis; the contract was not lifelong but annual. If a subscriber failed to continue his contribution, his right to benefits, including medical benefit, expired at the end of the current year. This anomaly was discussed in the House of Commons during the Committee stage of the National Insurance Bill in November 1911. 'The Post Office contributor has no benefit from the principle of insurance at all – absolutely none from beginning to end.'[13] For those in the working population of the Highlands and Islands who had a formal contract of employment the National Insurance therefore presented great difficulties. Even more were excluded from the scheme entirely; crofters were self-employed in the cultivation of their land and rarely had formal contracts for any other employment they could find.

There were those in the working population in other parts of Britain who shared these objections to the National Insurance Act.[14] But in one vital circumstance the people of the Highlands and Islands were unique. As was pointed out in the House of Commons, even when 'they pay their contributions weekly they will not be able to derive any medical benefit whatever.'[15] The necessary local general practitioner services were not to be found in the Highlands and Islands.

Since the eighteenth century the old military Gaelic society and its clan structure had been dissolved and transformed. A new society had grown up in the Highlands and Islands without a middle class, the class that in other societies 'held a middle station by which the highest and lowest orders were connected.'[16] It was at last acknowledged that the traditional concept that the lands occupied by a clan were the common property of the people was no more than a myth. In reality it had long been a case of ruler-owns-all. Clan chiefs were now recognised as landed gentlemen, legal owners of vast estates. However, it soon became apparent that the estates were grossly overpopulated and burdened by an obsolete agricultural economy. Many estates were bankrupt and almost all urgently required new investment to make them commercially viable. Some of the old aristocratic families raised the necessary funds by selling part of their estates; others sold out

13 Sir A. Cripps. *Hansard*, 21 November 1911, *op. cit*, col. 923.
14 The problems as experienced in the Lowland farming community were illustrated by the incident of the 'Turra Coo.' A. Fenton, *The Turra Coo* (Aberdeen, 1989).
15 *Hansard*, 21 November 1911, *op. cit.*, col. 919.
16 Samuel Johnson, in A *Journey to the Western Highlands of Scotland*.

completely, usually to men who had made fortunes overseas or in the new industries of the south. This new generation of owners introduced modern agricultural practices to the best of their arable land and gave over other vast acres to profitable sheep runs. In this restructured agricultural system there was a place only for landowners, their large tenants and a greatly reduced agricultural workforce. Employment could only be found for the few; the great majority of the population of the Highlands and Islands was now redundant. A few of the minor gentry stayed to become large tenant farmers but most found that they could only maintain their lifestyle by moving away. A very few of the ordinary people became large tenant farmers and many more – those who could find the means – emigrated in the hope of a new and better life in the south or in North America.[17] However, the mass of the population, unwanted in the new agricultural economy, were allowed to remain as small crofters or cottars on the least productive land on the margins of the great estates.

As the middle classes disappeared from the Highlands and Islands, so also did their medical attendants. By the end of the eighteenth century the people 'of education and considerable endowments'[18] were too few to provide employment for more that a very small number of medical practitioners. The ordinary people were very often obliged to look to the few educated men of the parish – the minister, the schoolmaster or the factor – for medical aid.[19] Most educated families owned a copy of William Buchan's *Domestic Medicine* and many parish ministers had prepared themselves for the role of irregular medical practitioner while at university. This amateur aid was willingly given and often valuable in the absence of professional medical help.

Medical Services Before 1913

Toward the end of the nineteenth century, as communications improved and commercial contacts with the south brought some degree of prosperity, professional medical men began to find their way to the Highlands and Islands. For a time it was possible to establish modest practices, at least in the market towns and larger villages. Then, in the economic depression that came with the end of the Napoleonic wars, poverty in the

17 In 1803, Dorothy Wordsworth found that 'they talked of emigration as a glorious thing for those who had money.' D. Wordsworth, *Recollections of a Tour in Scotland* (Yale, 1997), p. 91.

18 Samuel Johnson, *op. cit.*

19 'My own means have been considerably tested in the way of giving medicine to my poor practitioners – and not only medicine but food for the nourishment of the sick,' Rev. Augustus Macintyre of Kinlochbervie, letter to Dr. J. Coldstream, Royal College of Physicians of Edinburgh, 8 April 1851. RCPE Archive.

Highlands and Islands deepened once more. Numbers of medical practitioners could no longer make ends meet and were forced to leave. In 1845, Sir John McNeil hoped the Poor Law (Scotland) Amendment Act – which required parochial boards to provide medical attendance for the paupers on their Poor Rolls – would ensure that there would be at least one doctor in every parish.[20] However, many parishes could not afford to employ a medical officer and the exodus of doctors continued. From 1848 the scheme based on the Poor Law received financial encouragement from central government. An annual Treasury grant of £10,000 (Medical Relief Grant) was made available in Scotland to subsidise any parishes hoping to appoint a medical officer. This again proved unsuccessful in reversing the drift of doctors from the Highlands and Islands.[21] In 1851 an inquiry by the Royal College of Physicians of Edinburgh found that only 62 of the 170 parishes in the Highlands and Islands had a resident medical practitioner. Many parishes were precariously served by practitioners travelling from some distance and '41 were never, or almost never visited by any regular practitioner and could therefore be regarded as destitute of medical aid.'[22]

In the second half of the century, opportunities for private practice continued to decline and payment received for parochial duties soon came to make up the greater and the essential part of the Highland medical practitioners' income. New Public Health legislation increased the scope of their parochial employment. Parish practitioners could become vaccination officers,[23] public health officers[24] and, from 1908, there were opportunities in the new School Medical Service. In recognition of these expanding local services the Medical Relief Grant had been increased to £20,000 in 1882. But even with these additional possible sources of income, new doctors could not be attracted to the Highlands and Islands and many parishes still went without the medical services they so obviously needed.

In 1883, when the Napier Commission investigated the living conditions of over 300,000 people scattered over the 14,000 square miles of the region, they were served by only 103 qualified medical practitioners, 30 fewer than in 1851.[25] The following decades brought no improvement and it was this

20 Sir John McNeil, letter to the Royal College of Physicians of Edinburgh. Quoted in the Report of a Committee of the College, 3 February 1852. RCPE Archive.
21 M. McCrae, 'The Great Highland Famine; The Lack of Medical Aid,' *Review of Scottish Culture*, 14, 2002, pp. 58–73.
22 Royal College of Physicians of Edinburgh, *Statement Regarding the Existing Deficiency of Medical Practitioners* (Edinburgh, 1852).
23 Vaccination (Scotland Act), 1863.
24 Public Health (Scotland) Act, 1867; Local Government (Scotland) Act, 1894.
25 Report of the Inquiry into the Condition of the Crofters and Cottars of the Highlands and Islands of Scotland, 1884 Cmd. 3980 (Napier Report).

persisting scarcity of doctors in the Highlands and Islands that led Cathcart Wason[26] to protest, during the Committee stage of the National Insurance Bill, that contributors in the Highlands and Islands would be unable to benefit from the NHI scheme 'simply because of the impossibility of getting medical officers.'[27]

While the British Medical Association (BMA) in London was in very public and acrimonious dispute with the Treasury as it campaigned to secure the financial position of its more prosperous general practitioners in the south,[28] the lack of sufficient numbers of general practitioners in the Highlands and Islands was being overlooked. As the *Edinburgh Medical Journal* explained:

> In all the criticism which has been showered on the National Insurance Bill we have not observed any dealing with the exceptional position of the medical men in the Highlands and Islands of Scotland. It may be that those who are familiar with the conditions of practice in those remote districts recognise that no feasible amendments of the proposed Act would really touch the question. There are districts where no capitation grant which, even in his most conciliatory mood the Chancellor could agree to, would keep body and soul together and the smallest wage limit which has been suggested would have no terrors for the ordinary crofter. He has no employer and his employees are his own family. The whole contribution, then, would fall directly on him and he has no sevenpences to spare. If there ever was a case for exceptional treatment the Highlands provide it. The districts are enormous, the population very thin and very poor, and means of communication are few. The present conditions are terribly hard on those members of the profession who do their best in difficult circumstances. When conditions are exceptional, remedies must be exceptional too.[29]

On 11 July 1912 the Chancellor of the Exchequer set up a committee to consider 'how far the provision of medical attention in districts situated in the Highlands and Islands of Scotland is inadequate and to advise on the best method of securing a satisfactory medical service therein.'[30] The members of the committee (Dewer Committee) all had personal knowledge and

26 Member of Parliament for a Glasgow constituency.
27 *Hansard*, xxx, HC 1 November 1911, col. 919.
28 The BMA, afraid of mass defection of patients from the private practices of its more prosperous members, proposed that the service should be limited to those earning less that £140 per annum.
29 *Edinburgh Medical Journal*, vii, 1911, p. 100.
30 *Report of the Highlands and Islands Medical Service Committee* (Dewer Report), 1912, Cd. 6559.

experience of conditions in the Highlands.[31] Of its nine members, Dr. Leslie Mackenzie had been largely responsible for the investigations of the Royal Commission on Physical Training in 1903, and Dr John McVail had provided much of the medical evidence for the Report of the Royal Commission on the Poor Law of 1909.

As evidence of the inadequacy of medical services, the Dewer Committee quoted the large number of uncertified deaths in the Highlands and Islands. In many parishes the proportion was over 40% and in one parish it reached 80%. The Dewer Committee was in no doubt that this 'high percentage of uncertified deaths is due to lack of medical attendance, and that no medical service can be regarded as adequate where such neglect still obtains.' It reported that 'on account of the sparseness of the population in some districts, and its irregular distribution in others, the configuration of the country, and the climatic conditions, medical attendance is uncertain for the people, exceptionally onerous or even hazardous for the doctor, and generally inadequate.'

In 1912, the problem was getting worse. While the number of doctors in the Crofting Counties had not increased in the previous thirty years, for the parishes, the cost of even that number had become a more and more pressing problem. The annual Treasury grant to Scotland's Medical Relief Fund was still being made but increasingly the resources of the Fund were being diverted to improve the appalling conditions in the cities. The subsidy to support services in rural parishes was being correspondingly diminished. Faced by a decreasing income and the increasing expenditure demanded by new mandatory public health measures, ratepayers in the Highlands and Islands were becoming less willing to subsidise the treatment of patients who were not the registered paupers for whom the parish was legally responsible. Parishes could afford fewer rather than more doctors. Parish funds could certainly not provide the subsidies that would be required to support the number of doctors necessary to ensure the provision of the medical benefit of the NHI Scheme to the whole working population of the Crofting Counties.

The most radical solution proposed to the Dewer Committee came from the Highland doctors themselves. They were in general agreement that 'the present moment is ripe for the inauguration of a complete State medical service. Such a scheme is a coming event all over the country in the near

31 The Committee members were Sir John Dewer, MP for Inverness; the Marchioness of Tullibardine; J. C. Grierson, Convenor of the County of Shetland; A. Lindsay, Convenor of the County of Sutherland; Dr. Leslie Mackenzie, Medical Member, Local Government Board for Scotland; Dr. J. McVail, Deputy Chairman, Scottish Insurance Commission; Dr. A. Miller, Medical Officer for the Parish of Kilmallie; C. Orrocks, Chamberlain of the Lews; J. Robertson, Senior Chief Inspector of Schools for Scotland.

future ... The starting of such a service in the Highlands could be done with less opposition and much less friction than in the more densely populated parts of the country ... Both doctors and the public would favour such a form of medical service.'[32]

However, the Dewer Committee looked to less radical but more pragmatic and ingenious measures. It recognised that the inadequacy of medical provision was not due to an absolute shortage in the total number of general practitioners, though there were obviously too few in some districts. (The Highlands and Islands, with 6% of Scotland's population, had 5.6% of Scotland's doctors.[33]) However, the geography of the region made it impossible for this number of doctors to have effective access to a very scattered population.

The Dewer Commission was critical of the quality as well as the number of the medical practitioners. Over the years there had been many eager recruits from Scotland's eight medical schools but the turnover had been rapid. In the more remote parishes in particular, doctors often remained perhaps only for a year before moving on. The Committee took a somewhat unsympathetic view of those who chose to remain. In its judgement the majority of the doctors seemed to fall into two classes:

a) Young men recently out of college who make the appointment merely a stepping stone to something better, who remain only a year or two and b) Older men, who after perhaps a chequered career, fall back on such places as a last resort and harbour of refuge. While to the capable man, who, from inclination or perhaps the force of circumstances, elects to spend his life in these regions, the most hopeful outlook before him is to die in harness, in case he dies of starvation when old age and decrepitude render him incapable of work.

The Dewer Committee attributed the failure to recruit adequate numbers of competent and reliable doctors to the 'defective means of locomotion and communication and to the variety of conditions vitally affecting the welfare of the profession, which conditions in turn are calculated to discourage the average practitioner in the exercise of his profession and to prevent him from rendering services commensurate with the need of the people.' No doctor in the Highlands could easily afford to buy a car or a motor boat although in many cases he needed both.[34] There was no reliable telephone service. Doctors' houses were unsatisfactory 'both as regard accommodation

---

32 Dewer Report. Minutes of Evidence, 1913, Cmd. 6920, Minute 19,718.
33 M. W. Dupree and A. Crowther, 'A Profile of the Medical Profession in Scotland', *Bulletin of the History of Medicine*, lxv, 1991, p. 209.
34 It had long been the practice of many doctors to hire a horse, a horse and buggy or a boat only when required.

and situation.' Doctors had no security of tenure; 'the Parish Council has absolute power of dismissal and cases were cited where the Council appears to have acted harshly.' 'That the average income of the medical profession was low, those who know the Highlands and Islands intimately were well aware, but we were not prepared to hear that so many medical men were eking out a living, and some of them trying to educate a family, on incomes well below the limit of income tax.' Incomes were so low that the average doctor could not take a holiday, or take advantage of post-graduate courses because the cost of a locum was beyond his means. In his evidence to the Commission the Statistical Officer at Register House, Dr. J. C. Dunlop, suggested that general practitioners should have a guaranteed net income of £400, with housing and travelling expenses, to bring them into line with medical officers in the Colonial medical services. ('It is as great banishment to go to some of these places as to go to Borneo. Being stranded at Barra for the winter, or at Coll or Tiree, is not very tempting to a man with ambition.') In 1912, there were many doctors in the Highlands and Islands earning less than £100 a year. In many cases 'in order to subsist he must continue in harness long after he is fit to discharge his duties efficiently.'

Shortage of good doctors was not the only deficiency. The Dewer Committee was impressed by the volume of evidence, both from doctors and members of the public, that 'no matter affecting the welfare of the people of the Highlands and Islands is more urgent than the provision of an adequate supply of trained nursing.' However, the total number of nurses at that time was quite inadequate and the efficiency of the existing nursing services suffered from an almost complete lack of organisation.

In the second half of the nineteenth century the formation of Nursing Associations had become a favourite charitable enterprise for the wives of landowners in the Highlands. For an annual subscription of between 2 shillings and 10 shillings members were entitled to free nursing services; the nurse's services were also available to non-members at a small fee. The nurses first recruited by the Associations were either Cottage Nurses, with at least six months' experience in a recognised hospital, or Maternity Nurses, usually widows who had received three months' training in midwifery. After 1897, nurses for these Associations were usually found through the agency of Queen Victoria's Jubilee Institute of District Nursing. The Institute required high standards of training; nurses were only accepted after three years' hospital experience and a further period of training in the care of the sick poor in their own homes. The annual cost to the local associations for the employment of a Queen's Jubilee nurse varied from £80 to £90 from which the nurse received a standard annual salary of £35. In some parishes a house was provided, otherwise the nurse was allowed 10 shillings a week for lodgings. A bicycle was provided for transport. Special effort was made to find nurses for the parishes rarely visited by a doctor. In these remote parishes they served an important educational function, teaching basic sanitation and nutrition, as well as performing the practical nursing duties of caring for the sick and injured. However, in 1912, very few parishes could afford a nurse trained to this standard.

The Dewer Committee also found that the existing general hospital provision was quite inadequate even when used to its full capacity, which usually it was not. In spite of the known inadequacies in medical and nursing services most treatment, whether of illness or injury, had to be managed at home. In 1850 the only hospitals serving the crofting counties had been at Kirkwall and at Inverness, both at the periphery of the area and accessible to only a very few of its people. Later in the century, the cottage hospital movement had established 16 small hospitals across the Crofting Counties, each with an average of eight beds. Two larger hospitals of 22 beds had been opened at Oban and at Lerwick, and at Inverness (the town was not officially in the Crofting Counties) the Northern Infirmary of 68 beds provided services for the Crofting Counties of the northeast. But travel to hospital was difficult and patients were reluctant to leave home for treatment of uncertain benefit and in an alien environment. As a result the few hospital beds available in the Highlands were very often left empty. Only the most desperately ill were willing to travel. In 1912 patients from the West Coast requiring modern hospital treatment had to endure the sea journey to Greenock or Glasgow Royal Infirmaries and patients from the Orkneys and Shetland faced the long journey to Aberdeen or Edinburgh. The majority in need of hospital treatment opted to remain in their own part of the world in spite of its lack of modern hospital services. The Dewer Committee's answer to this problem was that the local hospitals should be improved.[35] More cottage hospitals should be built 'a) to bring near to the doctor a distant case requiring frequent visits. b) to provide for the removal of patients from conditions that render medical treatment largely futile. c) to reduce the cost and danger of travel entailed in removal from outlying parts to the existing hospitals. d) to provide a home for the district nurse and a local dispensary for the doctor.' It was also suggested that there should be more provision for the treatment of tuberculosis.

The Dewer Committee did not review local authority services in spite of their obvious relevance to the distribution of local financial resources on health. Until the end of the nineteenth century the Highlands and Islands had been almost without public health services. There were no sanitary

35 This recommendation which would have continued the dispersal of hospital beds in small local units was rejected by the Highlands and Islands (Medical Service) Board.

programmes of any kind before 1867. Then under the Public Health (Scotland) Act of 1867 the parochial boards across Scotland became the responsible sanitary authorities with powers for the prevention and mitigation of infectious disease by the provision of hospitals and by improving sanitation. In the Highlands and Islands the Act remained in these respects almost a dead letter. In 1885 the Inspector for the North Highland District complained that 'The Public Health Act, passed eighteen years ago, can hardly be said to be in operation except in a few places.'[36] To the local authorities, the installation of systems of drainage, sewage and water supply, for which there was clearly no pressing need in the Highlands and Islands, was regarded as an unjustifiable expense. The demolition of substandard housing, as required by the Act, threatened to become an impossible burden on the local rates by increasing the numbers of the homeless destitute to be supported under the Poor Law. Also there was little point in building isolation hospitals that would inevitably be remote and inaccessible to the majority of the population and would therefore be little used.

By 1912 Government legislation had made no special concession to the problems of the medical services in the region in spite of the fact that the region had been recognised in the Crofters Act of 1886 as so idiosyncratic as to require special administration. The recent Education (Scotland) Act of 1908 had added to the difficulties of the local authorities in the Highlands and Islands by introducing a school medical service. This new service had been set up following a report by a Royal Commission appointed in 1902 to assess the heath and welfare of school children in Scotland.[37] Investigations were carried out for the Commission in Edinburgh and in Aberdeen. The Commissioners were appalled by the obviously poor physical state of the pupils in these urban populations and deplored the absence of any medical inspection or medical help. Government then set up an Interdepartmental Committee to study the problem further. It concluded that the causes of the poor physique and medical problems of the young people of Scotland were:

1. Increasing urbanisation of the people had brought with it overcrowding.
2. The pollution of the atmosphere with the lack of sunlight that it produced, together with the absence of fresh air, was a potent cause.

36 The inspector suggested that 'the poisons arising from so many forms of pollution, within and without the houses are counteracted by the constant burning of the open fire burning in the centre of the houses and by the abundance of mountain and sea air which is admitted by the open and ill-fitting doors. It is also possible that the dense clouds of peat smoke in which the people continually live may have some salutary antiseptic effect.' Day, *op. cit.*, p. 291.
37 *Report of the Royal Commission on Physical Training (Scotland)*, 1903, Cd. 1507.

3. There was insufficient inspection of workplaces. The Factory Act of 1901 had not been fully implemented.
4. The drinking habits of the women had deleterious effects on their children and were a most potent and deadly agent of physical deterioration.
5. The depletion of rural areas.
6. The tendency of the better stocks to breed less.
7. The excessive use of tea and white bread.[38]

These were not the problems of the Highlands and Islands. Nevertheless the medical provisions of the Education (Scotland) Act, devised to correct them, applied to the Highlands and Islands as much as to the cities, placing another seemingly unnecessary burden on the finances of the parishes. The School Medical Service created by the Act also added to the commitments of local doctors recruited as medical officers in the new service, but to little effect. The medical problems discovered in the pupils at school medical inspections might be duly reported to the parents as required by the Act, but in most cases the general practitioner services that could have remedied them were not available. For decades health legislation, devised with Scotland's urban population in mind, had drained the Highland parishes of the resources to fund the improvements of which they were most in need – medical primary care.

In December 1913, the Dewer Committee found that the medical services in the Highlands and Islands were very near to collapse. 'Local resources are, in many parishes, well-nigh if not wholly, exhausted.' The medical services were already unsatisfactory and unable to support the National Health Insurance Scheme. Any ameliorisation of the existing deficiencies could not be achieved without further government intervention. In an Appendix to the report, Leslie Mackenzie, one of the Commissioners, set out a *Scheme for the Administrative Consolidation of Medical Services for the Highlands and Islands.* Six months later McKinnon Wood, the Secretary for Scotland, announced in the House of Commons:

It is expedient to make provision for improving Medical Services in the Highlands and Islands of Scotland and for other purposes connected therewith and to authorise for these purposes the payment out of moneys to be provided by Parliament of a) a Special Grant to be called the Highlands and Islands (Medical Service) Grant and b) the salaries or remunerations of the secretary and of the officers of a Board to be called the Highland and Islands Medical Board and of any expenses incurred by the Board in the execution of their duties.[39]

38 *Report of the Inter-Departmental Committee on Physical Deterioration*, 1904, Cd. 2175.
39 *Hansard*, iv, HC 12 July 1913, col. 1816.

The Highlands and Islands Medical Services

The Highland and Islands (Medical Services) Board appointed in 1913 had eight members, six of whom were doctors.[40] Every member was familiar with the way of life in the Highlands and Islands and had first-hand experience in the administration of contemporary medical services. Dr. Leslie Mackenzie, Dr. John McVail, Sir Donald MacAlister and Dr. Norman Walker had already made important contributions to the reform of medical services in Scotland.

The Board accepted Leslie Mackenzie's *Suggested Scheme* as the basis for the new service. The area to be served was defined by the Secretary for Scotland. 'There is no statutory definition of the Highlands and Islands but there is a definition of the Crofting Counties.'[41] The area to be served by the Highlands and Islands Medical Service (HIMS) was therefore set to coincide with the special administrative area designated as the Crofting Counties in the Crofters Holding (Scotland) Act of 1886. The new Board accepted responsibility for the provision of medical care for some 285,000 people scattered over 14,000 square miles of difficult country.[42] The annual Highlands and Islands (Medical Service) Grant of £42,000 to support the new service was equivalent to one shilling and sixpence for each member of the population.

The first objective of the HIMS was to provide general practitioner services for every member of the community. The Board found an imaginative way in which to make the best possible use of a very limited budget. Payment of general practitioners by capitation fee – the system recently adopted for the NHI scheme – was seen as inappropriate; it would operate to the unfair advantage of doctors in the more populous areas who had easy access to comparatively large numbers of patients without heavy expenditure on travel. Payment by salary would have been difficult to adjust to reflect the unequal demands of very different practices and, for some doctors, would act as a disincentive to effort and initiative, especially in caring for their most remote patients. The system adopted recognised that

40 Sir John Dewer, Bart., MP; Lady Susan Gilmour; Sir Donald MacAlister, Principal of Glasgow University, President of the General Medical Council; Dr. Leslie Mackenzie, Medical Member of the Local Government Board for Scotland; Dr. John Macpherson, Senior Medical Commissioner in Lunacy for Scotland; Dr. John McVail, Deputy Chairman of the Scottish Insurance Commission; Dr. J. L. Robertson, Senior Chief Inspector of Schools in Scotland; Dr. Norman Walker, BMA Representative for Scotland on the General Medical Council.

41 *Hansard*, 12 July 1913, *op. cit*, col. 1817.

42 The Registrar General, who counted heads per acre to the nearest whole head, demonstrated that the Highlands were not inhabited at all. M. Crosfil, 'The Highlands and Islands Medical Service,' *Vesalius*, ii, 1996, p. 120.

the chief disadvantage for doctors practising in the Highlands and Islands was the very high level of practice expenses. Travel to visit patients at home was expensive; it was also time-consuming, restricting the time available for other paid work. Medicines were provided free as an expense on the practice. Suitable practice accommodation was scarce and, although often less than adequate, always costly.

In the scheme adopted by the Board, Treasury funds were used to subsidise practice expenses rather than to contribute directly to the doctor's income. A grant was made to each practice that was calculated to reflect its particular operating expenses such as the distribution of free medicines and the cost of travel. Where necessary the doctor was assisted in buying his own motor car, motor boat or whatever means of transport seemed appropriate. Provision was also made either for the improvement of the houses already occupied by doctors or to build new ones. In calculating the grant for each practice, care was taken to ensure that the doctor's income would not fall below a reasonable minimum.[43] In return doctors were required to 'visit systematically those requiring medical attention, including Poor Law and insured persons, and also to undertake such Public Health duties as may be required.' For patients not insured or entitled to treatment under the Poor Law, doctors were allowed to charge fees of 5s for a first visit and 2s 6d for any subsequent visit; the fee for midwifery was set at £1, although, based on previous experience in the region, there was little expectation that fees would be paid. The Highlands and Islands Medical Board also undertook to refund 70% of all approved expenditure of the District Nursing Associations[44] and to make additional grants to provide appropriate houses for the nurses. Grants were also planned to meet the cost (almost entirely the cost of travel) of specialist services in Aberdeen, Glasgow or Edinburgh.

The full implementation of these plans was interrupted by the outbreak of war in 1914. Doctors were quickly recruited in 1913 but many soon left to join the armed forces. Only three houses for doctors and nine for nurses were completed before the war at a total cost of £5,730. In each of the war years the grant of £42,000 was underspent and by 1919 the Highlands and Islands Medical Service funds had accumulated to £57,000.

In August 1919 the administration of the service was taken over by the newly created Scottish Health Board and the Highlands and Islands (Medical Services) Board was disbanded. The new administration added a new scheme; arrangements were made to allow practitioners to attend refresher courses. Dr. A. Shearer, given early demobilisation from the army specifically for the purpose, was employed full-time by the HIMS Fund on

43 The minimum recommended in 1913 was £300 per annum.
44 Including nurses' salaries.

a salary of £500 per annum to act as a rotating locum.[45] The scheme to provide suitable houses for doctors in the new service, first drawn up in 1916, had been abandoned during the war. When the war ended, building costs had increased by as much as three times.[46] In 1920 the Scottish Health Board launched a revised scheme. Architects produced plans for suitable houses for doctors at a cost that the Board estimated that it could afford.[47] This removed the last of the major disincentives to medical practice in the Highlands.

The HIMS now offered secure employment by central government, a small but secure income, a decent house, periods of leave and subsidised practice expenses. These terms of employment proved attractive to doctors being released from military service and the end of the First World War. The number of doctors employed in the Crofting Counties quickly increased to 155, many of them young men with excellent training and experience, and by 1924 the Scottish Board of Health was satisfied that the deficiencies in the general practitioner services in the Crofting Counties had been largely remedied.[48] General practitioners were available even in the most inaccessible mainland districts and the most remote islands and it seemed that there were no remaining barriers which might prevent even the poorest from obtaining medical assistance. In 1929, when responsibility for the HIMS was transferred to the Department of Health for Scotland, general practice services were considered to be so satisfactory that they could be allowed to 'continue without material alteration.' There were then over 160 doctors employed in 150 practices; incomes and housing arrangements had been accepted as adequate; the HIMS locum scheme had allowed up to 40 general practitioners to enjoy periods of leave each year and attendance at refresher courses was being actively encouraged by the Board. Recruitment of doctors into the Highlands and Islands was no longer a problem.

The Effects of the HIMS

As statistical evidence of improvement in general practitioner services, the *Annual Reports of the Department of Health* showed that by 1936, on average, each general practitioner had a list of some 1,900 patients, a doctor/patient ratio that compared very favourably with the prevailing in the rest of the United Kingdom. In the past the high number of uncertified deaths had been taken as an index of the inadequacy of the general practitioner service. In 1911 the proportion of deaths going uncertified in the Crofting Counties

---

45 NAS HH/65/1.
46 *First Annual Report of the Scottish Board of Health* 1919, Cmd. 825, p. 79.
47 The estimated cost of each house was £746. NAS HH 65/24; NAS HH/52/1.
48 *Annual Report of the Scottish Board of Health*, 1924, Cmd. 2156.

had been 10.5%; by 1931–33 this had been reduced to 4.5%. The first full review of the HIMS was included in the Cathcart Report[49] in 1936. Cathcart concluded:

> This Service has revolutionised medical provision in the Highlands and Islands. It is now reasonably adequate in the sense that for all districts the services of a doctor are available on reasonable terms. Our witnesses informed us also that the Highlands and Islands were now attracting medical men of a quality superior to the bulk of practitioners who found their way to the Highlands before this service was instituted.

General practice owed much of its success to the improvement in domiciliary nursing services. As a witness before the Dewer Committee in 1912, Lord Lovat, Convenor of Inverness County Council,[50] had predicted that the medical salvation of the Highlands would lie in the provision and organising of nursing services. This proved to be the case. The end of the war released large numbers of nurses from wartime service and the number of fully trained Queen's nurses employed in the Crofting Counties leapt to 123. Most parishes were soon able to have a resident nurse. Suitable houses were built, usually with small hospices of two or more beds attached.[51] The introduction of an automated telephone service in the West Highlands made them more readily available to their patients – although they still had to rely on bicycles as their only means of transport. By 1929, 73 District Nursing Associations were being subsidised to employ a total of 175 nurses. Their living accommodation had been further improved and pushbikes were being replaced by motor bikes. When the Cathcart Committee reported in 1936, the number of fully qualified nurses employed in the Crofting Counties had risen to 200. As predicted by Lord Lovat, the employment of district nurses had proved to be crucial. In 1936 the Cathcart Report commented:

> The combination of doctor and nurse is extraordinarily impressive. Many of the doctors say that practice in their areas would be impossible without the services of the nurses, and everywhere we are told that co-operation between doctor and nurse leaves nothing to be desired. The nurse is in a position to establish intimate contact with the people and so help in detecting illnesses at an early stage. She

49 *Report of the Committee on Scottish Health Services* (Cathcart Report), 1936, Cmd. 5204.
50 Lord Lovat was the owner of a Highland estate of 181,800 acres.
51 As planned by the Scottish Health Board a nurse's house cost £228, a house with a small hospice of two beds £390 and with a larger hospice £750. NAS HH/65/24; NAS HH/65/25.

attends at the periodic school medical examinations and does what follow up may be arranged. In some areas the nurse also visits the schools every month to inspect the children. Not the least part of the value of the nurse lies in her work in health education. It appeared to us that she is at present the main agency for educating the people in hygiene ... We are told by most witnesses that the people were improving in personal and household hygiene and most of the doctors attribute this improvement largely to the nurse.

A parish minister, the Rev. John MacLeod, had described the problems in treating patients at home as they had been before the introduction of the HIMS:

It is only in extreme cases that medical aid is usually sought. When we consider that his [the doctor's] stay is necessarily short, that his visits, if repeated at all are so only at distant intervals and that his prescriptions, if administered in his absence, are given unsatisfactorily and partially under much injudicious treatment calculated to counter-act their efficiency, the medical attendant can be of little service and the people have but too generally lost confidence in medical aid.[52]

The nursing services of the HIMS remedied these and other deficiencies, adding very greatly to the effectiveness of general practice. Without the support of efficient. nursing services the Department of Health for Scotland could not have found that the Crofting Community was being adequately served by only 165 doctors.[53]

Extending the Service

Satisfied that the deficiencies in general practice had been met, in 1929 the HIMS turned its attention to hospital services, introducing a new regional policy for the Crofting Counties. Cottage hospitals, small and poorly equipped, had been randomly dispersed across the counties with each parish ambitious to have its own small complement of hospital beds. The Dewer Committee had recommended that reliance on local small cottage hospitals should continue and their number increased. This policy was reversed almost at once by the HIMS Board which decided that without centralisation it would be neither practically nor economically possible to develop modern specialist services. Improvement grants were given on an ad hoc basis to the existing hospitals that were judged to be of a useful size. In

---

52 Rev John Macleod of Morven. Letter to Dr John Coldstream, 9 January 1851.
53 The number of practices reached 155; the number of additional assistants varied from time to time.

1924 a full-time consultant surgeon was appointed at Stornoway on a trial basis. The results of the experiment were impressive. In addition to the care of inpatients, the consultant was able to offer an outpatient service. Before his appointment, the total number of outpatients seen at Stornoway each year had been seven; six years later that number had grown to 1,690. It was soon appreciated that admission to hospital offered advantages in treatment that outweighed the reluctance of the sick to be moved from their homes. At Stornoway alone admissions more than trebled between 1915 and 1923 and the number of operations more than doubled.[54]

In 1929 the HIMS came under the direction of the Department of Health for Scotland. The annual grant of £42,000 was continued indefinitely along with 'such sum as may be voted annually.' Since the general practitioner service was judged to be well founded, it was decided that it should continue 'without material alteration'[55] and that all new money could be devoted to extending specialist services. Improvement grants were made to the managers of the hospitals at Lerwick, Kirkwall, and Stornoway, to the local authorities in Ross and Cromarty and in Caithness in respect of hospitals in Wick and Thurso, and to the trustees of the Belford Hospital at Fort William. The Royal Northern Infirmary at Inverness[56] was given financial encouragement to act as an up-to-date and fully equipped centre for all specialist services for the whole region so that only cases of unusual difficulty need be referred out of the region to the teaching hospitals of Glasgow or Aberdeen. The Inverness Infirmary had received intermittent subsidies from the beginning but in 1930 this support was confirmed as an annual grant of £5,000 for ten years. Staffing of the local hospitals within the Crofting Counties had originally been by GP specialists. In 1929 the trial appointment of a specialist surgeon at Stornoway was made permanent and other appointments followed. By 1934 there were full-time consultant surgeons in Shetland, Orkney, Caithness and Lewis. In 1935 a consultant physician was appointed at Inverness, contracted to provide consultant outpatient services on a regular basis at all the HIMS hospitals. To facilitate and encourage the use of the expanding hospital and specialist services, additional grants were made to local authorities to promote and support ambulance services.

Glasgow became the preferred centre for tertiary referrals following the setting up of an Air Ambulance service in 1933. This service sprang from the initiative of a general practitioner on Islay who, 'despairing of the life of a patient too ill to stand the long journey to hospital by sea and road,'

---

54 Crosfil, *op.cit.*, p. 124.
55 *Annual Report of the Department of Health for Scotland*, 1929, Cmd. 3529, p. 114.
56 Although the Royal Northern Infirmary served the region, the town of Inverness was not formally within the Crofting Counties.

persuaded a pilot of Midland Scottish Air Ferries to fly his patient to Glasgow. This led to requests for similar help from other doctors in other parts of the Highlands and Islands. The Air Ambulance, now operated on a regular contract basis by Scottish Airways Limited, soon became an essential part of the hospital service. In 1935 there were eight emergency Air Ambulance Service flights and by 1938 this had increased to 34, all financed by the local authorities with two thirds of the cost refunded by the HIMS. Until 1939 the Air Ambulance was based at Renfrew, serving only airfields in Kintyre, the Hebrides and Orkney but during the war years the service extended as more airfields became available. By 1948 the annual number of flights had increased to 245 carrying 275 patients over a total distance of 65,000 miles.[57]

The Highlands and Islands Medical Service was finally absorbed by the National Health Service in 1948. But in effect it had begun to lose its separate existence during the preparations for the Second World War. By that time it had already been judged an outstanding success. It had been conducted

> ... in an atmosphere of sympathy and understanding between the central department and the doctors, nurses and other parties, and to the satisfaction of all concerned ... The Highlands and Islands area is the only part of Scotland which has in effect a complete general practitioner service available for all classes and the Highland and Islands Medical Service works on the basis of co-operation between the State and doctors.[58]

The HIMS had succeeded in all its primary objectives. In the Crofting Counties, subscribers to the National Health Insurance scheme were able to receive the full medical benefit to which they were entitled. The gross deficiencies in the medical services available to the population had been made good. The acute distress that throughout previous centuries had been caused by the lack of medical help at times of crisis had been relieved.

The HIMS As a Pilot Study

In his *Suggested Scheme for the Administrative Consolidation of Medical Services*, Leslie Mackenzie, recognised that the creation of a comprehensive medical service for the Highlands and Islands presented an opportunity 'to show how far it is possible to bring about an administrative consolidation that would result in increasing the efficiency of the present services in devel-

---

57 J. Smith, 'The Scottish Air Ambulance Service,' *The Practitioner*, clxx, 1953, p. 67.
58 Cathcart Report, p. 227.

oping the resources of the present services, in demonstrating what additional service is necessary and in preparing the way for any legislation afterwards found to be expedient.' Mackenzie clearly saw the potential of the HIMS as the pilot for the later creation of a comprehensive state medical service.

The terms of the Highlands and Islands (Medical Service) Grant made this entirely possible. They were framed to make certain that the services of a general practitioner would be freely available to all without any financial barrier, thus opening the way for the development of a demand-led service. The terms of the Grant also made it possible for the Highlands and Islands Medical Service Board to expand the scope of general practice by incorporating domiciliary nursing services in the structure of general practice and making it possible for patients from the Highlands and Islands to have access to specialist services at every level, including services that were not available within the administrative area of the Crofting Counties. The HIMS came to include all the elements of that 'comprehensive medical service for every citizen covering all treatment'[59] envisaged in the Beveridge Report in 1942 and provided the full range of 'the resources of medical skill and the apparatus of healing' that Aneurin Bevan aimed to organise after 1945.[60]

However, what impact a 'comprehensive medical service for every citizen covering all treatment' might have on the health of the community was still quite unknown. Nor was it possible to foresee the financial implications of making 'the resources of medical skill and the apparatus of healing.'[61] The experience of the HIMS, over some twenty years, had it been studied as a pilot trial, should have indicated the answers to these unknowns.

The Population

In 1913 the unique population of the Crofting Counties offered the best available model for the population of Scotland as it was to become 30 years later when decisions were being made that would determine the success or failure of the future NHS.

In 1913 the age and sex structure of the population of the Highlands and Islands was quite dissimilar from that of Scotland as a whole.[62] However, in

---

59 *Report of the Commission on Social Insurance and Allied Services*, 1942, Cmd. 6404.
60 Aneurin Bevan, *In Place of Fear* (London, 1952), p. 75.
61 *Ibid.*
62 M. Anderson and D. J. Morse, 'High Fertility, High Emigration, Low Nuptuality: Adjustment Processes in Scotland's Demographic Experience,' *Population Studies*, xlvii, 1993, p. 324.

the first decades of the twentieth century, different levels of fertility and different patterns of migration and emigration had brought the two communities together in their social structure by the first years of the NHS (Table 1)

Table 1. **Population Structure: Crofting Counties in 1911 & Scotland in 1911 and 1951**

	Aged (0–14)%	Aged 65+ (%)	F/M Ratio
Scotland – 1911	32	5	106
Crofting Counties – 1911	28	12	109
Scotland – 1951	25	10	109

Source: Calculated from *Census of Scotland*, 1911 & 1951

In the middle years of the nineteenth century the people of the Highlands and Islands, in spite of their poverty, were healthy. Their health and longevity were remarked upon in almost every report to the *First Statistical Account of Scotland.* They enjoyed the benefits of space, fresh air and sunlight and, provided harvests were normal, an excellent diet. The traditional diet of the crofting community was superior, both in calorific value and in first-class protein, to that of the great industrial populations of the United Kingdom.[63] Housing conditions, although primitive, were not the threat to health so often supposed by casual visitors. The Napier Report commented:

> Among the various inconveniences which the people of the Highlands and Islands suffer in connection with their position as occupiers of land, the one which strikes the stranger as the most deplorable, and which affects the natives with the least impatience is the nature of their dwellings ... In the main his house does not make him unhappy, for he does not complain; it does not make him immoral, for he is above the average standard of morality in his country; it does not make him unhealthy, for he enjoys an uncommon share of vigour and longevity.

The people of the Highlands and Islands had escaped the disturbance of physical growth and the debilitation so evident in the people subjected to the living conditions of the Lowland industrial centres.[64] They were some

63 Napier Report, p. 74; E. P. Cathcart and A. M. T. Murray, *A Study in Nutrition: An Inquiry into the Diet of Families in the Highlands and Islands of Scotland* (London, 1940).
64 W. W. Knox, *Hanging by a Thread: The Scottish Cotton Industry* (Preston, 1995); C. A. Whatley, 'Women and the Economic Transformation of Scotland,' *Scottish Economic and Social History*, xiv, 1994.

inches taller.[65] In 1860 the proportion of the population surviving longer than 75 years was four times greater in Argyll than in Glasgow. Crofting families suffered less from the infectious diseases that were so fatal in the industrial communities of the south. This was reflected in the different death rates of children under 5 years, the chief victims of the acute infectious diseases. A child in Glasgow was ten times more likely to die than one in Shetland; a child in Dundee was more than seven times more likely to die than one in Sutherland. In the Highlands and Islands the Infant Mortality Rate was 85; for Scotland as a whole it was 121.

From the middle years of the nineteenth century, improved living conditions allowed the industrial population of Britain to begin a gradual recovery from the diseases and debilitating effects of almost a century of ruthless urbanisation. At the same time greater social intercourse between the two populations led to the importation of some of the diseases of the Lowland industrial population – notably tuberculosis – into the Highlands and Islands. By 1913, the death rate from pulmonary tuberculosis had become almost as great in the crofting community as in Scotland's large towns.[66] Towards the end of the century improved transport brought 'shop food' within reach of crofting families; the quality of the diet of the Highland population thereafter began to lose its advantage over that of the majority in Scotland. As the health of the Lowlander improved, that of the Highlander began to decline. When the HIMS was launched, the great differences in health had become insignificant.[67]

In 1913 the population of the area served by the HIMS was eminently suitable for a social experiment. It was stable and well defined geographically. It had the same sex and age structure as the population of Scotland. There were no significant health problems that were not shared by both communities and no other health systems that might have influenced health trends within the area over the 'trial period' from 1913 to 1948.

Cost Effectiveness

Between 1913 and 1945 health improved both in the Highlands and Islands and in Scotland as a whole. As judged by the accepted health standards of

65 In the Boer War the Highland regiments were able to maintain their standards while, in order to find sufficient numbers in the industrial south, the general limit for recruitment to the British army was reduced from 5ft 3ins. to 5 ft. 'The industrial Lowlanders had bent backs and rounded shoulders . . . in the Highlands the men walked as erect as noblemen.' *The Scotsman*, quoted by K. Fenyo, *Contempt, Sympathy and Romance* (East Linton, 2000), p. 62.
66 Death Rates from pulmonary tuberculosis in 1913 were: Crofting Counties, 1.17; Lowland Large Burghs, 1.27; Scotland 1.04. *Annual Report of the Registrar General for Scotland.*
67 Appendix III.

the time, there is no convincing evidence that HIMS conferred any special advantage on the people of the Highlands and Islands or had any significant impact on the continuing trend of improvement over these years. While the Death Rate in Scotland fell by 14.8%, in the Highlands and Islands it fell by 14.7%. The Infant Mortality Rate, then accepted as the best single indicator of the health of any community,[68] fell by 45.3% in Scotland and only 28.3% in the Highlands and Islands.[69]

The decrease in the Infant Mortality Rate between 1913 and 1945 was largely due to the decline in fertility and a reduction in the birth rate which occurred in both communities but was greater in the overall population of Scotland (by 33% in Scotland and by 14% in the Highlands and Islands). Smaller families increased the chances of infants surviving as the number of children to be fed and cared for by the mother decreased.

The standards of health of the population of the Highlands and Islands showed steady improvement after 1913 but this was a continuation of a trend already established. The medical care provided by the Highlands and Islands Medical Service caused no discernible break in that continuing trend.[70]

The major improvements in health that occurred in every part of Scotland were essentially the result of general social change. The most rapid improvements were in those parts of Scotland that had suffered most from the appalling urban deprivation and physical degeneration of the early nineteenth century. With no comprehensive state medical service, it was in the industrial Lowlands of Scotland that the statistical indicators of 'health' improved most rapidly. Over this period a universal and free system of medical care in the Highlands and Islands put the population there at no measurable advantage.

Although the success of the HIMS is not quantifiable in terms of crude health statistics, it was an undoubted success by popular acclaim. The experience of the HIMS demonstrated the interesting paradox that as the health of the population improved, the medical services were used more rather than less by the 'healthier' population. As new services became available, they were eagerly taken up. This had important financial implications. Figure I shows that the cost of general practitioner services increased but soon reached a plateau. As the potential of domiciliary nursing came to be more fully appreciated, more nurses were employed and the cost of nursing services increased before reaching a steady level. When limited specialist services became available in 1924 and were extended after 1929, it

68 Sir George Newman, Chief Medical Officer at the Ministry of Health from 1919 to 1935, first advocated its use for this purpose in *Health of the State* (London, 1907).
69 Appendix III.
70 Ibid.

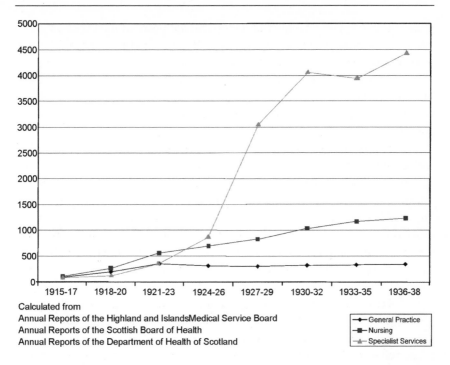

Calculated from
Annual Reports of the Highland and IslandsMedical Service Board
Annual Reports of the Scottish Board of Health
Annual Reports of the Department of Health of Scotland

● General Practice
■ Nursing
▲ Specialist Services

FIGURE I   HIMS Percentage Increases in Expenditure, 1915–1938

became evident that, in a demand-led system, the demand for more
sophisticated forms of investigation, new technical procedures in treatment
and the products of advances in medical science promised to be infinite but
without demonstrable benefit to the physical health of the community.
Whether a comprehensive demand-led service, provided out of public
funds, was of advantage to the state remains a complex question. Politically,
the HIMS may have helped to prevent disaffection in one corner of the
country. Administratively it undoubtedly solved a problem in social
management. But in serving the state by improving the health of the
population, by the conventional indices it could claim no measurable
success.

Administration

Recruitment – General Practitioners
The Highlands and Islands Medical Service Board found that, even in a
demand-led service, it was possible to determine an optimum complement
of doctors that would maintain general practice at its maximum level of
efficiency. Experience showed that in the circumstances of the Crofting
Counties in the late 1920s and 1930s this optimum number was approxi-

mately 170. A smaller number of doctors would have found it impossible to maintain a satisfactory standard of care and many would have been grossly overloaded; a larger number would have been unnecessarily expensive and would not have provided every doctor with a sufficient clinical load to allow him to maintain his clinical skills. It was found that on average each general practitioner, for maximum efficiency, should have the care of approximately 2000 patients.

It had soon become evident that there was no shortage of well-qualified and committed doctors eager to find employment in a state service administered by a central government department.[71] The attraction for doctors lay in security of tenure with guaranteed periods of subsidised study leave, the opportunity to attend their patients uninhibited by the cost of transport, the freedom to prescribe for their patients without crippling financial constraint and practice arrangements that included the co-operation of nursing staff and a full range of supporting services. Given such conditions, general practitioners were happy to be employed by the state.

The HIMS allowed general practitioners to take on private patients at modest fees. In the case of the lower-income patients, who made up the great majority of patients in the crofting communities, fees were neither requested nor received provided the doctor had a secure income from some other source. General practitioners were not debarred from entrepreneurial private practice but the Scottish doctors in this 'trial' did not find this essential to their standing as independent professional men. Employment by the state did not deprive them of clinical freedom provided they had security of employment and were not subjected to the vagaries and unpredictable demands of employment by local authorities.

In the last years of HIMS the average income from the state of its general practitioners was £800 per annum[72] and this had proved to be readily acceptable. Yet, in 1943, the leadership of the BMA refused to countenance any form of employment by the state that did not offer an annual income of over £1,000. The BMA leaders also continued to protest that employment by the state posed a threat to the 'traditional freedoms' of doctors and claimed that 'to convert at a stroke one of the oldest and most honourable professions into a public service, amenable to all the discipline which public service involves, is an operation quite without precedent.'[73] A precedent already existed in the HIMS which had shown that many doctors were more

71 The BMA in Scotland did not adopt the confrontational attitude that characterised the parent body in London over the introduction of the National Health Insurance Scheme in 1911. The BMA took no part in the founding of the HIMS but was consistently co-operative thereafter.

72 J. Ross, *The National Health Service in Great Britain* (Oxford, 1952), p. 66.

73 Webster, *op. cit.*, p. 38.

than willing to opt for state service in preference to a career in entrepreneurial practice, which for the great majority meant a financially precarious existence and little professional satisfaction. In the HIMS general practitioners found their terms of employment attractive and in return provided an excellent and committed service. The assumption made by the Ministry of Health, that it would be impossible to maintain discipline and to ensure a satisfactory standard of performance unless general practitioners were salaried employees of the state,[74] was also demonstrably unfounded.

Recruitment – Nursing Staff

For over thirty years the HIMS demonstrated that, together, general practitioners and nurses formed an efficient and cost-effective partnership. However, the importance of nursing to domiciliary medical practice was not recognised in the planning of the NHS nor was it recognised for many years as the service expanded and developed. Posts in the integrated general medical service of the HIMS had proved attractive to well-trained and experienced nurses leaving the forces at the end of the First World War. They would have proved equally attractive at the end of the Second World War.

Recruitment – Consultants and Specialists

The first full-time surgeon in the HIMS was appointed in 1924. There was no shortage of applicants for this salaried post or for those that were created in the following years. As the hospital service grew, the university medical schools saw a new opportunity for their specialists in training. Salaried posts in the HIMS offered opportunities for men who wished to develop a specialist career but who were unable to finance the traditional and inevitable waiting years at the teaching centres in the cities before they could become established. In 1931, a surgeon was appointed to the HIMS at Wick, nominated by the Professor of Surgery at Aberdeen for a limited tour while, as recorded in the *Annual Report of the Department of Health for Scotland*, 'his positions in relation to the University and the Infirmary were not to be diminished'. This and later similar appointments attracted highly skilled candidates and made good specialist services widely available outside the main medical centres. This early move to involve university medical schools in the state medical services was followed elsewhere in Scotland from 1932.[75] The value of this association between the teaching centres and

---

74 J. Pater, *The Making of the National Health Service* (London, 1981), p. 37.
75 Aberdeen University expanded its service to the Highlands and Islands. In 1932, the professors of Medicine, Surgery, Obstetrics and Gynaecology, and Child Life and Health became responsible for the care of patients in Edinburgh's three municipal hospitals. Similar arrangements were made in Glasgow and Dundee.

the peripheral services was recognised and exploited in the National Health Service (Scotland) Act to the great advantage of the NHS in Scotland. This lead was not followed in England where teaching hospitals were allowed to distance themselves from peripheral services. The Ministry of Health was not persuaded of the value of a fully integrated hospital service and in the years of negotiation in the 1940s the leaders of the BMA seemed oblivious to the new opportunities that a salaried state service offered to medical graduates who wished to make a career outside general practice.

Regionalisation of Hospital Services

In 1940 the Ministry of Health believed that the regionalisation of hospitals, organised at that time as a wartime expedient for the care of casualties, would be 'irrelevant to a peace time service'.[76] The Ministry held to the view that the proper administrative units for hospital administration in a state service were the countries and county boroughs. 'No government would wish such a service to be administered by the minister direct.'[77] By then the HIMS had been operating very successfully on a regional basis for 25 years. Local authorities had made it clear that they had no wish to take on the administration of an integrated hospital service. It had also been found that 'medical and other opinion is emphatically against it.'[78]

As early as 1941, the Ministry had decided that teaching hospitals should be given separate and special status.[79] In the Highlands and Islands it had been found that the teaching hospitals of the university centres and the local hospitals could work together to their mutual advantage. The HIMS had built up a sound hospital service on the basis of the existing voluntary and local authority hospitals. Policy decisions and consultant appointments were made by general agreement. In 1916 the HIMS Board had set up, in each of the Crofting Counties, a committee of County and District Medical Officers of Health, the School Medical Officers, representatives of Local Medical Committees and Panel Committees under the National Insurance Act, a representative from each of the Secondary Education Committees and the principal medical officer of each of the general hospitals to advise on general policy.[80] Each of these committees was chaired by the County Convenor. These committees continued to co-operate successfully until 1948.

76 Pater, *op. cit.*, p. 24.
77 *Ibid.*
78 Cathcart Report, p. 231.
79 Pater, *op. cit.*, p. 27.
80 *Annual Report of the Highlands and Islands Medical Service Board*, 1916, Cd. 8246, p. 15.

The Local Authorities in a Comprehensive Medical Service

From the beginning the Highlands and Islands (Medical Service) Board decided that no direct support would be given to local authority medical services. Nevertheless, these services benefited indirectly. The general practitioners established in the region by the HIMS became available to staff local authority clinics on a part-time basis.[81] Their presence throughout the region also ensured that the problems discovered by the Maternity and Child Welfare Clinics and the School Medical Service would be properly investigated and treated.

Co-ordination of Services

The HIMS demonstrated that the various health services operating in Scotland were ready to work together. The District Nursing Associations had been co-operative from the beginning. The Northern Hospital at Inverness, although not eligible for a grant from the Highlands and Islands Medical Service Fund,[82] agreed informally in 1919 to act as a secondary referral hospital for the HIMS.[83] From 1919 the St Andrew's Ambulance Service, a charity organisation, provided a motor ambulance at each of the general hospitals. The voluntary assistance of the Midland Scottish Air Ferries led on to the establishment of an air ambulance service.

The HIMS also offered new experience for civil servants as part of a successful organisation to which they could make a personal contribution. Those who administered the HIMS found opportunities for exercising management skills in addition to their usual duties of regulation. They 'built up by flexible central administration a system of co-operative effort, embracing the central department, private general practitioners, nursing associations, voluntary hospitals, specialists, local authorities and others to meet the medical need of the people.'[84] It was to Scotland's great benefit that this 'system of co-operative effort' was carried over in the administration of the NHS in Scotland.

---

81 Nevertheless, the Cathcart Committee found that the only medical services in the Highlands and Islands that had not reached a satisfactory level of performance were those which remained completely in the control of the local authorities.

82 A regular grant was later made by the Department of Health for Scotland after 1929.

83 T. C. Mackenzie, *The Story of a Scottish Voluntary Hospital* (Inverness, 1946), p. 225.

84 Cathcart Report, p. 232.

2

Collins, Cathcart and
the Distance from London

S ir Godfrey Collins and Professor E. P. Cathcart personified the
influences that separated the medical services of Scotland from those
of England and Wales in the 1930s. Sir Godfrey Collins, Secretary of State
for Scotland and an advocate of devolution of the administration of
government, appointed a committee to review the health services of
Scotland, a review that had no counterpart in England and Wales. Professor
Cathcart, who chaired that committee, typified the leadership of the medical
profession in Scotland, a profession with traditions and an approach to the
practice of medicine quite different from those of the medical profession in
England and Wales.

Collins and the Political Will

On introducing the National Health Service (Scotland) Bill for its Second
Reading on 10 December 1946, the Secretary of State for Scotland, Joseph
Westwood, stressed that his was a Scottish Bill and that he would keep it as a
Scottish Bill. Its details would be 'threshed out'[1] in debate within the
Scottish Grand Committee. Although he acknowledged that over many
months there had been 'many interesting and valuable discussions . . . on the
English Measure',[2] he made it clear his Bill was nevertheless still based on
the recommendations made by the Scottish Health Services Committee
(Cathcart Committee) in 1936 and on the 33 years of practical experience of
the administration of the comprehensive Highlands and Islands Medical
Service. In presenting his Bill, Westwood quoted frequently and at length
from the *Report of the Scottish Health Services Committee*[3] of which he himself
had 'had the honour and privilege to be a member.'[4]

The Committee had been appointed in June 1933 when Britain had not yet
begun to recover from the Depression, and its industrial communities still
suffered massive unemployment, poverty, malnutrition and disease. But it
was Britain's fiscal problems rather than the particular urgency and severity of
the health problems in Scotland that had caused the appointment of a

1 *Hansard*, xlxxxi, HC 10 December 1946, col. 1002.
2 *Ibid.*, col. 1001.
3 *Report of the Committee on Scottish Health Services*, 1936, Cmd. 5204. (Cathcart Report)
4 *Hansard*, xlxxi, *op. cit.*, col. 996.

committee to review Scotland's health services. The brief post-war boom had come to an end in the early 1920s and the downturn in world trade had soon led to recession in industry in Britain and deepening problems in the country's balance of payments. In 1929, the Wall Street Crash caused an international slump, exacerbating Britain's troubles. National income could not support existing commitments. A third of government spending was already taken up in repaying charges on debts accumulated during the First World War. In itself this was an enormous problem but it was made worse by the spiralling cost of supporting the increasing numbers of the unemployed. By January 1931 the government deficit had almost doubled since 1928; the United Kingdom was in financial crisis. The Labour Government, having failed to find a formula to meet the crisis, was replaced by a National Government in August. The emergency budget devised by Snowden, the Labour Chancellor of the Exchequer, in September again failed to improve matters. Following the election of 5 November, Snowden was replaced as Chancellor by the Conservative Neville Chamberlain.

Among the possible strategies for recovery, Chamberlain gave first priority to protection behind a barrier of tariffs in an attempt to reduce the adverse balance of trade. But there was also to be a rigorous tightening of the belt at home. Chamberlain looked for a reduction in public expenditure. He wrote to the local authorities both in England and Wales and in Scotland, requiring them to form committees to 'consider the whole field of local expenditure and make recommendations at the earliest possible date for securing reduction in such expenditure whether defrayed by Exchequer Grant, Rates or other sources, whether or not imposed on local authorities as a duty by statute, order or regulation.'[5] A time limit of three months was set for their replies.

Two separate committees – for England and Wales and for Scotland – were formed as directed but neither was able to find answers as quickly as the Chancellor had demanded. Finally, in November 1932, the committees produced two very different documents. The Report of the Committee on Local Government Expenditure in England and Wales, after careful review of spending on the various local authority services, indicated possible scope for economy only in very general terms and set no financial targets. On spending on health this committee recommended only that:

1. There should be an immediate inquiry into building costs of institutions and, when suitable standards had been determined, action should be taken to secure that they are observed.
2. Careful consideration should be given to the feasibility of establishing standards of maintenance costs.

5 *Report of the Committee on Local Expenditure (Scotland)* (Lovat Report), 1932, Cmd. 4201, p. 1.

3. Institutional treatment should be reserved for cases that could not adequately be treated otherwise.
4. Large economies could be secured in expenditure on hospital supplies by simplifying and standardising the articles required and by central purchasing.
5. Persons able to pay should be required, as a rule, to contribute to the costs of the service provided for them.
6. Comparative statements of costs were of real value but the function of the Ministry of Health should not be limited to collecting and publishing them.[6]

The responsible minister in England and Wales,[7] Sir Hilton Young, the Conservative Minister of Health, took no action in response to these recommendations.

In Scotland the response to the Chancellor's directive was quite different. The Committee in Scotland was formed by three representatives each from the Association of County Councils of Scotland, the Royal Burghs of Scotland, and the Association of the Counties of Cities, with Lord Lovat as Chairman.[8] This committee (the Lovat Committee) examined the public services in detail, making specific recommendations and setting financial targets for each one. On education the Committee identified possible savings of £950,000 with a further reduction on yearly capital commitments of £500,000; on roads annual savings of £1,250,000 were recommended and on police services annual savings of £250,000. On housing £153,500 could be saved (£117,000 accruing to the Exchequer and £36,500 to the rate-payers). From Public Assistance savings of £400,000 were possible and on administration, £529,800 (£527,000 accruing to the ratepayers and £2,800 to the Exchequer).

On spending on health the Lovat Committee reached a decision very different from the very broad and accommodating suggestions made by the Committee for England and Wales. After the most careful scrutiny the Scottish committee was forced to conclude that 'no real savings can be achieved in relation to health services until they are submitted to a comprehensive enquiry that would take into account modern medical knowledge and the prevailing financial condition.' The Committee en-dorsed and quoted the views of one Medical Officer of Health:

6 *Report of the Committee on Local Expenditure (England and Wales)* 1932, Cmd. 4200.
7 At that time the Ministry of Health was responsible for all local government.
8 Lord Lovat, KT, DSO (Inverness-shire); Ian Carmichael, DSO, MC, MA (Lanarkshire); J. M. Hodge (Perthshire); Sir Henry Leith, LLD, JP (Hamilton); Provost J. R. Rutherford, JP, FICS (Kirkintilloch); Provost Henry Smith (Kilmarnock); Treasurer L. S. Gumley (Edinburgh); Treasurer M. Lunan (Aberdeen); Treasurer G. D. Morton (Glasgow).

The health policy of the nation has never been completely reviewed since the latter half of the last century- over 50 years ago – and since then statutory health services have branched out in many different directions. No attempt has been made to relate these diverse activities to a clear purpose. And it is the absence of the clear purpose and the failure to correlate all health activities to serve it that is at the root of the tragic lag between established knowledge and its application in promoting fitness.

The Lovat Committee had found no opportunities for the reduction in the range of local authority health services that would lead to worthwhile economies. However, their investigation had revealed inefficiencies in the organisation and administration of the existing services with much over-lapping of responsibilities and waste of resources. The Committee therefore recommended that 'an independent enquiry into the whole subject of Public Health from every standpoint – health, social and financial – be at once instituted.' The Lovat Report was presented to the House of Commons in November 1932 by Sir Godfrey Collins, the recently appointed Secretary of State for Scotland. Within a few months he had appointed the Committee on Scottish Health Services.

Collins had been in office for only two months when he received the report of the Lovat Committee.[9] For the future development of health services designed specifically for Scotland, his was a singularly fortunate appointment. His term of four years as Secretary of State for Scotland was a brief Indian Summer for the New Liberalism that had influenced political thinking in the early years of the century. Sir John Simon recorded the great delight of the Liberals in the Commons that, in 1932, Collins' opportunity had come at last.[10] Collins grasped his opportunity and at once embarked on a programme of social reform for Scotland. By an accident of timing, the Lovat Committee's recommendation for an inquiry into Scotland's health services became caught up in Collins' overall programme for Scotland.

Collins had been attracted to national politics in 1910 by the social reforms which Asquith and Lloyd George were then carrying through Parliament. His support for social reform was in keeping with his family tradition. Through several generations the family had been active in philanthropy, in the temperance movement and in local government. The family publishing house, of which Collins was then the very successful

---

9 Sir Archibald Sinclair had been Secretary of State for Scotland in the National Government since August 1931 but was unable to accept its tariff policy. He resigned from the Government in September 1932.

10 *The Times*, 14 October 1936.

managing director,[11] had been established by his great-grandfather to publish the sermons of his close friend, the evangelical reformer Dr Thomas Chalmers. Later generations of the family promoted their company to become the only publisher of Bibles and the principal publisher of educational material in Scotland.

Collins was already well known in the West of Scotland for his advocacy of New Liberalism when he was asked to stand for Parliament as a Liberal in 1910. From his first election until his death in 1936 he represented Greenock, a town which, in its poverty, ill health and slum housing, was among the worst in Scotland. His constituency was part of Red Clydeside where, especially in the years of the First World War, there was considerable unrest due to 'a convergence of Marxist political theory with industrial fact.'[12] Collins was a conscientious Member of Parliament, seen always to be active in the interests of the deprived in his constituency. He was a popular and effective campaigner in the backcourts and greens of Greenock. In seven general elections he retained a comfortable majority against strong opposition from Communist and Labour candidates. Throughout his long parliamentary career he served a working-class constituency that shared in full all the social ills of the 1920s and 1930s. In his last election in 1935, shortly before his death, he had his highest-ever majority.[13]

Within months of his arrival in the House of Commons in 1910, Collins had been appointed as a Parliamentary Private Secretary to the Secretary of State for War. As a young man he had served in the Royal Navy; on the outbreak of the First World War he volunteered for service in the army and served with distinction in Gallipoli and in Mesopotamia. On his return to the House of Commons, he was made a Junior Lord of the Treasury in 1919 but in office he soon became disheartened and disillusioned by the Government's failure to secure the strict control of public expenditure that he believed to be essential. In the end, it was his refusal to accept government policy for Ireland that led to his resignation in 1920. In 1921, he crossed from the government side of the House to join the Asquith Liberals. Now openly in opposition, he was free to speak against Government policy on reparations, believing that they would destabilise Germany and eventually lead to war. On home affairs he argued that a continuing excess of

11 Collins had expanded the company's list. He launched the *Collins Illustrated Pocket Classics*, *The Nation's Library*, and *The Sevenpennies*. He published H. G. Wells, Rose Macaulay and Walter de la Mare. He introduced Agatha Christie, Dorothy L. Sayers and Ngaio Marsh as authors of his series, 'Crime Club'. His final venture as a publisher was to produce the 'Westerns' so much enjoyed by Lloyd George.
12 C. Harvie, *No Gods and Precious Few Heroes* (Edinburgh, 1981), p. 16.
13 It had been widely expected, and forecast in the press, that as a Liberal National, he would lose his seat in an election in which a large Conservative majority was expected and Liberals of all groups seemed almost irrelevant.

government bureaucracy would inhibit the recovery of the country's economy. For almost all of his remaining years in Parliament, he had remained excluded from any position of influence. When he was suddenly and unexpectedly invited to become Secretary of State for Scotland, he received the invitation with 'utter amazement.'[14] But he was more than ready to accept the appointment.

From the beginning he made it clear that his objective as Secretary of State for Scotland was to reduce Scotland's material deprivation in all its forms. His cause was, as always, essentially humanitarian but in 1932 he had an additional motive. By improving social conditions he hoped to dampen the rising spirit of nationalism and silence the crescendo of calls for Home Rule. Within weeks of his appointment he wrote to the Chancellor of the Exchequer:

> I think you are aware that in recent months the agitation in certain quarters for a measure of Home Rule for Scotland has assumed considerable proportions. My opinion is that the ranks of the supporters of the movement at the present time are greatly swelled by the prevalence of a belief that Scotland is not obtaining a fair return for her contribution to the national revenue.[15]

In the years until his death in office Collins set about securing that 'fair return' for Scotland by laying the foundations for improvements in the economy, in housing and, not least, in health.

To ensure the effective management of his schemes for Scotland, he at once proceeded to devolve the relevant administrative authorities from London to Scotland. Having been a believer in reduced government in 1920, he had become a convert to a new faith in 1932. He set about creating a commanding centralised, but devolved, Scottish administration. First, he began a reorganisation of the Scottish Office. A substantial part of its work was transferred from Dover House in London to various departmental offices sited in Edinburgh. On 15 February 1934 he opened the Edinburgh Branch Office of the Scottish Office as a temporary headquarters until a new building could be built on Calton Hill to house all the Scottish Departments together on one site. At the opening of the Branch Office, he announced his intention to set up a Committee[16] to 'inquire into and report upon the responsibilities and organisation of the Scottish administrative Departments under the control of the Secretary of State, the distribution of duties amongst these Departments, their relationship to the central executive

---

14 G. Pottinger, *The Secretaries of State for Scotland* (Edinburgh, 1979), p. 54.
15 NAS HH 1/791.
16 This committee was still at work at the time of Collins' death in June 1936.

Government, and the arrangements under which liaison is maintained between Edinburgh and the central executive government.'[17] The Department of Health for Scotland, which had previously conducted its business in Edinburgh with little or no reference to the Scottish Office in London, became part of a new integrated Office of the Secretary of State for Scotland.[18] This office was established in Edinburgh as a confederation of the four large Departments – Home Department, Department of Health, Department of Agriculture and Fisheries and Department of Education. As a result of Collins' initiative, the Department of Health for Scotland, with its responsibility for housing as well as health, was made part of a devolved administration in Edinburgh, answerable only to the Secretary of State for Scotland and not to the Minister of Health in London

In 1918 Collins had complained of the inadequacies of the staff of the Scottish Office.[19] In office as Secretary of State he set out to find 'officers of suitable quality, education and otherwise'[20] to replace the civil servants of executive grade who had previously made up the staff of the Scottish Office. In 1935 he obtained Treasury approval to recruit administrative-class officers into the Department of Health. Among the first to be recruited, through Class I open competition, was T. D. (later Sir Douglas) Haddow. He and the other able and ambitious civil servants who came together in the Department of Health were later to play a vital role in the establishment of the National Health Service in Scotland.

Having begun the reorganisation of the Scottish Office, Collins increased its powers to influence the Scottish economy. Under the Special Areas (Development and Improvements) Act of 1934 schemes were designed to aid the recovery of those parts of the United Kingdom that had been most severely affected by the Depression. Although one of these distressed areas was centred on Lanarkshire, in the original drafting of the Bill it had been intended that there should be only one Commissioner for all the Special Areas in the United Kingdom who would answer to the Minister of Labour. Collins persuaded Chamberlain that this would not be acceptable to public opinion in Scotland. Cabinet reluctantly agreed that there should be a separate Scottish Commissioner within the jurisdiction of the Scottish Office with a budget twice the 'Goshen formula.'[21] This new capability for the promotion of industry was the beginning of a new economic

17 NAS HH 45/61.
18 'The clean method of overcoming difficulties is to make one fold, as there is one shepherd, by a general transfer of the power and the duties of Departments to the Secretary of State.' NAS HH 1/799.
19 *Hansard*, cvii, HC 4 July 1918, col. 1974.
20 Sir G. Collins, quoted by I. Levitt, *The Scottish Office* (Edinburgh, 1992), p. 16.
21 A calculation made in 1888 that Scotland was entitled to share in grants in the ratio of 11 parts to England's 80 as recognition of her share of taxation.

development function for the Scottish Office. Before his death Collins had sanctioned the formation of the Scottish Economic Committee that was to be developed by his successor as Secretary of State, Walter Elliot.

Collins also acquired additional powers for the Scottish Office to cope with Scotland's longstanding problems in housing. For more than a century it had been widely recognised that housing conditions in Scotland were worse than in England and worse than in most other parts of Europe. But it was the report of the Royal Commission on Scottish Housing[22] in 1917 that had revealed the full appalling extent of the problem. The Royal Commission recommended that the state must accept direct responsibility for the housing of the working class. In 1919 the National Government announced its intention to promote house building as part of post-war reconstruction, building 'homes for heroes.' In the 1920s and into the 1930s, housing in the United Kingdom remained high on the agendas of successive governments. But, as had been admitted in 1917, there were particular problems in Scotland

Successive Scottish Secretaries before Collins had argued in Cabinet for special consideration for Scotland's greater needs but with no success. In 1920, Robert Munro had been unable to prevent the suspension of the Scottish building programme. His successor, Lord Novar, had failed to persuade Neville Chamberlain that Scotland's housing problems justified special treatment in his Housing Act of 1923. John Wheatley, as Minister of Health in the Labour government, though himself an MP for a Clydeside constituency, had made little concession to Scotland's special problems in his Housing (Financial Provisions) Act of 1924. In 1925 Walter Elliot, as Parliamentary Under Secretary of State at the Scottish Office in the succeeding Conservative government, made an ingenious attempt to win concessions for Scotland. He out-manoeuvred the denial of special aid for Scotland by the Minister of Health, Neville Chamberlain, by inviting the Prime Minister, Stanley Baldwin, to visit the slums of the Gorbals[23] and Cowcaddens. Following his visit, Baldwin announced a subsidy of £40 per house to Scottish local authorities for the erection of steel prefabricated houses. The manoeuvre backfired; the steel houses found no favour with the local authorities and Chamberlain announced that in future he would be extremely watchful that the Scottish Office got no more out of Government than its fair share.[24] Sir John Gilmour, as Secretary of State, continued to

---

22 *Report of the Royal Commission on the Housing of the Industrial Population of Scotland Rural and Urban*, 1917, Cd. 8731.
23 Walter Elliot had personal experience of the Gorbals as a medical student and while working on nutritional problems with Professor Cathcart in the Department of Physiology of Glasgow University.
24 J. Gibson, *The Thistle and the Rose: A History of the Scottish Office* (Edinburgh, 1985), p. 71.

maintain that the British housing policy 'barely touched the fringe'[25] of the problems in Scotland but, either in spite of, or because of, his Under Secretary's activities, no concessions were forthcoming. By 1932 the gap between Scotland and England in the supply of houses had widened further than ever. With interest rates and other costs falling, England was beginning to enjoy a housing boom that was not matched in Scotland. Sir Hilton Young, the Minister of Health, felt justified in withdrawing housing subsidies except for those aimed specifically at slum clearance. It was now that Collins won the first real concession for Scotland; the general subsidy was retained in Scotland and Collins went on to consolidate this success. In 1934, when the cabinet agreed that the Housing Bill for England should make provision of a basic subsidy of £3 for each house for twenty years, Collins successfully argued that considerable modification of this scheme would be required for Scotland. The Housing (Scotland) Act 1934 negotiated by Collins allowed for a basic subsidy of £6.15.0 for forty years with an additional £4 per house in areas where extensive redevelopment was required.[26]

Collins was equally determined to pursue an independent line for Scotland in improving the state of the country's health. By increasing the strength and potential of the Department of Health for Scotland, he created a suitable instrument. The Lovat Committee provided the occasion. While in England the responsible minister, the Conservative Sir Hilton Young, took no action in response to the recommendations of the Committee on Local Expenditure (England and Wales), Collins, the Liberal reformer in Scotland, seized on the recommendation of the Lovat Committee as the opportunity to improve all medical services in Scotland – including those for which his department was not yet responsible. In June 1933, Collins appointed the Committee on Scottish Health Services:

> To review the existing health services of Scotland in the light of modern conditions and knowledge and to make recommendations on any changes in policy and organisation that may be considered necessary for the promotion of efficiency and economy.[27]

The Cathcart Committee

Collins brought together in the Committee on Scottish Health Services the best and widest spectrum of advice available. He did not ask the public bodies in Scotland, state and voluntary, with responsibilities for providing

25 Quoted by Levitt, *op. cit.*, p. 43.
26 Levitt, *op. cit*, p. 272.
27 Cathcart Report, p. 3.

health care to appoint a delegate to represent their various interests. The records of the British Medical Association and the Royal Medical Corporations in Scotland show no evidence that the medical profession was formally consulted about the constitution of the Committee. Invitations to take part in the work of the Committee were made to individuals chosen as those most likely to be useful in shaping new health services for Scotland.

The Chairman chosen for the Committee was Sir John Dove Wilson, a senior servant of the Crown with experience of chairing such bodies.[28] Nicol McColl of the Administrative Section of the Department of Health was appointed as Secretary. Three senior officials of the Department of Health attended (J. Vallance, Assistant Secretary, James Brownlie, Chief Medical Officer, and John Jardine of the School Medical Service).

Although not formally represented by delegates, the principal organisations with an interest in the existing health services each found a voice from among the eighteen members of the Committee. There were voices from:

Local Government: Provost David Fisher of Hawick, Sir Andrew Grierson, Treasurer of Edinburgh, and Violet Robertson, Convenor of Glasgow Corporation Health Committee.
Insurance Committees: W. M. Marshall, Scottish Association of Insurance Committees.
Trade Unions: Joseph Westwood, Political Organiser, Scottish Miners.
Public Health: Alexander Macgregor, President of the Royal Sanitary Society.
British Medical Association: R. W. Craig, Scottish Secretary.
Royal Medical Corporations: Alexander Miles, President of the Royal College of Surgeons of Edinburgh.
University Medical Schools: E. P. Cathcart, Professor of Physiology, Glasgow University.
Nursing: Mrs Chalmers Watson, Queen's Institute of Nursing.

Each Committee member was more than a voice from the body to which he or she belonged. Every member had already made a significant contribution to the improvement of public service. Following the precedent of the Scottish Board of Health in 1918, the Committee included women members. These were not token members.[29] Mrs A. M. Chalmers Watson MD,

28 Sir John Dove Wilson was a retired Judge President of the Natal Division of the Supreme Court of South Africa and currently Chairman of the Committee on Recurrent Offenders.
29 In spite of their achievements, while their husbands are listed in *Who's Who*, the women themselves are not.

CBE,[30] the wife of the senior physician at Edinburgh Royal Infirmary had been the first woman medical graduate of Edinburgh University and was a recognised authority on nutrition. (She was later appointed to the Government's Advisory Committee on Diet.) She was President of the British Medical Women's Federation, editor of the *Encyclopaedia Medica* and a founder of the Edinburgh College of Domestic Science. In the First World War she had been the first Controller of the Women's Army Auxiliary Corps. At the time of her appointment she was Hon. Secretary of the Queen's District Nursing Association. Lady Mackenzie, CBE was the wife of Sir Leslie Mackenzie who, as the first Medical Inspector of the Local Government Board for Scotland, had been prominent in public health reform since his researches for the Royal Commission on Physical Training in 1903; Lady Mackenzie had been her husband's assistant in his researches. When appointed to the Committee she was Director of the Edinburgh College of Domestic Science and author of several works on child welfare, special schools and mental deficiency. Baillie Violet Robertson CBE was a graduate of Queen Margaret College, Glasgow and the University of Dresden. For many years she had been Convenor of Glasgow Corporation Health Committee, the first woman in Britain to hold such a post. (After the Second World War she was to be awarded the St Mungo Prize for her work in child health.)

Of the men, R. W. Craig had played a prominent part in drawing up the BMA's proposals for reform in its pamphlet *A General Medical Service for the Nation*, published in 1930.[31] Ian Carmichael DSO, MC, Convenor of Lanarkshire County Council, had been a leading member of the Lovat Committee that had first recommended that health services in Scotland should be reviewed. David Fisher was a member of the Empire Marketing Board that had initiated John Boyd Orr's famous trial of the nutritional value of milk in 1926.[32] Alexander Gray, Professor of Political Economy at Aberdeen University, was a former member of the Royal Commission on National Insurance and Chairman of the Consultative Council on National Health Insurance. Sir Andrew Grierson, Town Clerk of Edinburgh had, for several years, been an outspoken advocate of administrative reform

30 Mrs Mona Chalmers Watson, the first woman medical graduate of Edinburgh, was a member of a distinguished family. Her brothers Sir Eric Geddes and Sir Auckland Geddes had both been members of the Cabinet in the Coalition Government 1916–1922. Elizabeth Garret Anderson, the first English woman medical graduate, was a cousin.
31 *BMJ*, i, 1930, p. 165.
32 Sir Leslie Mackenzie was chairman of the Empire Marketing Board; Tom Johnston, Secretary of State during the wartime planning of the NHS, was also a member. Its successor, the Milk Marketing Board, was set up in 1933 by Boyd Orr's friend and Collins' successor as Secretary of State, Walter Elliot.

by extension of local government. Alexander (later Sir Alexander) Mac-gregor, as Medical Officer of Health for Glasgow, had established a reputation by making maximum use of the existing enabling legislation to expand the local authority health services in Glasgow further than had been attempted by any other authority in Scotland. Alexander Miles was editor of the *Edinburgh Journal of Medicine*, a member of the General Medical Council and a Curator of Patronage of the University of Edinburgh. Joseph Westwood had been briefly Under-Secretary of State for Scotland in 1931 and was later to be the Secretary of State at the time of the National Health Service (Scotland) Act in 1947.

During his few years of political influence before his death in 1936, Sir Godfrey Collins was determined that social condition in Scotland must be improved and was convinced that improvement could best be achieved by a devolved administration. In the Department of Health for Scotland he created a devolved bureaucracy to administer health services separately in Scotland. In the Cathcart Committee he created an authoritative body to advise on how these services should be shaped.

Cathcart and Medical Leadership

The dominant personality on the Committee, and the inevitable choice as its chairman on the death of Sir John Dove-Wilson in April 1935, was Professor Edward Cathcart. His background, his career and his philosophy made him an outstanding leader of the medical profession in Scotland and an appropriate choice as a guide in the planning of future health services for Scotland. That he should represent the leadership of the medical profession in Scotland provides an insight into the nature of the differences between the Scottish medical tradition and the tradition in England, a gulf that was to complicate the creation of a National Health Service in the United Kingdom. Cathcart qualified in medicine in Glasgow in 1900, intending to make his career in clinical medicine. It was then usual in Scotland for ambitious clinicians to complete their training in Germany or in one of the other great continental centres of medical science.[33] Cathcart went first to Berlin and then to Munich for postgraduate experience in the clinically useful science of bacteriology. It was a chance meeting with the physiologist, Karl Voit, in Munich that diverted his interest from bacteriology to the new science of nutrition and diverted him from a career as a clinician with special interest in bacteriology to a career as a medical scientist with close links to clinical practice.

---

33 After the war the link with Germany was lost. Before the Second World War the United States had already begun to take Germany's place in postgraduate training in medicine.

Germany was then at the forefront of medical science. In the reconstruction of Germany after the Napoleonic Wars the universities had been become state institutions instructed 'to redirect the emphasis from pedagogy and encyclopaedic learning to independent research.'[34] The German states were intent on producing graduates ready to tackle the problems of the industrialising economy of Germany in the middle of the nineteenth century. Almost every university in Germany established new research institutes to produce work in the interest of the state. Germany became perhaps the foremost centre of scientific research in the nineteenth century.

The medical sciences were of particular interest to the state. While it was accepted that the state had a duty to promote the wellbeing of the citizen, it was also accepted that the citizen had a duty to the state to maintain his fitness for labour in industry and for service in war, and fitness required an adequate diet.

Karl Voit, Cathcart's mentor, having established his reputation by developing quantitative methods for determining the food requirements for the maintenance of a 'normal' life, was required by the state to use these methods in advising on the control of food intake in such institutions as prisons and workhouses and in the military services. Employers in German industry were also interested in sound nutrition with a view to securing the fitness and efficiency of their workers. Their interest was expressed by *Kölnische Zeitung.*

> To create, maintain and support industrious workers, that is the unavoidable requirement for the future of industry. Countries such as England, France and Belgium owe their superiority in certain branches of industry partly to the greater productivity of their workers. We must endeavour to grant the worker all he needs for his and his dependants' subsistence.[35]

It was in this context that Cathcart was introduced to the study of nutrition in Munich. His later work derived from this training and experience. His nutritional research was on food as a source of energy and on the design of diets to maximise human capacity for work. (Cathcart eventually published his corpus of work in 1929 in his book *The Human Factor in Industry.*)

After working for a time with Francis Benedict in the United States, Cathcart returned to Britain in 1915 as Professor of Physiology at the London Hospital. He was quickly recruited into the Royal Army Medical Corps to investigate the energy requirements of army recruits and, later, to advise on the dietary requirement of soldiers in the field. Cathcart con-

34 A. M. Tuchman, *Science, Medicine and the State in Germany* (Oxford, 1993), p. 5.
35 *Kölnische Zeitung,* 29 December 1880.

tinued to be consulted by government after the war and after his return to Glasgow as Professor of Physiological Chemistry at Glasgow University. As the *BMJ* later said of him, 'few men can have served on so many expert committees.'[36] He was at some time a member of the Medical Research Council, the League of Nations Technical Advisory Committee on Nutrition, the Army Hygiene Advisory Committee, the National Advisory Committee on Physical Training (Scotland), the Ministry of Health's Advisory Committee on Nutrition, the Committee on Nutrition in the Colonial Empire, the International Labour Office's Committee on Industrial Hygiene, and Chairman of the Industrial Health Research Board. His experience as a regular adviser to governments and his eminence as a medical scientist made him an obvious choice to serve on the Committee on Scottish Health Services. As an eminent advocate of the principle that medical practice and medical science were inseparable, Cathcart was respected by members of every branch of the medical profession in Scotland. That he had held a university chair for twenty years established his authority in Scotland where the medical profession traditionally looked to the universities for leadership.

The medical profession in England did not draw its leaders from the universities. In England and Wales the leaders of the profession belonged to a body of elite clinicians who kept medical science and the medical scientists of the universities at a careful distance. In the 1930s Lord Horder, royal physician and physician to St Bartholomew's Hospital, London, was perhaps the most prominent member of that elite. In 1936, Lord Horder was invited to give the opening lecture of the Bicentenary Session of the Royal Medical Society in Edinburgh.[37] He was at pains to make it clear to his audience of Scottish medical students that he was not of 'the tradition in your country.' While he expressed his respect for the tradition of Cullen, Syme, Lister, Bright, Addison and Simpson, he was proud to belong to another, English tradition. This, Horder held to be the tradition of Hippocrates, realised in England by the great William Harvey, Thomas Sydenham, Edward Jenner and Samuel Gee. In the early years of the twentieth century (while Edward Cathcart was completing his training in physiology in Munich), Samuel Gee, Horder's mentor at St Bartholomew's, was instructing his students: 'When you enter my wards, your first duty is to forget all your physiology. Physiology is an experimental science and a very good thing in its proper place. Medicine is not a science but an empirical art.'[38] In the English tradition the ideal physician was a gentleman-scholar, devoted to literature

36 *BMJ*, i, 1954, p. 532.
37 Published later in Lord Horder, *Health and a Day* (London, 1937), p. 42.
38 Quoted by Sir Henry Dale, *BMJ*, ii, 1950, p. 1187.

and natural history, caring conscientiously and empirically for his patients in patrician style with his mind uncluttered by scientific theory.[39] In the English tradition, as Horder informed his student audience in 1936, the personality, personal experience and 'horse sense' of the doctor were the fundamental elements in the management of patients. The study of medicine was to be regarded as an extension of natural history rather than of experimental science. Clinicians were advised to be cautious of 'laboratory methods and the exploitation of instruments of precision.'[40] While the information provided might add to his careful observation of the patient, Horder denied that the physician's work required the sanction of science. The practice of medicine must be inductive and empirical.

By the beginning of the twentieth century an English medical elite in this tradition had become institutionalised in the London teaching hospitals, in Harley Street, at the Royal College of Physicians of London and the Royal College of Surgeons of England.[41] The position of the Colleges was challenged in 1815 when a licence from Apothecaries' Hall became recognised as the essential qualification for general practitioners in England. Faced by this competition, in 1860 the Royal College of Physicians extended its area of jurisdiction beyond London, granting licences to practice elsewhere in England and Wales. However, many public appointments now required a qualification in both medicine and surgery; in 1884 the Royal College of Physicians of London and the Royal College of Surgeons formed a Joint Board examining for a combined qualification[42] 'to prevent candidates from crossing the border to Scotland.'[43]

At that time the only universities granting degrees in medicine in England were Oxford, Cambridge and Durham. 'By 1890 to these had been added the complex of colleges and medical schools comprising the Victoria University centred on Manchester',[44] and by the early years of the new century the provincial universities all granted degrees in their own right. Nevertheless, large numbers of those intending to make their careers in general practice across England and Wales continued to take only the qualifying examination of the Joint Board.[45] Even as medical education

---

39 Christopher Lawrence has set out an excellent critique of the English tradition in 'Ornate Physicians and Learned Artisans', in W. F. Bynum and R. Porter (eds.), *William Hunter and the Eighteenth Century Medical World* (Cambridge, 1985).
40 Horder, *op. cit.*, p. 48.
41 The evolution of this elite is discussed in Chapter 8.
42 MRCS, LRCP.
43 C. Newman, *The Evolution of Medical Education in the Nineteenth Century* (London, 1957), p. 298.
44 *Ibid.*, p. 292.
45 The examinations of the Joint Board were thought to be easier than those of the universities. Many students took the MRCP LRCP as a bird in the hand.

expanded, London continued to be the head and heart of the English system, and its patrician clinicians remained in charge.

In the 1930s, in essentials, nothing had changed. Graduates of Oxford and Cambridge still dominated the Fellowship of the Royal Colleges in London and the consultant clinicians to the English teaching hospitals were, without exception, Fellows of the Colleges. In the 1930s this elite, practising privately among the wealthy and adopting the lifestyle and leisure activities of their plutocratic patients,[46] dominated the medical profession in England and set the style of practice. (It was their commitment to the empiric clinical individualism that later, during the struggles for the National Health Service, was to be disguised as 'clinical freedom' and claimed as a right for the whole medical profession.) In London, the patrician doctors, practising, and to some extent living, in the society of the most wealthy, aristocratic and influential in the country, made up the most powerful medical interest in Britain in the 1930s.[47]

In Scotland there was no counterpart of the London entrepreneurial medical elite nor was there a society in Scotland that could have supported such an elite. The transfer first of the Crown, and later of Parliament, from Edinburgh to London in 1603 on 1707 respective had drawn generations of the aristocracy, the wealthy and the politically powerful to London.[48] Medicine and the other distinctively Scottish institutions of civil society, the church, the parish schools, the law, and the universities, had survived the Union of the Parliaments. Over two centuries, the medical profession had flourished but had not developed a hierarchical structure as in England where the structure of the medical profession reflected the structure of the hierarchical society it aimed to serve. In Scotland, trained with different objectives, the medical profession developed in close association with the universities.

From the beginning of the eighteenth century, and in contrast to the free-for-all of the London teaching hospitals where training was conducted by individual clinicians,[49] the Scottish university medical schools had a set curriculum and teaching was firmly under the control of the professors. While the practice of medicine was acknowledged to be an art, that art was based on the systematic study of natural philosophy, botany, anatomy, experimental chemistry and physiology, pathology and materia medica. In

46 Bertrand (later Lord) Dawson found it necessary to have dancing lessions before becoming physician to Edward VII. F. Watson, *Dawson of Penn* (London, 1950), p. 35.
47 They exerted their influence quietly. Since the activities of the BMA were noisier and better documented, historians have tended to exaggerate its relative importance.
48 N. T. Philipson, 'Nationalism and Ideology', in J. N. Wolfe (ed.) *Government and Nationalism in Scotland* (Edinburgh, 1969), p. 170.
49 Discussed in Chapter 8.

teaching clinical medicine, Edinburgh gave the lead in following the Boerhaave 'system.'[50] At that time, there was a division in the medical world between those who, as in England, were content with the observation of facts (empirics) and those, like Boerhaave, who sought explanations (dogmatists). In the Boerhaave system adopted in Scotland, the subjects to be taught in the medical schools were clearly defined and the relevant facts and theories were brought together and studied with 'sceptical dogmatism.' In the dogmatic nosology, diseases were grouped together according to a single outstanding characteristic (e.g. 'fever') and studied in relation to 'proximate cause' to give guidance on rational treatment and in relation to 'ultimate cause' to guide on prevention. By the middle of the century the Boerhaave system had been developed by William Cullen to a pattern that was followed thereafter in Edinburgh and Glasgow and adopted in North America.[51] Although Cullen's system was dogmatic, it remained open to change in the light of new evidence. 'No man can go much further than the state of science at his particular period allows him,' and it was only 'the combination of philosophy with the facts of physic that could make any considerable change to the state of the art.'[52]

Cullen made certain that no student at Edinburgh or Glasgow could graduate without attending the set classes[53] and satisfying the examiners.[54] (Cullen tried without success to persuade government to introduce Royal Commissioners to inspect all medical schools in the United Kingdom, to correct abuses and to ensure that medical degrees were given only after two years' student training and after rigorous examination. His recommendations were eventually incorporated in the Medical Act of 1858.)

Although education in the Scottish medical schools was progressively modified in the nineteenth century, in its principles it continued unchanged. While a few Scottish graduates went on to achieve great success in entrepreneurial private practice in Harley Street or elsewhere, they continued in the systematic science-based Scottish tradition. The most ambi-

50 M. Barfoot, 'Cullen's Medical Teaching; An Analysis of the Pedagogical and Epistemological Meaning of 'System' by Philosophy and Method', in A. Doig, J.P. Ferguson, I. A. Milne, and R. Passmore (eds.), *William Cullen and the Eighteenth Century Medical World* (Edinburgh, 1993), p. 110.

51 A. Doig *et al*, 'Cullen's Influence on American Medicine,' *ibid.*, p. 40.

52 W. Cullen quoted by Barfoot, *op. cit.*, p. 119.

53 Lectures could be attended by those with only limited interest in medicine and who did not intend to graduate. Church of Scotland ministers often attended medical courses in preparation for taking up their parish duties.

54 Until the nineteenth century St Andrews University; King's College, Aberdeen; and Marischal College, Aberdeen offered almost no training and conferred medical degrees on personal recommendation and the payment of a fee. This was thought by some to undermine the reputation of the high-quality Scottish degrees from Edinburgh and Glasgow.

tious and, in due course, the leading Scottish physicians strengthened their roots in medical science by extending their postgraduate training in the leading institutes in Europe. In 1935, most physicians at Edinburgh Royal Infirmary[55] had received part of their training in Vienna, Freiburg, Berlin, or Heidelberg; in Glasgow, the physicians of the Western Infirmary, with only two exceptions had postgraduate experience in Paris, Vienna, Berlin or Strasbourg.[56] This contrasted with the relative neglect of postgraduate scientific interest and training among the physicians of England who remained deliberately committed to empiricism. In 1935 none of the physicians of the London Hospital, St George's Hospital or St Mary's Hospital had received any training outside Oxbridge and the London teaching hospitals. St Bartholomew's, St Thomas's, St George's, Guy's, Middlesex, and Westminster Hospitals each had one physician with post-graduate scientific training (in, respectively, Munich, Berlin, Frankfurt, Munich, Vienna and Vienna). King's College Hospital had two (Gothen-burg and Freiburg). The only physician on the staff of University College Hospital with postgraduate scientific training (Freiburg) was a Glasgow graduate. Charing Cross Hospital also had two, one an Edinburgh graduate (Munich) and the other a Dublin graduate (Berlin and Frankfurt).

In London, the leaders of the medical profession did not owe their position to their place in medical science but to their place in society. They exercised their considerable influence with government through personal contact with their wealthy and influential patients and through the London Royal Colleges that they dominated.

In Scotland there was no such medical elite with established and continuing private access to the country's leading figures. While private practice flourished at a certain level in Scotland, it was not linked to an hierarchical society that could, at its top, support a body of elite and influential doctors. In consequence, in Scotland, there was no influential medical elite to confer privately with members of the government. Unlike the Royal Colleges in London, the Scottish Royal Corporations were not traditionally consulted by government.[57] The medical profession in Scot-land had no voice 'at court' to compare with that of the institutionalised elite in London. The medical members of the Cathcart Committee, chosen to advise on the future of health services in Scotland, were not drawn from a body of successful patrician clinicians. They belonged to a profession that looked for its leadership among those who had distinguished themselves in public service or in medical science.

55 Edinburgh Royal Infirmary and Glasgow Western Infirmary are cited since they were the main teaching hospitals in Scotland's largest medical schools.
56 *Medical Directory*, 1935.
57 'Who Should Speak for the Medical Profession,' Appendix I.

Cathcart and his Philosophy

In the 1930s, Professor Cathcart was respected and his position as a leader of the medical profession in Scotland was unquestioned. However, outside Scotland, and especially among medical scientists, he had become a controversial figure, caught up in two contemporary disputes.[58]

In the early years of the twentieth century, a group at Glasgow University[59] led by Noel Paton, the Professor of Physiology, and Leonard Findlay, Lecturer in the Disease of Childhood, had established a reputation for their work on nutrition and on the aetiology of rickets. For them, and in the Scottish tradition, physiology was one of the Institutes of Medicine[60] to be studied in association with clinical observation and practice. In 1918, their position was challenged by the emergence of a new generation of laboratory-based medical scientists. Frederick Lowland Hopkins had been appointed to the foundation chair at Cambridge in 1914, the first Professor of Biochemistry in the United Kingdom. Since there was then only a small medical faculty at Cambridge and no clinical teaching, Hopkins' work was confined to the laboratory. He had established his reputation in the investigation of the 'accessory food factors' initially in relation to beri-beri, not then or since a clinical problem in man in the United Kingdom. His interests widened to include the study of other animal models of disease and in 1918 one of his group, Edward Mellanby, working with pups, claimed to have shown that rickets was caused by a lack of an accessory food substance in the diet.[61]

Leonard Findlay, on the basis of his extensive experience of what was then a very common condition in Glasgow, had already published his conclusion that rickets was not a dietary problem but was probably caused by lack of exercise and time spent in the open.[62] In 1918, Margaret Ferguson, another member of the Glasgow Group, had again reached the conclusion that 'inadequate air and exercise seem to be potent factors in determining the onset of rickets.'[63] However, the Medical Research

58 These controversies have been discussed by D. Smith and M. Nicolson and by M. Mayhew as listed in the bibliography.
59 Often referred to as the 'Glasgow School' following the publication of L. Findlay, 'A Review of the Work Done by the Glasgow School on the Aetiology of Rickets,' *Lancet*, i, 1922, p. 825.
60 In earlier times, the sciences relating to medicine, such as physiology, were known as the Institutes of Medicine and were taught by clinical professors who might expect to be promoted later to be Professors of Medicine.
61 E. Mellanby, 'The Part Played by an 'Accessory Factor in the Production of Experimental Rickets,' *Journal of Physiology*, lii, 1918, xii and liii.
62 L. Findlay, 'The Aetiology of Rickets: A Statistical and Experimental Study,' *BMJ*, i, 1908, p. 965.
63 M. Ferguson, 'Social and Economic Factors in the Causation of Rickets,' *Medical Research Council Special Report Series No. 20* (London, 1918), p. 94.

Council (MRC) had been persuaded by Hopkins that 'accessory factors' (vitamins) were of vital importance in nutrition and had accepted Mellanby's experimental evidence of their role in the aetiology of rickets. A memorandum for famine relief workers produced by the MRC's newly appointed Accessory Food Factor Committee in July 1919 included recommendations based on the dietary deficiency theory of rickets.[64]

Paton was dismissive of Mellanby's work and scornful of all those who wished to separate medical science from medical practice:

> They indeed become a real danger to the advance of knowledge. Starting from nowhere and going no-whither, generally ignorant of what has to be done and not seeing what to do, they flicker their silly lamps in all directions and only obscure the path of real progress.[65]

The Glasgow Group continued to argue that rickets was not essentially due to a deficiency in the diet[66] although, by 1920, Paton was willing to concede that feeding might play some part in its control.[67] However, scientific opinion strongly supported Mellanby and Glasgow lost its position as a major centre for MRC-funded research on rickets.[68] Findlay moved to private practice in London and Paton died an embittered man in 1928.[69]

Cathcart, who succeeded to the Glasgow Chair of Physiology on Paton's death, had no difficulty in accepting the laboratory evidence that accessory food factors had a role in nutrition but he remained sceptical of the clinical importance attributed to them. In relation to rickets his views were vindicated in 1973 when it was discovered that the form of vitamin D essential for the prevention of rickets was produced by the action of sunlight on the skin.[70] But in the 1930s he was on the wrong side of the argument and, in the later judgement of historians, thought to be exhibiting an unfortunate 'conservative style of thought.'[71]

64 *Some Facts Concerning Nutrition for the Guidance of those Engaged in the Administration of Food Relief to Famine Stricken Districts* (London, 1919).
65 D. N. Paton, *Edinburgh Medical Journal*, xxxv (1928), p. 10.
66 D. N. Paton, L. Findlay, and A. Watson, 'Observations on the Cause of Rickets,' *BMJ*, ii, 1918, p. 625.
67 Smith and Nicolson, 'The "Glasgow School" of Paton, Findlay and Cathcart,' *Social Studies in Science*, p. 202.
68 *Ibid.*, p. 204.
69 *Ibid.*
70 In 1973 it was shown that even in subjects taking oral supplements of vitamin D, over 80% of the circulating vitamin D was in the 25 OHD form produced in the skin by the irradiation of ergosterols by ultraviolet light. J. G. Haddad and T. J. Hahn, 'The Natural and Synthetic Sources of Circulating Hydroxyvitamin D in Man,' *Nature*, ccxliv, 1973, p. 515.
71 Smith and Nicolson, *Social Studies in Science*, *op.cit.*, p. 197 and p. 223.

Although he had differed so publicly with the MRC,[72] Cathcart retained the confidence of the Ministry of Health and in Parliament the Minister, Sir Kingsley Wood, quoted him as a preferred authority.[73] It was this that once again involved him in controversy and led to criticism of his attitude to the health of the urban working class.[74]

By the end of the nineteenth century there were growing fears that as a consequence of the industrialisation of the nation and the urbanisation of the great mass of its people, the population of Britain had been afflicted by physical degeneration. Over a third of the men who presented themselves for recruitment to the army during the Boer War were found to be poorly grown and underweight. To many commentators it seemed evident that the urban working class was badly fed and that this must be attributed to poverty.[75] The evidence produced by John Boyd Orr at the Rowett Institute in the 1920s[76] and in his *Food, Health and Income*[77] in the 1930s was widely thought to have put this conclusion beyond doubt.

Government, however, was content to believe that the state welfare measures in place – old age pensions, National Insurance, maternity and child welfare schemes – had abolished poverty. The Ministry of Health did not 'wish to know about other evidence that equated undernourishment with low income.'[78] As early as 1906 government had blamed any deficiencies in diet on ignorance and carelessness.[79] This had been the conclusion of Paton and his colleagues after surveys in Edinburgh in 1901[80] and in Glasgow in 1913.[81] That poor feeding was due to 'fecklessness' had become identified as the view of the Glasgow Group. By 1931, Cathcart had modulated the language but still believed that lack of education, poor marketing skills and bad cooking were to blame rather than poverty.[82]

When pressed in the House of Commons by claims that in Britain in 1936 there was still widespread malnutrition due to poverty, the Minister of Health found it useful to quote Cathcart:

---

72 *Ibid.*, p. 204.
73 *Hansard*, cccxiv, HC 8 July 1935, col. 1243.
74 Smith and Nicolson, *Social Studies in Science, op.cit.*, p. 215.
75 These arguments and the supporting evidence are reviewed by Mayhew, *op.cit.*
76 Rowett Research Institute, *Family Diet and Health in Pre-War Britain* (London, 1955).
77 J. Boyd Orr, *Food, Health and Income* (London, 1937).
78 Mayhew, *op. cit.*, p. 455.
79 Smith and Nicolson, *Social Studies in Science, op. cit.*, p. 219.
80 D. N. Paton, J. Dunlop, E. Inglis, *A Study of the Diet of the Labouring Classes in Edinburgh* (Edinburgh, 1901).
81 D. E. Lindsay, *Report upon the Dietary of the Labouring Classes of the City of Glasgow* (Glasgow, 1913).
82 Smith and Nicolson, *Social Studies in Science, op. cit.*, p. 218.

We often hear Sir John Boyd Orr quoted rather incompletely, but there is an equally eminent member of the Ministry of Health Committee who can, I suppose, be regarded equally as an authority, and that is Professor Cathcart. He says that malnutrition is due not so much to poverty as to ignorance and other causes of the same kind.[83]

The Minister omitted to inform the House that, by 1936, Cathcart and John Boyd Orr were working together, that Cathcart had contributed to Boyd Orr's *Food, Health and Income* and had modified his views.[84] Although in 1936 Cathcart continued to attach particular importance to education, he may be excluded from the judgement by David Smith and Malcolm Nicolson that the Glasgow Group 'advocated policies that served the interests of the professional and middle classes as against those of the working class.'[85] Cathcart belonged to that layer of Scottish society – comfortably off, well-educated, professional men and women – which felt an obligation to improve the lot of the less fortunate. His attitude was undoubtedly paternalistic, and in seeking to improve the health of the people he intended, as Smith and Nicolson have observed, 'to preserve the forms of medical and scientific education which had become traditional in the Scottish universities.'[86]

Professor Cathcart was therefore eminently qualified to speak for medical practice in Scotland. Soon after succeeding Noel Paton as Professor of Physiology at Glasgow in 1928 he had begun to devote much of his energy to the work of a number of advisory bodies, both national and international. He became respected as a medical philosopher and statesman who promoted the new concept that the practice of clinical medicine should be primarily the promotion and maintenance of the 'constructive physiology' of the individual. This concept had emerged from the new discoveries of physiology, then the discipline at the forefront of medical science. Fuller understanding of the body's mechanisms seemed to offer the prospect that they could be successfully manipulated to correct abnormalities and maintain normal health. This new form of preventive medicine for the individual was particularly welcome at a time when specific cures were still virtually unknown.

In Scotland, Sir Donald MacAlister,[87] in *A Scheme of Medical Service for*

83 *Hansard, op. cit.*
84 Sir John Brotherston, 'The Development of Public Medical Care 1900–1948,' in G. McLachlan (ed.), *Improving the Common Weal* (Edinburgh, 1987), p. 82.
85 Smith and Nicolson, *Social Studies in Science, op. cit.*, p. 223.
86 *Ibid.*
87 Chairman, Consultative Council on Medical and Allied Subjects, Scottish Board of Health; Principal of the University of Glasgow; President of the General Medical Council.

Scotland in 1920,[88] had already set out an 'exposition of some general principles' which should govern the future practice of medicine. In addition to Public Health measures and the medical treatment of individual patients, greater attention should be given to 'safeguarding of the individual health.' This view was promoted in all the Scottish medical schools. In his lectures at Glasgow in 1932, A. K. Chalmers[89] argued that general practitioners should not confine themselves to the treatment of recognisable ailments but should actively promote the health of their patients. In his lectures, which were published in the *Glasgow Medical Journal*, Chalmers quoted Aristotle – 'health is no quiescent state, but a condition of unstable equilibrium maintained by continuous struggle.'[90]

This emphasis on maintenance of normal physiology represented a radical shift of ideas. In the second half of the previous century, physicians had been guided by the sciences of morbid anatomy and bacteriology. Without curative medicines the expertise of the physician lay in the diagnosis and the mitigation of the symptoms of disease.[91] His reputation, within the profession, was determined by his success in predicting the precise morbid changes that would be found in the post-mortem room. This was 'Mortuary Medicine', academically satisfying but of limited immediate benefit to the patients.[92]

In the 1930s, with progress in the science of physiology and the increasing understanding of the maintenance of normality, the perspectives of the medical profession were already changing. Supported by a growing canon of research, it was possible to look on the practice of medicine as 'constructive physiology,' the promotion or restoration of normal function. The treatment of disease, although still continuing to form the bulk of practice, could be regarded as secondary. Professor Cathcart, as an eminent physiologist, was an advocate of the widest interpretation of this constructive physiology. 'His interest in physiology was broad based. He was concerned with the Nature of Man and not with a mere corner of the human organism.'[93]

---

88 *A Scheme of Medical Services for Scotland*, 1920, Cmd. 1039 (MacAlister Report).
89 Medical Officer of Health for Glasgow.
90 A. K. Chalmers, 'Our Provision for Treating the Sick,' *Glasgow Medical Journal*, cxvii, 1932, p. 1.
91 In this period, the surgeon's skill was based on anatomy and he was occupied by the new opportunities following the introduction of aseptic surgery and more sophisticated anaesthesia. The obstetrician was still taken up by the unsolved problem of puerperal sepsis.
92 J. S. Fairbairn, 'Changes in Thought in a Half Century of Obstetrics,' *Edinburgh Medical Journal*, xvii, 1935, p. 63.
93 Minute of Council, Royal Faculty of Physicians and Surgeons of Glasgow, 1 March 1954.

In June 1933, the month of his appointment to the Committee on Scottish Health Services, he set out his ideas in an address at the Anderson College of Medicine in Glasgow. He described how the practice of medicine should be reshaped, not only in the interest of the individual but also in order to promote the fitness of the nation. He predicted that the future of medicine was in prevention:

> I do not anticipate, of course, that disease will vanish, that epidemics will cease, that immortality is within our grasp; in other words that the practice of medicine, as ordinarily conceived, will be exterminated in the near future. To hold such views would be the height of folly; but what will surely happen is that the earliest divergences from the so-called normal physiological state will be more readily detected, that, wisely or unwisely, the expectation of life will definitely be increased, that epidemics will be nipped in the bud, before, that is, they assume gross proportions. The aim of investigation will be the narrowing of the present gap which exists between perfect physiological normality and openly confessed disease. The difficulty, as I see it, will not so much be the detection of the earliest manifestation of disease, but the fixation of what is true normality, of the perfect physiological state.[94]

This perfect physiological state included not only the efficient functioning of the bodily systems – 'circulatory, digestive, and so on' – but the mind, since it was clear that the healthy happy mind was intimately related to the functioning of every other physiological system. Cathcart regretted that psychology had alway been divorced from physiology. 'What medicine wants today more than anything else is a true conspectus of the state of health.'

In giving priority to the maintenance of health over the treatment of disease, Cathcart proposed a change in the role of the general practitioner:

> Until it is thoroughly appreciated that unless and until your ordinary medical attendant knows perfectly your condition when you are well and fit, it will be impossible for him to detect the earliest signs of unfitness or disease. The doctor should not be regarded as one of the necessary evils of the sick-bed, as a man who has to be called in when you are stricken with disease, be it slight or severe, but as one who has your health and fitness in his charge and who can advise you as to the best measures to adopt in order to maintain your individual normal or to assist in restoring you to that normality.

94 E. P. Cathcart, 'Preventive Medicine and Public Health,' *Glasgow Medical Journal*, cxix, 1933, p. 185.

In giving prevention priority over palliation of disease, the state would be faced with difficult questions of ethics and morality:

> Immediately allied to preventive medicine is Public Health, – the application of preventive medicine to the community at large. Right and proper though this application of preventive medicine to the community may be, it may also, when looked at from another angle, be regarded as a deadly menace to the State. It is no doubt a good thing to applaud this manifestation of philanthropy as given by the State and the communal authorities at the cost of the taxpayer but there is a reverse side to this shield which, not being very attractive, is rarely looked at. Remember it is promiscuous philanthropy which is practised, general not selective. Look, for instance, at one of the many applications; the perpetuation of the unfit, the prolongation of the lives of the insane. It is, of course, difficult in cold blood to condemn these earnest endeavours, but why look askance at birth control and the sterilisation of the unfit.

Above all, the maintenance of a healthy race would require the active participation and co-operation of every individual member of the community. Cathcart believed that this could be achieved by educating the public:

> The progress of the future will be slower because the object to be attacked is man. Material things, no doubt, offer resistance, ordinary physical resistance, but they can always be overcome given time, patience and money. But man, feeble, pliable and of limited life as compared to the material obstacles of Nature, is resistant, conservative and stubborn. Time, patience and money may do much to overcome this human barrier to progress, but there is no certainty in the efficacy of any of these weapons. Of the three, time, not counted in days or months but in decades, is the weapon of choice in this duel *à outrance*. Not because time is like an abrasive that will wear away any form of recalcitrant material, but because it will give the needed opportunity for education. Education and good will on both sides and faith are the only solvents of the difficulty ... but it is a matter of supreme difficulty to convince ill-educated man in the mass ...
>
> The outlook of the man in the street, especially those least well endowed, has to be broadened. It is not merely that he, and far more important than the normal wage earner is the housewife, has to be educated as regards his nutrition and his housing, but he has to be educated in the proper use of his life.

Cathcart went on to emphasise that there are hazards to health other than from disease and that these must be taken into account in the education of the public:

All around us we hear the cry for rationalisation of industry. This means the better fitting out of shops with up to date machinery for the more economic production of goods. The aim of all modern machinery designers is to make machines automatic. What necessarily follows is that fewer and fewer workers are employed or shorter shifts will be worked. And hence the average working man will have more and more compulsory leisure. Is man at present fitted to utilise in proper fashion, to utilise to his good and not his detriment, his leisure hours? As Dean Inge has well said – 'A man's soul is coloured by the colour of his leisure thoughts.' The right use of leisure will become in the end as urgent and dominant a cry as the right use of machinery. It is infinitely easier to degenerate through excess of leisure than through the excess of work. Hard work never killed a sound, healthy man, but too much leisure may easily ruin him physically and spiritually. The majority of people have not yet grasped the dangers of leisure, its soul-destroying evils – gambling, drink and the rest. Those in control of the community must take thought to this gigantic problem, the insidious dry rot of the community and the State.

In this exposition of his ideas Cathcart made it clear that, for a healthier nation, he looked essentially to the creation of a more enlightened society. At the same time, the process of improvement would also require greater intervention by government in personal health care. It was equally clear that he intended that that intervention and control should be for the benefit of the whole population and should not be confined only to those defined sections of society recognised as having special needs.

Professor Cathcart accepted without question that the state should accept the role of *paterfamilias*. In this he was neither original nor unique in 1933. That the state should intervene to show people how to live and be healthy was accepted across the political spectrum of inter-war Europe.[95] It represented a view that had been growing in strength in Scotland for some years and was shared by the medical members of the Cathcart Committee and sat easily with a Scottish tradition of medicine based on science and system. Intervention by the state was inevitably less acceptable to the medical profession in England whose leaders held that the individual patient must be 'king'[96] and that health did not 'depend on science at all.'[97] The Committee on Scottish Health Services began work with a set of assumptions that were natural in Scotland but alien to the most influential leaders of the medical profession in England.

95 M. Mazower, *Dark Continent* (London, 1998), p. 78.
96 Lord Horder in an address to Westminster Hospital Medical School, 28 September 1936. Horder, 1937, *op. cit.*, p. 30.
97 Lord Horder in a BBC talk, 5 April 1937. *Ibid.*, p. 104.

The Cathcart Committee was an appropriate instrument in Sir Godfrey Collins' policy of taking an independent Scottish line in making state provision for the health of the people of Scotland. Collins had shown that, in the 1930s, there was the political will to have health services appropriate to social conditions as they were then in Scotland. In his re-structuring of the Scottish Office, he had created a bureaucracy to administer those services. In appointing the Committee on Scottish Health Services, he had brought together people well qualified to advise on how that should done as a development of existing Scottish practices and in accordance with Scottish values in the practice of medicine. The Committee had found in Edward Cathcart an eminent spokesman who could present the consensus view and articulate the philosophy on which it was based.

3

The Cathcart Report: The Context

The Cathcart Committee was commissioned to carry out an urgent
'review of the health services in Scotland in the light of modern
conditions and knowledge and to make recommendations in policy and
organisation that may be considered necessary.' The Committee saw that
the review could not be confined only to statutory health services. An
adequate assessment of the problems of the 1930s would be 'impossible
without taking account of the work of the general medical practitioner in
private practice, the voluntary hospitals and the many other private and
voluntary agencies that are concerned with health.'

While the immediate need was to repair the deficiencies of the past, there
was also an ultimate purpose to 'promote the health of the people.' In inter-
war Europe other countries were reshaping their health services with the
same objective. The promotion of sound health and well being of the
individual citizen was a humanely desirable objective. In the insecurity of
the time, when nation-states were in dangerous rivalry with each other, the
state also had a vital interest in the health and strength of its people. Across
the political spectrum in a number of countries in Western Europe there
was pressure for the state to intervene in private life to show people how to
live in order to be fit to serve the nation.[1] The potential benefits of the
collective management of the health of the human stock of a nation were
unquestionable, both to the individual and to the state. However, giving first
place to the interests of the state raised moral and ethical problems. It could
be argued that, in the biological management of the people, the removal of
the genetically unfit, the mentally defective, the chronically disabled and
the criminal was rational and desirable and therefore ethically acceptable. In
the 1930s, sterilisation schemes were introduced in Germany, Switzerland
and Sweden and continued for many years. By 1936, Germany was already
going to extremes in creating a racial welfare state. In the 1930s it had
become common currency that, in addition to providing preventive health
services, the state should intervene to guide and assist the individual in
promoting his own health, both in his own interest and in the interest of the
state. The Cathcart Report did not explicitly relate its search for a new
health policy to this European movement but, given the associations of its
medical members with universities in Europe, it may be assumed that the

1 M. Mazower, *Dark Continent* (London, 1998), p. 78.

Cathcart Committee was alive to the possible advantages in taking the same line.

In the 1930s there was clearly no point in continuing in conformity with England. In the fiscal crisis of the time central government had raised tariff barriers to protect a failing economy and to contain the soaring costs of social welfare. (The idea that the tariffs could finance social reform was an illusion.) In England the health services were not under review and their reform was not being contemplated. The Westminster administration of the 1930s was eager to show that, even during the Depression, state pensions and National Insurance had abolished poverty and that the health of the people was being well maintained by local authority services and the medical benefits of the National Health Insurance Scheme. Such satisfaction found some justification in the evidence from London itself and from that part of England, to the south and east of Birmingham, where a level of prosperity was maintained by new light industries and an associated building boom. But in the industrial North and in Wales the problems of unemployment and social distress were undeniable. There the old heavy industries had been in decline since the end of the war. In its original form the National Insurance Scheme and the associated health benefit could not cope with the rising numbers of unemployed and their deteriorating health. Between 1920 and 1926 there had been no fewer than fifteen Insurance Acts in response to a volume of unemployment that had not been foreseen, and in the process the insurance principle had been almost entirely abandoned. In the 1930s, the problem in the industrial North increased as the cyclical short-term employment, for which the National Insurance Scheme had been planned, changed to deep-seated long-term unemployment; the level of unemployment rose to heights beyond the capacity of the original National Insurance scheme. In 1924–29, economic depression had brought an end to any forward movement in social reform; in the 1930s social policy in England was on the defensive, struggling to contain the cost of the massive unemployment in the North and in Wales. England was two nations, and voters in the prosperous Southeast were in the majority and not necessarily willing to make sacrifices to relieve the problems in the industrial provinces. The preoccupation of Government and the Ministry of Health in the 1930s was to persuade the public that, in a time of financial difficulty, there was no pressing need for great investment in a new programme for health. The public in London and in the Southeast could be easily persuaded of the soundness of government policy; in the industrial provinces of the North and West the government's benign assessment of the effectiveness of welfare services was demonstrably wrong and to the public the government's policy seemed unjust. On the need for reform of health and welfare services, England was divided.

There was no such division in Scotland. Industrial decline and unemployment affected every area and the effects on the wellbeing of the people were visible everywhere. There was no prosperous and flourishing community with interests in conflict with those of the mass of the country's population in the industrial central belt. The Cathcart Committee had to plan for one people, united in the social distress of the 1930s. Unlike the Ministry of Health, the Department of Health for Scotland had made no attempt to disguise or to minimise the problems; the evidence was set out year by year in its Annual Reports. The Secretary of State and a devolved administration looked to the Cathcart Committee for a new policy for health, clearly necessary for Scotland at that time, while the Ministry of Health remained determined to justify and maintain its existing policy for England and Wales. In the London administration there 'existed a consensus to prevent anything unusual from happening.'[2] In Britain, in the 1930s, there was general need for reform of the health services. It was in Scotland, where that need was frankly acknowledged, that a committee was set up to devise a scheme for reform. But it was not the intention of the Cathcart Committee that the policy it put forward should be so idiosyncratic that it could not be followed elsewhere in Britain.

The Cathcart Committee reviewed the histories of the existing health services 'to discover the purposes for which they were instituted and whether there were any leading principles that have determined their development and may be taken as a guide for the future.'

The development these services began in a British context. At the beginning of the twentieth century Sir George Newman drew attention to a change then taking place in the concept of public health in Britain. 'The centre of gravity of our public health system is passing from the environment to the individual and from the problems of sanitation to the problems of personal hygiene.'[3] For more than a century, the crowding of a growing population into the country's industrialised centres had exposed the people, particularly the poor, to new risks of contagious disease and sudden and early death. These risks had been contained by the sanitary measures in the second half of the nineteenth century. But nothing had been done to relieve the effects of chronic poverty on the physical and mental wellbeing of a very large proportion of the population. The problem of poverty may not have become worse at the end of the nineteenth century but there was by then a growing consciousness of the evils of unemployment and poverty. Sensational publications such as 'The Bitter Cry of Outcast London', serialised in the *Pall Mall Gazette* in October 1883, and General William Booth's *In*

2 P. Addison, *The Road to 1945* (London, 1994), p. 14.
3 Sir G. Newman, *The Health of the State* (London, 1907), p. 7.

Darkest England[4] in 1890, had drawn public attention to this social problem and its extent had been measured in the surveys of Charles Booth in London in 1889[5] and by Seebohm Rowntree in York in 1901.[6] Dispassionate concern was heightened to interested alarm by the inadequate performance of the British Army during the Boer War. The effectiveness of British institutions was questioned and a cult of Efficiency was taken up for a time by politicians of both main parties and by the management of many public and private bodies. However, it was the strength of the population that caused greatest concern. It was generally accepted that national strength depended on the size of the population and the fitness of its individual members. The problems immediately identified were, first, the decline in the size of the population, attributed to a falling birth rate, and an appallingly high death rate among infants during the first year of life that seemed to threaten the strength of the nation. ('Our successors will be unable to bear the burden of empire' as 'the human reservoirs of the country dry up.'[7]); second, the lack of physical fitness of the individual members of this diminishing population made all too clear in the medical examinations of those presenting themselves for recruitment into the army during the war. A third and later concern was for the health and welfare of the workers in the country's essential industries.

These were the problems addressed by government legislation in the few years before investment in social reform was halted by the First World War and by the economic decline in the 1920s. In 1902, a Royal Commission was appointed to discover whether the 'physical education' of children and adolescents would 'contribute to the national strength.'[8] The results prompted the appointment of the Inter-Departmental Committee on Physical Deterioration;[9] the creation of the School Medical Service followed both in Scotland and in England and Wales. It was soon pointed out in Scotland that, in the promotion of the health and development of the country's progeny, more could be achieved by directing resources to the care of infants and pregnant mothers.[10] This became widely understood throughout Britain. Maternity and child welfare schemes were added to those few already established by charity organisations and some local authorities. Central government increased the efficiency of these schemes in the Notification of Births Act of 1907 and the Notification of Birth

4 W. Booth, *In Darkest England* (London, 1890).
5 C. Booth, *Life and Labour of the People of London* (London, 1902).
6 B. S. Rowntree, *Poverty: A Study of Town Life* (London, 1902).
7 Earl Grey, *The Times*, 26 February 1901.
8 *Report of the Royal Commission on Physical Training (Scotland)*, 1903, Cd. 1507, p. 7.
9 *Report of the Inter-Departmental Committee on Physical Deterioration*, 1904, Cd. 2175.
10 *Glasgow Herald*, 7 December 1906.

(Extension) Act of 1915. The Royal Commission on the Poor Laws and the Relief of Distress had reported in 1909. While its Majority Report gave support to the *status quo*, its Minority Report recommended the abolition of the Poor Law and the creation of a more unified and more comprehensive system of health care. The recommendations of the Minority Report were set aside until after the First World War, but they had increased the momentum for the creation of a new government department to rationalise the organisation of the country's health services, leading to the later creation of the Ministry of Health and the Scottish Board of Health in 1919.

Scottish experience had played an important part in making to make the case for change in Britain in these early years of the century, but the resulting initiatives were British initiatives.[11] The new services – the School Medical Service and Maternity and Child Welfare Services – did not call for new administrative structures but were grafted on to existing Scottish organisations, the Scotch Education Department, the Scottish local authorities and Scottish charity organisations. The creation of a new welfare bureaucracy in Scotland came a few years later.

A Separate Welfare Bureaucracy

The health services of Scotland would not have been separately reviewed in the 1930s and a new policy for health would not have been devised had there been no separate administration in Scotland:

> The argument is not that Scotland had control over its own legislation, although it could influence that. The key point is [that] the politics that mattered were those of the bureaucracy, in the sense that the autonomy and distinctiveness of any country in the mid-twentieth century rested more on the way its bureaucracy interpreted legislation than on the legislation itself. Scotland had its own welfare state bureaucracy.[12]

The crucial event was a last-minute amendment carried at the final stage of the National Insurance Bill in 1911. At that time, a movement for Home Rule for Scotland was still being kept alive by both the Liberals and by the new Labour Party in Scotland. However, for the Government, Home Rule for Ireland was a much more pressing issue. During the 1910 election, Asquith had given an explicit pledge to introduce Home Rule for Ireland.[13]

---

11 The investigations of the Royal Commission on Physical Training were carried out by Leslie Mackenzie in Leith and Matthew Hay in Aberdeen; the medical evidence to the Royal Commission on the Poor Laws came largely from John McVail, MOH of Stirlingshire.

12 L. Paterson, *The Autonomy of Modern Scotland* (Edinburgh, 1994), p. 103.

13 J. Grigg, *Lloyd George: The People's Champion* (London, 1978), p. 241.

This added a late complication for Lloyd George in his long and difficult struggle over his National Insurance Bill. As a Treasury Bill, it was initially designed to apply to all parts of Great Britain and Ireland, but there was great pressure, in the expectation of Home Rule, for separate arrangements to be made for Ireland. Lloyd George made it clear in May 1911[14] and again in June that the Government had 'no intention of excluding Ireland from the benefits of the National Insurance Bill.'[15] However, at a meeting at Maynooth in November 1911, the General Council of the Irish County Councils and the Catholic Archbishops and Bishops of Ireland all agreed that the National Insurance Bill, however suited to an industrial population such as Great Britain, was quite unacceptable and even 'mischievous' in the wholly different conditions in Ireland.[16] In the House of Commons Lloyd George was asked to defer to this 'almost unanimous' expression of Irish opinion.[17] But Irish members were not, in fact, as united as claimed in rejecting the scheme completely. T. M. Healy, the Member for Louth, objected only to the proposal that 'the Commissioners are to be gentlemen residing solely in London.'[18] John Redmond asked only for amendments to the Bill that would make it more relevant to conditions in Ireland.[19] However, six months after the Bill had been presented to Parliament and three years after Lloyd George had begun work on his project, Irish members presented a last-minute demand for a separate Irish Commission and a separate Irish Insurance Fund.[20] 'The political position was such, with the Parliament Bill on hand and Home Rule in the offing, these demands had to be acceded to and incorporated in amendments to the Bill.'[21] The relevant amendments were therefore formally drafted for presentation to the House of Commons at a discussion of Clause 59 scheduled for 13 November.

Clause 58, dealing with minor adaptations of the Bill for application in Scotland, was also due for consideration on the same day. On Friday 10 November a meeting of some dozen Scottish Liberal members decided to follow the example of the Irish members and demand a separate Commission for Scotland. Their demand was immediately accepted by the Lord Advocate and presented as a Government amendment on Monday 13 November. The majority of Scottish members had their first warning of this

14 *Hansard*, xxv, HC 10 May 1911, col. 1342.
15 *Hansard*, xxvii, HC 29 June 1911, col. 567.
16 *Ibid.*, col. 699.
17 *Ibid.*
18 *Hansard*, xxx, HC 24 October 1911, col. 74.
19 *Ibid.*, col. 154.
20 The list also included the demand that the whole of Ireland should be excluded from the operation of that part of the Bill that provided Medical Benefit.
21 W. J. Braithwaite, *Lloyd George's Ambulance Wagon* (London, 1957), p. 223.

amendment only on the previous Saturday. Although several protested at the lack of time to consider, Lloyd George nevertheless agreed to the amendment because he 'thought that was the general view of Scottish members on the subject.'[22] 'The Government proposal was to have one Commission for the United Kingdom and so treat the matter here, as in Germany, as an Imperial matter ... All I can say is that I regret the conclusion they have come to.' According to Braithwaite,[23] Lloyd George had simply become impatient after years of struggle and was 'pressing on now to finish regardless of anything. He wanted have done with it.'[24] That same evening the amendment was passed by 171 votes to 89, 'the hastiest piece of legislation in the history of Britain.'[25] The Scottish Commission, with its supporting staff, took up its duties on 1 January 1912. A separate welfare bureaucracy for Scotland had not been contemplated by Government in the summer of 1911, but now one existed in embryo as an unforeseen by-product of the struggle over Home Rule for Ireland. Within two years a small increment had been added to the growth of that embryo bureaucracy by the creation of the Highlands and Islands Medical Services Board.

The Insurance Commission for Scotland and the Highland and Islands Board were significant precedents, but when the movement began for the formation of a Ministry of Health during the First World War it could not yet be assumed that there would be separate provision for Scotland. The movement to create a Ministry had begun in August 1914 with the appointment of Christopher Addison as Parliamentary Secretary to the Board of Education.[26] Assisted by Sir Robert Morant, Chairman of the Insurance Commission,[27] Addison prepared a memorandum arguing for the amalgamation of no fewer than 14 existing government health bodies to form a single health ministry. In 1915, he was moved to the Ministry of Munitions and for the moment his plan came to nothing. Then, in 1916, as one of the organisers of the coup that made Lloyd George Prime Minister, Addison was made a Minister in his new Coalition Government, and a year later became Minister for Reconstruction. He was now in a position to resurrect his plan

22 *Hansard*, xxxi, HC 13 November 1911, col. 64.
23 W. J. Braithwaite was the civil servant chosen to assist Lloyd George at the Treasury in preparing his Health Insurance scheme.
24 Braithwaite, *op. cit.*, p. 224.
25 *Ibid.*
26 Addison had been elected to Parliament in 1910 at the age of 41, having been Professor of Anatomy at Sheffield for the previous eleven years. As a leading medical member of the House of Commons he had assisted Lloyd George in the preparation of the NHI Bill; his chief contribution to the Bill was the clause which led to the foundation of the Medical Research Council.
27 Morant had recently been the Permanent Secretary of the Board of Education.

for a health ministry. There was strong resistance to his proposal from inside Government, especially from successive Presidents of the Local Government Board.[28] As he recorded in his diary, 'the struggle that went on behind the scenes for nearly two years to secure the establishment of the Ministry of Health is a good example of how difficult it is to secure the passage of an effective reform, even when, as in this case, it was supported by public opinion and by men of all parties.'[29] Addison's most effective support came from outside the official organisation of government, from Lloyd George's 'Kindergarten' (officially the Cabinet Intelligence Branch) and at informal meetings at Lloyd George's home in Wales. At these meetings the interests of the medical profession were represented by Major-General Sir Bertrand Dawson, Physician to the King and at that time Consulting Physician to the British Armies in France. (Significantly, in view of Lloyd George's experience of its recalcitrance in the setting up of his National Health Insurance Scheme, a representative of the BMA was not included in these unofficial meetings.) The purpose of these discussions was made public by Lord Astor (an 'Honorary Kind'[30]), first in April 1917 in his pamphlet *The Health of the People* and again on 13 October in an address to the Royal Institute of Public Health on *The Health Problem and a State Ministry of Health*. On 10th January 1918 he brought his case to wider public attention in a letter to *The Times*[31] in which he called for the establishment of 'a Ministry of Health to co-ordinate and develop measures for the health of the people throughout England and Wales.' In his letter he made only passing and obscure reference to 'necessary matters in relation to Scotland and Ireland.'[32]

In Scotland, the case for a separate Ministry was first made by the Royal College of Physicians of Edinburgh in a memorandum to the Secretary for Scotland on 6 December 1917.[33] This was followed by matching memoranda from the Royal College of Surgeons of Edinburgh on 5 February 1918,[34] and from the Royal Faculty of Physicians and Surgeons of Glasgow on 8 April 1918.[35] The Deans of the Faculties of Medicine of the Scottish

28 K. Morgan and J. Morgan, *Portrait of a Progressive: The Political Career of Christopher Addison* (Oxford, 1980), p. 75.

29 C. Addison, *Politics from Within*, i (London, 1924), p. 221.

30 C. Sykes, *Nancy: The Life of Lady Astor* (London, 1979), p. 198.

31 *The Times*, 10 January 1918.

32 'There is a general impression that the mere suggestion to establish a Ministry of Health has aroused so much departmental jealousy that whatever form any Bill will take it will meet with strenuous opposition from one department or another.' *BMJ*, ii (1917), p. 559.

33 The Minutes of the College include the statement supporting a separate Ministry for Scotland but neither the Minutes nor the Minutes of Council record the reason for the statement being made at precisely that time.

34 *Records of the Royal College of Surgeons of Edinburgh*, 16 May 1918.

35 *BMJ*, i, 1918, p. 519.

universities were informed of these memoranda and gave their support. The Court of St Andrews University declared its support for a separate Ministry in February 1918.[36] While each of these bodies acted separately, there had been open communication among them, establishing a clear consensus of view among the leaders of the medical profession in Scotland, the Royal Medical Corporations and the universities. (It is indicative of the relative unimportance of the British Medical Association in Scotland at that time that it was not included in the distribution of the many communications that passed between these various bodies.[37])

The Approved Societies in Scotland made their support for a separate Ministry known to the Secretary for Scotland in July 1918.[38] The views of the local authorities were presented by a deputation from the Convention of Royal Burghs, the County Council Association, and the Association of District Councils in Scotland to the House of Commons on 17 July 1918. In common with all other interested parties in Scotland the deputation

> ... desired a separate Ministry for Scotland. The deputation wished the Secretary for Scotland to be nominally the Minister for Health with a Parliamentary Secretary as the responsible person for dealing with questions arising under the Public Health Act. Instead of one Bill for the establishment of Ministries for Scotland and for England, the view of the public authorities was that they would prefer the Scottish Ministry to be dealt with in a separate Bill.[39]

That same evening in the House of Lords, the Government indicated that the case presented by the deputation had been accepted.[40] Next day, 18 July, the arrangements for Scotland were settled at a meeting of the Cabinet Home Affairs Committee.[41]

In contrast to the 'extraordinary opposition'[42] to the creation of the Ministry of Health in London and the conflicts which resulted,[43] the creation of the Scottish Board of Health had been achieved without dissent. From 1 July 1919 the Board assumed the powers and duties of the Local Government Board for Scotland, the Scottish Insurance Commissioners, and the Scotch Education Department (with respect to the medical

36 *Ibid.*, p. 243.
37 'Should the BMA Speak for the Medical Profession?', Appendix I.
38 NAS HH/1/469.
39 *The Scotsman*, 17 July 1918. The deputation said that 'their experience was that Scottish matters dealt with in an English Bill, with English phraseology, was unsuitable and difficult to deal with in Scotland.'
40 *The Scotsman*, 18 July 1918.
41 PRO CAB, 26/1 HAC 3rd: 2.
42 J. Macintosh, *Trends of Opinion about Public Health* (Oxford, 1953), p. 95.
43 F. Honigsbaum, *The Struggle for the Ministry of Health* (London, 1970).

inspection and treatment of children and young persons) and, on 1 September 1919, the powers and duties of the Secretary for Scotland on the Highlands and Islands (Medical Services) Board. Sir John Pratt was appointed as an Under-Secretary at the Scottish Office to head the Board, with the Secretary for Scotland, Robert Munro, as President and the responsible Minister.

The new Ministry of Health in England and Wales was formed on a model long established in Whitehall. The Minister of Health was supported by an hierarchical structure of civil servants headed by a powerful and influential Permanent Secretary. In Scotland the management structure was closer to that of a commercial enterprise. The Secretary for Scotland became President and a specially appointed Under-Secretary of State took the role of chief executive. Policy was determined by the Board, chaired by Sir George McCrae. The routine tasks of administration were carried out by a staff of 380 civil servants (279 previously with the National Insurance Commission, 94 from the Local Government Board, seven from the Highlands and Islands Board) without a head in the influential position of a Permanent Secretary in Whitehall. Policy was guided by a board of six (later reduced to three) – the Scottish Board of Health. Each Board member brought extensive experience in the management of one of the 'companies' taken over as a branch of the new organisation (Local Government Board for Scotland, Highlands and Islands Board, Scottish Insurance Commission, Friendly Societies, local authorities[44]). Both the Board and the executive were served by 'technical advisory boards' in the form of Consultative Councils.

The Scottish Board followed a pattern first devised for the administration of the Poor Law in 1885. Lindsay Paterson has described the relationship between these boards and society in Scotland.[45] The Scottish Board of Health, like other Scottish Boards, centralised state power, but remained more closely embedded in society than a professional civil service department in White-hall. It was made up of members brought to positions of influence through networks within the Scottish professional associations and the Scottish universities.[46] That part of Scottish society from which the members of the Scottish Health Board were drawn was small and those appointed were already well known to each other, both professionally and socially. Consensus on policy for Scotland was easily achieved by Board members who enjoyed a unity of purpose and maintained their links with society outside the immediate circles of government and public administration.

44 Appendix IV.
45 Paterson, *op. cit.*, p. 51.
46 Appendix IV.

The members of the Consultative Council on Medical and Allied Services were appointed in a way that was distinctively Scottish and that strengthened an existing predisposition to consensus. In England, four Consultative Councils were set up – for Medical and Allied Services; for National Health Insurance; for Local Health Administration; and for General Health Questions. The Chairman of the Scottish Board adapted this arrangement. By combining the committees on Local Health Administration and on General Health Questions he was able to accommodate a Highlands and Islands Consultative Committee while limiting the total number of committees to four in line with the arrangement in England.[47] Again attempting to conform as far as possible to a UK pattern, the Scottish Board consulted with the Permanent Secretary of the Ministry of Health, on setting up the influential Consultative Council on Medical and Allied Services. The Ministry had devised a complicated scheme for England and Wales under which no few than 32 bodies were to be asked to submit an unlimited number of names; from this very large number of candidates, 20 were to be selected by a panel drawn from the Royal Colleges and the British Medical Association.[48] This scheme was rejected by the Scottish Health Board which opted instead to appoint its Consultative Council on Medical and Allied Matters directly and strictly according to the provision in the Act that 'every Council should include persons of both sexes and should consist of persons having practical experience of the matters referred to the Council and that due regard should be had in constituting them to any special interest (including those of Local Authorities and of labour) which might be involved.'[49] The selection of members of the Consultative Council on Medical and Allied Services was therefore made without concession to the British Medical Association or the Medical Corporations or to any other outside body. From the beginning the Consultative Council in Scotland therefore had a very different character from its opposite number in London. The 20 members of the Consultative Committee in Scotland were drawn from general medical and dental practice, consultant and specialist practice, public health, industrial medicine, laboratory services, nursing, pharmacy, the General Medical Council, and the BMA. Significantly, seven of those appointed were also heads of university departments.[50]

This degree of importance and influence given to the Scottish universities, even within a very broadly based advisory body, created a precedent that was followed thereafter, establishing a continuing difference in the

47 NAS HH/1/469.
48 Ibid.
49 Ibid.
50 Appendix V.

route by which influential medical opinion was delivered to Government for Scotland and for England and Wales. For centuries before the creation of the Ministry of Health, the Privy Council and Whitehall had looked to the Royal College of Physicians of London for guidance on medical matters[51] and the BMA had won a position of influence during the struggles over the National Insurance Bill in 1911. The Royal Colleges in London and leaders of the BMA retained considerable influence in Whitehall even after the establishment of the Ministry of Health and they continued to exert pressure on Government from outside and in the interest of particular sections of the medical profession. In Scotland the influence of a much wider spectrum of the medical profession was presented from within the system through the statutory advisory bodies and was most powerfully articulated in these bodies by their university-based members.

By 1929, when the Scottish Health Board was replaced by the Department of Health for Scotland, there was already a well-established habit of co-operation within the health services. The distinctive health bureaucracy that served that consensus had grown with the years. In 1926 it was strengthened when the Scottish Secretary, Sir John Gilmour, became a Secretary of State with a seat in Cabinet. This conferred a useful increase in status on his civil servants. Their status was further increased two years later; in 1928, on the recommendation of the Royal Commission on the Civil Service, the Re-organisation of Offices Act replaced the Scottish Health Board and its idiosyncratic organisation of civil servants with a Department now brought within the ordinary civil service structure. The change was intended to ensure 'more effective responsibility for action and advice' and to facilitate 'the interchange of personnel between the Scottish Office [at Dover House in London] and Departments in Edinburgh.'[52] These new Departments, including the Department of Health for Scotland, were now hierarchical, each under a Permanent Secretary. The power and influence of Scotland's central bureaucracy was considerably increased. The new Departments offered an improved career structure, attracting higher-calibre entrants. They also allowed increased scope for the more ambitious civil servants in Scotland without need to shift their allegiance from Edinburgh to Whitehall. Under the Secretaries of State, Sir John Gilmour and Sir Godfrey Collins (and later Walter Elliot and Tom Johnston), greater authority was devolved to Edinburgh, establishing the new Scottish Office as the centre of effective governance in and for Scotland.

To succeed in persuading Cabinet to allow special provision to be made specifically for Scotland, the Secretary of State for Scotland had still to

51 Appendix I.
52 NAS HH 1/526.

present a strong case. 'When he could construct a Scottish consensus on social policy he could get his way, providing that the direction he was pursuing did not deviate too far from Government policy in London.'[53] The Secretaries of State for Scotland between the wars were all men of 'middle opinion'[54] fostering 'a kind of one-party state ethos bridging businessmen, professionals and collectivists.'[55] For the state to serve such potentially diverse interests, consensus was essential. The Scottish Office bureaucrats therefore exerted great influence 'since it was by means of their Committees and networks that [the Secretary of State] could sound out and mould Scottish opinion.'[56]

The Cathcart Committee was one of these committees. Its members were not delegates from outside bodies but chosen to ensure the strong consensus required by the Secretary of State in presenting a case for special consideration for Scotland. The Cathcart Committee could also draw on consensus views expressed in previous reports on the development of health services in Scotland – the MacAlister Report in 1920,[57] the Mackenzie Report in 1926[58] and the Walker Report in 1933.[59] These reports had made recommendations for the adaptation of British legislation for application in Scotland. The establishment of a separate bureaucracy and advisory structure for Scotland had not led to a separation of policies. It had ensured that the implementation of British legislation was achieved in Scotland efficiently and in a spirit of co-operation. In reviewing the history of the development of health services for guidance the Cathcart Committee able to draw on experience that was both Scottish and British.

The Policy and the State

The Cathcart Committee's aim was to secure 'the health of the people.' The policy to be followed was to be 'a positive one and not merely the removal of obstacles to health' and was to be developed with a 'higher degree of responsiveness and a finer sensitiveness, than was conceived by the legislature of the last century.' Policy was to take account of the contemporary 'concern for the quality of the race.' Mingled with other motives, this concern for the quality of the race had, in the Committee's view,

---

53 Paterson, *op. cit.*, p. 109.
54 Collins was a Liberal; Elliot was a nominal Conservative; Johnston was Labour; his radicalism as an ILP member had dissipated before he became Secretary of State.
55 C. Harvie, 'Scottish Politics', in A. Dickson and J. H. Treble (eds.), *People and Society in Scotland*, iii (Edinburgh, 1992), p. 247.
56 Paterson, *op. cit.*
57 *A Scheme of Medical Services for Scotland* (MacAlister Report) 1920, Cmd. 1039.
58 *Report of the Hospital Services (Scotland) Committee* (Mackenzie Report), HMSO, 1926.
59 *Report on the Hospital Services of Scotland* (Walker Report), HMSO, 1933.

inspired new developments in health care and led to a new conception of health policy. Health, physical fitness and the prevention of invalidity were to be promoted by the state and primarily in the interest of the state. With this in mind the best means for procuring health and curing disease were to be made available to every citizen. 'Best means'[60] were at that time only available to the small proportion of the population that could afford to provide the full range of medical services for themselves. A greater part of the population could afford only limited medical care but could also rely for further help on insurance schemes, club schemes and the services of voluntary hospitals. A section of society was completely dependent on charity or the Poor Law. There was great disparity across society in the deficiencies in 'best means' that should be made good by a national health policy. While it was generally accepted that, in principle, Government should ensure that every member of the public should have access to whatever medical services were necessary, the extent to which these services should be financed by local or Treasury funds was still to be determined. While the officials of the Ministry of Health continued to assume that state medical services should be administered by local authorities, for the Cathcart Committee this was an open question.

There was also the important question: to what extent would the public welcome government intervention in personal health care? A large section of society had at first disregarded the Maternity and Child Welfare Services and had resented the School Medical Service as an intrusion on privacy. At the beginning of the century it had seemed appropriate that the state should impose only on the poor and the delinquent who made up a recognised social problem group. But the First World War had undermined individual confidence and changed attitudes.[61] The massive loss of life during the war and the even greater loss in the influenza epidemic that came after it, had been suffered by all sections of society. For the great mass of people the 1920s and 1930s were times of continuing uncertainty. During the war years they had come to accept the loss of a degree of personal freedom in return for a share in collective security. (This was perhaps particularly the case in Scotland with its 'penchant for state corporatism as a means to social reform.'[62]) In the Brave New World intervention by the state might be accepted in the expectation of scientific expertise, professional skill and administrative competence.[63] It is implicit in the Cathcart Committee's brief assessment of the history of state health

60 This phrase has been borrowed from the Sir Bertram Dawson who used it frequently in the years after the war.
61 T. C. Smout, 'Scotland 1850–1950', in F. M. L. Thompson (ed.), *The Cambridge Social History of Britain*, i (Cambridge, 1993), p. 210.
62 Paterson, *op. cit.*, p. 109.
63 Mazower, *op. cit.*, p. 92.

services that it accepted that it was appropriate in those years that health policy had been dictated by the managers of the country and imposed for the benefit of the nation.[64] It is also implicit in its Report that the Committee assumed that state health services should continue to be paternalistic. Although this issue was not discussed in these terms, it is clear that Cathcart contemplated only a health system that would be continue to be supply-led.

In 1933 the Cathcart Committee could assume that the role of the state in health care would increase and that every member of the public would be affected by government health policy. But the nature of the relationship between the state and the individual had to be determined.

The Application of Medical Science

The Cathcart Committee was required to view medical services in the light of modern knowledge at a time of change both in medical science and in the politics of medicine. In the first half of the twentieth century the medical sciences were experiencing a period of shift in priorities and ambitions. The gains in health of the mass of the people had been achieved by engineering rather than medical science. Systems of drainage, water supply and general sanitation had contained the infections that had still been the chief threats to life and health at the middle of the nineteenth century. Surgery had advanced over these same decades. Having been based on little more than a study of anatomy, surgery had benefited from advances in pathology and the assistance of anaesthesia. Medicine, on the other hand, had changed relatively little. The pharmacopoeia was hardly more effective in 1933 than it had been for centuries. Chemistry and the brewing and viniculture industries' interest had led to the isolation of micro-organisms and the understanding of their role in disease. For a time the science of bacteriology promised to revolutionise the practice of medicine and bacteriology was studied by rising clinicians such as Edward Cathcart. But by the turn of the century understanding of bacteriology had been of direct benefit to very few patients. (Sir Godfrey Collins was to die of septicaemia following minor surgery although he had the attention of a leading physician of the time.) Bacteriology was not living up to expectations and Edward Cathcart was not alone in turning from bacteriology to physiology. Even in 1933, when the Cathcart Committee was convened, specific cures and effective medical treatments were still years away. Insulin and diphtheria anti-toxin[65] had

---

64 Since Professor Cathcart left no papers and all papers relating to the Cathcart Committee, other than the Minutes of Evidence, have been destroyed, it is only possible to offer conjecture.
65 The anti-toxin was only effective if given early in the course of the illness; it was rarely available or administered in time.

come into use but they were regarded only as minor additions to digitalis, quinine and morphine, then the chief items in the small range of helpful but non-curative medicines available in the pharmacopoeia.[66] For the Cathcart Committee and their contemporaries, curative medicine, as we now know it, was still inconceivable. Physiology (including psychology) rather than therapeutics seemed to offer the best option as the basis for progress in medicine. For even the most progressive doctors in the 1930s the emphasis could not be on the cure of disease, but only on its alleviation or, whenever possible, on its avoidance. An ability to control and maintain normality suggested a whole new approach to the practice of medicine. A full understanding of the mechanisms controlling the body made it seem possible that these mechanisms might be manipulated to maintain or restore health. Physiology in the early 1930s was the commanding medical science of the day, occupying the place enjoyed by genetics in the 1990s. It was therefore appropriate that a Committee to advise on medical services in the 1930s should be led by a physiologist and inevitable that the Committee, in planning 'in the light of modern conditions and knowledge,' should look to the exploitation of the potentials of physiology.

The Population

The Cathcart Report presented an assessment of the size and constitution of the population to be served by future health services in Scotland. However, the Committee acknowledged that its assessment left certain important questions without a clear answer and that it would be necessary to make a number of important assumptions.

In the first years of the century, the quantity, the total number, of a population was still taken as a valid measure of its strength. In 1936, the population of Scotland was falling. In the past this would have been regarded as sure evidence of racial decline but there had been a change in emphasis. There was now greater concern about the quality and strength of the people, and it was beginning to be understood that the structure of the population had important implications for the physical and mental health of its members. 'Changes now occurring in the rate of growth of the population and its distribution, not only between urban and rural areas but also by age and sex, are effecting far reaching changes in the problems of public health.'

---

66 Although the early forms of sulpha drugs had been introduced in 1935, they were seldom used because of their side effects. More easily tolerated derivatives, effective against a limited range of bacteria, came into general use after the Cathcart Committee had reported. They were first used in Glasgow in the winter of 1937. *Bulletin of the Royal College of Physicians and Surgeons of Glasgow*, xxix, 2000, p. 13.

Scotland had shared in the explosion of population that had occurred across Western Europe from the middle of the eighteenth century. But as the nineteenth century progressed into the twentieth, the rate of increase in Scotland had tended to slow down. The natural increase in the population declined from 12.4 per thousand in 1870 to 6.3 in 1930, and when the Cathcart Report was published it had fallen further to 5.1 per thousand. This was a reflection of a steady fall in the birth rate from 34.6 per thousand in 1870 to 18 in 1934. But over that period the trend in the size of the population had become less regular due to the fluctuating rate of loss by emigration. In the 1920s the rate of emigration had been high. Since then emigration had slowed but was still large enough to convert the natural increase of the population into an actual net loss of 39,517 (0.8%) between 1921 and 1931.

In this changing situation, the Cathcart Committee attempted to forecast the population trends on the basis of a) the birth rate; b) the death rate; and c) migration. Cathcart was obliged to make crucial assumptions. His first assumption was that 'by far the most important of these factors is the birth rate. It has now declined to a point at which, leaving migration out of account and assuming no great changes in the death rate, it cannot for any length of time maintain the population at its existing level.'

> Whether the falling trend in the birth rate may be arrested, and ultimately reversed, or whether it will continue is a matter of speculation. The answer to be given depends on what may be considered the underlying causes; and these are obscure and the subject of much controversy. It depends also on how far these causes, if ascertainable, may be affected by future events.

The dominant theory among geneticists was that the fundamental cause of the fall in the birth rate was a decline in man's natural fertility. Two of Britain's leading experts on fertility gave evidence to the Committee. Their theories were not reproduced in the Cathcart Report but were set out at length in their books. Carr-Saunders,[67] in *The Population Problem: A Study in Evolution*,[68] and Professor Crewe[69] in *Organic Inheritance in Man*,[70] both accepted the contemporary theory that all inherited characters were carried by the sperm and the ova (the germinal constitution) but that these characters were predispositions only and subject to modification (germinal change) by environmental conditions. Both experts postulated that the ability of the foetus to survive until birth was itself an inherited character-

67 A. M. Carr-Saunders, Professor of Social Science, University of Liverpool.
68 A. M. Carr-Saunders, *The Population Problem: A Study in Evolution* (London, 1922).
69 F. A. E. Crewe, Professor of Animal Genetics, University of Edinburgh.
70 F. A. E. Crewe, *Organic Inheritance in Man* (Edinburgh, 1927), p. 175.

istic and therefore open to influence by external factors at some stage in the development of the foetus. Both expert advisors thought it probable that the falling birth rate must be the result of some factor or factors in the environment adversely affecting the ability of the foetus to survive; in effect, the natural fertility of man was being gradually eroded by his environment.

In the absence of factual evidence, Cathcart rejected the views of the experts in favour of his own reasoning. First, it was inherently probable that a change in natural fertility, if it was occurring at all, would manifest itself only slowly and cumulatively over a long period of time. It seemed highly improbable that such a change in the nature and constitution of men and women could, in only two generations, account for the fall in the birth rate from 35 per thousand in 1871 to 18 in 1934. Cathcart therefore dismissed a decline in natural fertility as the cause of the decrease in the birth rate.

It was a common assumption in the 1930s that the main cause of the fall in the birth rate was an increase in the average age at marriage. At Cathcart's request, this possibility was investigated by Dr. McKinlay, the statistician of the Department of Health for Scotland. He showed that the average age of all persons marrying in Scotland had varied only between 27.3 years in 1861 and 27.8 in 1930 and that there was no correlation between these small changes and the decline in the birth rate.

With no evidence to support changes in natural fertility or in the age at marriage as the explanation, Cathcart concluded that the fall in the birth rate must be attributed to an increasing knowledge and practice of birth control. While this must be the immediate mechanism, Cathcart believed that 'deeper-seated causes are operative, of which the widespread adoption of contraceptive methods are but the outward manifestation.' Cathcart declined to speculate on any possible political or religious factors and confined discussion to the economic considerations that might motivate parents to limit their families.

Cathcart noted that the decline of the birth rate had proceeded for decades through times of relative prosperity and times of depression and in countries unaffected by the revolutions of the trade cycle. Cathcart found no evidence that family size was influenced by the state of the national economy. The most striking observation was the marked difference in the birth rate between social classes, the highest rates being found in the poorest sections of the community. Cathcart recorded that 'it has been a matter of frequent observation that one of the first effects of an improvement in the standard of life is to evoke a desire to maintain that standard, with, as a means thereto, a consequent restriction in the size of the family.' Cathcart therefore suggested that a continuing general increase in the country's standard of living would inevitably lead to a progressive fall in the birth rate of the poorer classes and that the trend towards a decline in the population would continue. Cathcart concluded 'that the main immediate cause of the low birth rate is deliberate prevention of births, that this cause will probably continue to operate and that for purposes of social policy a continued low birth rate may be assumed.'

The Cathcart Committee was more confident in reaching a conclusion on death rates. Death rates had declined less dramatically than birth rates, falling from 22.7 in 1871 to 12.92 in 1934. Any appreciable further fall was thought to be unlikely; indeed as the average age of the population increased, death rates would probably show some small increase. However, 'we may rule out any movement of the death rate in considering future numbers.'

Cathcart also ruled out migration (emigration/immigration) as a factor that would materially affect the size of the population. For long periods of the nineteenth century and early twentieth century there had been emigration of large numbers of Scottish people balanced in part by immigration from other parts of the United Kingdom, chiefly from Ireland. Cathcart offered no figures but stated firmly that in the preceding few years this balance had changed. 'There has been some movement of Scottish people to the midlands and South of England, but overseas emigration has practically ceased and the immigration of Irish people has considerably slowed down.' The return of some emigrants from overseas during the world recession was discounted as a passing phenomenon. Cathcart assumed that in the future migration would not be a substantial factor in modifying the size of the Scottish population although it might have some slight influence tending to diminish rather than increase the population. Based on this assessment of trends in birth rate, death rate and migration, Cathcart concluded that 'the population of Scotland will almost certainly not expand much further and is likely to decline.'

Cathcart forecast that the Scottish population would continue to become more urban. In 1931 a third of the total population already lived in the four large cities of Glasgow, Edinburgh, Dundee and Aberdeen. At the 1931 census over 80% of the population lived in urban areas (57.7% in 1861) and only 20% in the rural areas (42.35% in 1861). 'On the geographical distribution, the salient fact is to be found in the concentration of population in a small part of the total area, namely in the industrial belt between the Forth and the Clyde with strips of lower density along the east and south-western coasts.' This was not seen as a threat to health in 1936. 'There is not now the discrepancy that used to exist between the health of the town and the country. The great sanitary improvements, above all by a plentiful supply of water and by sewerage, have chiefly affected the towns, and the experience has demonstrated that those elements in an urban environment that are harmful can to a large extent be removed or "neutralised."'

Cathcart, while not worried by increasing urbanisation, feared that Scotland was facing the reciprocal problem of depopulation. This was most obvious in the Highlands and Islands where the population of the area served by the Highlands and Islands Medical Service had fallen by 14.6% between 1911 and 1931. In 1936 the depopulation of certain areas of Scotland was 'now raising acutely the question of the capacity of the area to provide, through the present units of administration and from present financial resources, the services that are demanded by modern standards.'

The increasing proportion of old people in the population promised further difficulties. The average age of the population had increased from 26.5 years in 1861 to 31.3 in 1931. While the proportion of those in the 'early years of industrial life' (15–45 years) had remained almost constant (44.4%–45.6%), the proportion of younger people had fallen from 36% to 27%, and of those older than 45 years the proportion had risen from 19% to 28%. Since the increase in the average age of the population had been increasing since 1881–1891 and the increase had accelerated since then, Cathcart concluded the 'it may be assumed that the proportion of older people will increase and the average age rise correspondingly.' It was forecast that the broad effect would be that the diseases of later life would come to represent a larger, and those of earlier life a smaller, proportion of the sum-total of the diseases of the whole population. This would undoubtedly affect health policy and would have a profound effect on 'the outlook of medicine.' The fact that people were living longer would increase the overall demands on personal and domiciliary services as the people made increasing efforts to maintain fitness throughout a longer span of years. Hospital services would also be affected as more and more institutional facilities were required by a growing number of old people. 'The increased numbers who survive to the later ages of life have made this problem of the aged, whether in health or in sickness, one of the dominant factors in the provision of general hospitals, mental hospitals and public assistance.'

The increasing age of the population was expected to continue to affect the sex ratio (females/males) of the population. This had remained almost constant at around 1.08 in the fifty years before 1931, showing only slight falls during wars and at times of high emigration. However, as a consequence of the disproportion of the number of women surviving into old age the sex ratio had shown some increase, particularly in the older age groups; in the age group over 85 there were already two women for every man. However, Cathcart took the view that 'the sex ratio is probably not a matter of fundamental importance for health policy.'

Cathcart's assessment of trends in population was entirely credible in the circumstances of the first half of the 1930s. But these forecasts made in the early 1930s were of little help in the planning of medical services in the later

1930s and 1940s. The population of Scotland had already begun to increase even while the report was being prepared. Between 1933 and 1938 the population increased by almost 2%. The increase continued to 5% in 1948. At its peak in the late 1960s, the population of Scotland was 6.5% greater than when the Cathcart Committee was appointed.

As forecast by Cathcart, the death rate played little part in these changes, falling steadily from 13.2 in 1933 to 11.8 in the 1948. However, contrary to Cathcart's expectation that the birth rate would not be influenced by changes in the national economy, between 1931 and 1934, when unemployment and poverty were at their worst, the birth rate fell from 17.6 to 16.3. The subsequent improvement in the economy was followed by a slow rise in the birth rate to 17.8 in 1938, an increase which continued to 19.4 in 1948.

However, this natural increase did not result in a corresponding rise in the total population. Cathcart had been wrong to assert that 'migration may be ruled out as a factor materially affecting population.' Emigration had indeed almost completely stopped during the 1930s. But after Cathcart had reported, the recovery in the economy, both in North America and in the United Kingdom, revived both emigration and migration from Scotland. Between 1931 and 1951 net emigration/migration reduced the natural increase of the Scottish population by 49.6%. This was a modest figure compared with what was to come in later decades. By 1971–81 net migration was more than twice the natural increase in the population.

The Cathcart Committee's assumptions proved to be mistaken. But there can be no doubting Cathcart's prediction that contraception would be the most important factor in determining the size of the population. Cathcart was convinced that, on that basis, the population would continue to shrink. 'In submitting proposals that involve increased expenditure from the rates and increased contributions from insured persons, we are conscious that these, as sources of additional income for public service, are nearing exhaustion.'

Cathcart accepted that the urbanisation of Scotland would continue. Anderson[71] has demonstrated that this was indeed the case. Since 1931, the distribution of the people was changed only by the continuing movement from the rural areas, the expansion of existing towns, and the emergence of new towns. Where there had been some apparent evidence of rural increase, it 'turns out on close observation to involve expansion of single towns within parishes dominated by rural depopulation.'[72] In the process of expanding,

71 M. Anderson, 'Population and Family Life,' in *People and Society in Scotland*, (eds.) A. Dickson, and J. H. Treble, *op. cit.*
72 *Ibid.*, p. 16.

Scottish towns were becoming more 'rural,' perhaps evidence in support of Cathcart's contention that urban living was no longer to be regarded as necessarily a hazard to health.

Cathcart was also proved to be correct in his prediction of an ageing population. In 1961 the proportion of the population in 'the early years of industrial life' had fallen to 34.2% (45.6% in 1931) and children younger than that age to 27.6%. Those over 45 years of age now formed the largest proportion at 38.2% (28% in 1933). The effect of this change on the cost of medical services was complex, and as became clear later, the proposition that the ageing of the population would necessarily result in an increase in the cost of medical service was not as certain as assumed by Cathcart.

Overall, Cathcart's assessment of the demographic changes to be expected in Scotland were only correct in the most general terms and were not reliable as a guide to the planning of future health services. Given the changes that took place in society as the Scottish economy unexpectedly began to recover in the late 1930s and in the unforeseeable circumstances of a Second World War, this was inevitable.

4

Social Conditions and Health

The Cathcart Committee was appointed to review the 'existing health services in the light of modern conditions.' Scotland was then in the depths of the Depression. But over three years the Committee turned the focus of its attention from the crisis situation of 1933 to concentrate on planning for the long-term future of health services in Scotland, and by implication in Britain. For that plan to be successful would require the support of the Government and those responsible for the management of the country's welfare services. The Committee was therefore circumspect in offering judgments that were in conflict with those being put forward at that time by Government and careful to distance itself from the current controversies over the effectiveness of the welfare services during the distress of the Depression.[1]

The Cathcart Report included only the briefest account of social conditions as they were in Scotland in the 1930s. Of a total of eight pages, four were completely taken up by the personal views of only six witnesses. In these few pages Cathcart did not attempt to disguise the extent of poverty and deprivation in Scotland, but by setting its assessment in the context of the changes that had taken place over several decades the Cathcart Committee was able to present social conditions in the best possible light.

In a hundred years, Scotland had advanced from 'insanitary squalor to decency.' As the stimulus for this very satisfactory improvement the Committee identified the evidence submitted to the Poor Law Commissioners in 1842:

> The general impression left, after reading these reports, is that, among informed people of the time, there was serious alarm over the widespread physical and moral deterioration that was taking place and that poverty and lack of sanitation were regarded as primary and interacting causes.

Since then, the standard of living and the habits of the Scottish people had been transformed. The Report briefly acknowledged the vital part played by the sanitation schemes – drainage, sewerage and water supply – put in place in the nineteenth century. At greater length the Report gave particular

---

1 C. Webster, 'Healthy or Hungry Thirties?', *History Workshop Journal*, xiii, 1982, p. 111.

credit to the relief of poverty, recalling the observations of Professor Robert Cowan[2] and Professor W. P. Alison[3] who had accompanied Chadwick on the inspections carried out by the Poor Law Commissioners. Cowan, in a paper read to the British Association in 1840, had observed that 'the prevalence of epidemic disease depends upon various causes but the most influential of all is poverty.'[4] Alison, in his *Observations on the Management of the Poor*,[5] had attributed the appalling living conditions discovered by the Commissioners to 'pauperism, or destitution worse than pauperism, which had demanded relief but had failed to find it.' He had concluded that this poverty was

> . . . not only much greater in Scotland than in any other European countries similarly situated, but that it was greatly increasing, and that this increase, together with the influx of rural and Irish pauperism into our great towns, had brought them into a condition greatly more favourable than they had ever been before to the spread of epidemic disease, and accordingly raised their mortality far above the level of corresponding towns in England or the Continent.

In the middle years of the nineteenth century wages in Scotland were low and the cost of living relatively high. Women and children, from the age of seven or eight, were employed in the mines for 10 or 12 hours a day. Accidents in the workplace were common and in the absence of legislation for workmen's compensation or social insurance there was no organised assistance for the unemployed. Poor Relief, the only form of public assistance, was scanty and uncertain. Cathcart noted that since then

> . . . the standard of living has risen and, apart from increases in real wages, the minimum standard of subsistence below which the community does not allow any of its members to fall is higher than any previous time and certainly much higher than during the last century. A wide range of social services – workmen's compensations, health and employment insurance, widows' and old age pensions, public assistance, etc – has abolished destitution as it was understood and described in the Sanitary Inquiry Reports of 1842.

The working environment had also improved. Industrial machinery had reduced the wear and tear of physical exertion. Leisure time had increased.

2 Professor of Medical Jurisprudence and Medical Police at Glasgow University
3 Professor of Medicine at Edinburgh University.
4 Cathcart Report, p. 38.
5 This and the quotations in the following two references paraphrase Alison's views but are not direct quotations from W. P. Alison, *Observations on the Management of the Poor in Scotland* (Edinburgh, 1840).

Public transport had made it possible for workers to live at a greater distance from their place of work. The development of transport had also brought a greater range of food and other commodities within the reach of the people. Increased leisure time had encouraged the 'cult of gardening and facilitated all kinds of open-air recreation.' Gas lighting had reduced the risk of accidents at home and in the streets. Electric power had created a healthier atmosphere by reducing the burning of coal. Extended education, reinforced by the influence of the cinema and wireless broadcasting, had changed the outlook of the people, heightening their 'capacity and . . . will for healthy living.'

As evidence that health had indeed improved, the Cathcart Committee pointed to the reduction in death rates.[6] As evidence of a new and more enlightened life style, Cathcart cited the decrease in the number of court convictions for drunkenness; one witness had assured the Committee that 'alcoholism has decreased enormously . . . delirium tremens is never seen and the sequelae of chronic alcoholism are rarely found.' Cathcart concluded

. . . that the social and economic background has changed so as to allow immeasurably greater possibilities of healthy living for the mass of the people, that the habits of the people from whatever cause or combination of causes – improved sanitation, higher standard of living, more general education, quicker communications, increased and more varied facilities for recreation and so on – are in fact healthier.

On the very limited evidence it had solicited, the Cathcart Committee felt able to make an optimistic projection of future trends:

Improvement in working and living conditions during the period of greatest development of the health services has combined with the results of these services to produce changes in the health of the people, their habits and outlook, and in the problems of health policy and organisation. Changes have occurred or are still in progress, for example, in diet, in leisure and recreation, in housing, in severity of labour and in working conditions, and so on. The sum-total of these changes, viewing them together, has altered the general attitude and outlook of the people in ways that are specially significant for health policy.

Although 'no witness suggested that there was not great room for improvement', the Cathcart Committee was confident that, as a result of many years of improvement in social conditions in Scotland, in the 1930s 'health is

6 Appendices II and III.

prized' and the people were prepared to 'lead ascetic lives' to preserve it.

It was only by taking the long view that the Cathcart Committee could be so confident about the attitudes of the public and so optimistic about a continuing progress towards healthy living. Those who were more focused on the immediate problems of the 1930s were far from unanimous in sharing this confidence.

In *The Condition of the Working Class in Britain*, the Communist Harry Pollit wrote that 'in 1933, for the mass of the population, Britain is a hungry Britain, badly fed, badly clothed and badly housed.'[7] This same bleak assessment was more famously presented by George Orwell in *The Road to Wigan Pier*.[8] Statistical evidence of severe deprivation was published by a Medical Officer in the North of England.[9] However, later historians have claimed that these and other similar accounts were prejudiced and that the 'Hungry Thirties' were 'a myth sedulously propagated'[10] – a view that has, in turn, been vigorously debated.[11] At the time, the Government professed confidence that the economic crisis of the 1930s was no more than a passing phenomenon during which the health and strength of the people were being well protected by the state. In the House of Commons on 17 July 1935 the Minister of Health, Sir Kingsley Wood, claimed that 'the nation has learned and is learning today, in many ways, the supreme art of Living.'[12] In 1935, the Prime Minister, Stanley Baldwin, reassured a concerned public that the social services were proving 'wonderfully well maintained'[13] and fully effective.

His claim rested on evidence supplied by the Ministry of Health. In 1930 the Minister had commissioned surveys of state medical services 'to satisfy himself that the Local Authorities were achieving and maintaining a reasonable standard of efficiency and progress in the discharge of their functions relating to public health services.'[14] Visiting Medical Officers

---

7 H. Pollitt, Introduction to A. Hutt, *The Condition of the Working Class in Britain* (London, 1933).
8 G. Orwell, *The Road to Wigan Pier* (London, 1937).
9 G. M. McGonigle and J. Kirby, *Poverty and Public Health* (London, 1936).
10 C. L. Mowatt, *Britain Between the Wars* (London, 1968), p.432.
11 That the 'myth' was false-Mowat, *op.cit*, D. H. Aldcroft, *The Interwar Economy in Britain* (London, 1970); J. Stevenson and C. Cook, *The Slump* (London, 1974); J. M. Winter, *The Great War and the British People* (London, 1986). That the distress of the 1930s was real – C. Webster, 'Healthy or Hungry Thirties?', *History Workshop Journal*, xiii, 1982, p. 110; C. Webster, 'Health Welfare and Unemployment During the Depression', *Past and Present*, cix, 1985, p.204; L. Bryder, 'The First World War; Healthy or Hungry', *History Workshop Journal*, xxiv, 1987, p. 139.
12 *Hansard*, ccciv, HC, 15 July 1935, col. 1061.
13 PRO MM 55/688, quoted by C. Webster, 'Health, Welfare and Unemployment During the Depression', *op. cit.*, p. 204.
14 *Annual Report of the Ministry of Health, 1931–32*, Cmd. 4113, p. 43.

from the Ministry of Health found no 'cause for criticism' and commended the high quality of the work being carried out by local services. The Ministry also showed that, although the numbers included in the National Health Insurance Scheme had risen steadily, the total amount of support required had fallen.[15] Reports on housing were also satisfactory. In 1931 the Ministry reported that there was no overall shortage of houses in England although there was a need to 'replace houses that ought to be demolished.'[16] A scheme was launched to build 300,000 houses to replace the slums.[17] By 1935 the Ministry was able to report that since the end of the war, apart from slum clearance schemes, 1,213,397 low-cost houses[18] had been built in England with state assistance.[19] Less reassuring was the report that the numbers receiving aid under the Poor Law had increased by 64% between 1930 and 1935,[20] suggesting that there had been some increase in poverty. However, there was no proof that this had resulted in hunger or malnutrition.[21] The Ministry concluded that England was enjoying a period of 'very signal development and improvement in many directions, valuable in themselves and so conceived as to lay sound foundations for the future.'[22]

While the Ministry of Health in London was reassuring government ministers and denouncing local reports of poverty and ill health as 'socialistically motivated stunts,'[23] the Department of Health for Scotland was taking a very different line. It made no secret of the extent of the problems in Scotland or that the deficiencies in the welfare services 'are only now being thrown into prominent relief.'[24] The Department therefore welcomed the appointment of a Committee to review services in Scotland.

The Cathcart Committee no doubt fully shared the Department of Health's appreciation of the situation but, as we have seen, wished to avoid impolitic confrontation with the administration in London. Nevertheless, it did allow that in 1917 the Royal Commission on Housing had been able 'to point to much poverty, bad working conditions, slums and overcrowding although to nothing quite so gross as any of the typical conditions described in the reports of the first half of the last century.'[25]

---

15 From £29,231,000 in 1929 to £25,637,000 in 1934. *Annual Report of the Ministry of Health 1934–35*, p. 329.
16 *Annual Report of the Ministry of Health 1931–32*, p. 96.
17 *Annual Report of the Ministry of Health 1934–35*, p. 147.
18 Rateable value less than £78.
19 *Annual Report of the Ministry of Health 1934–35*, p. 157.
20 From 720,547 in June 1930 to 1,183,166 in March 1935.
21 *Annual Report of the Ministry of Health 1934–35*, p. 137.
22 *Ibid.*, p. 14.
23 Webster, 1982, *op. cit.*, p. 112.
24 *Annual Report of the Department of Health for Scotland*, 1935, Cmd. 5123, p. 21.
25 *Ibid.*, p. 40.

The Committee accepted that there was a danger that 'people at large may come to accept as a matter of course the sanitary achievements of these latter days and may fail to realise how recently that standard has been attained and how necessary it is to maintain them at their full efficiency.'[26] By going no deeper into the poverty and poor living conditions in Scotland, the Cathcart Committee failed to emphasise how much urgent improvement was still required or to explore what were the fundamental causes of Scotland's persistently bad record of health.

A Long-Term Problem in Scotland

In Scotland there was little confidence that the social and economic misery of the 1930s was a passing phenomenon. Commentators at the time saw little prospect of industrial recovery in Scotland.[27] The heavy industries of Scotland's Economic Miracle had been in decline since the end of the First World War, and in the mid-1930s there were still no signs of any new industrial activity which might stimulate an economic recovery. The loss of income and the hardship that had accompanied the decline in the economy over more than a decade had been exacerbated by the massive unemployment of the Depression. In the House of Commons, Walter Elliot described Scotland's cities as 'heaped up castles of misery.'[28] The misery was not confined to the cities but was widespread and severe across the country. Edwin Muir wrote of his journey through Scotland in 1934:

> My impression was one of emptiness, and that applied even more to the towns than the countryside. Scotland is losing its industries, as it lost over a hundred years ago a great deal of its agriculture and most of its indigenous literature . . . Now Scotland's industry, like its intelligence before it, is gravitating to England, but its population is sitting where it did before, in the company of disused coal-pits and silent shipyards.[29]

The industrialisation of Scotland had left 'its mark on several generations of men, women and children by whose work it lived, in shrunken bodies and trivial and embittered minds.'[30] The statistical evidence of the effect of poverty and dreadful living conditions was reported year by year by the Department of Health for Scotland. There was less formal, but equally

26 *Ibid.*
27 A. Maclehose (ed.), *The Scotland of Our Sons* (London, 1937); J. A. Bowie, *The Future of Scotland* (Edinburgh, 1939).
28 Walter Elliot, quoted in Maclehose, *op. cit.*
29 E. Muir, *Scottish Journey* (2nd ed., Edinburgh, 1996), p. 243.
30 *Ibid.*, p. 42.

persuasive, evidence in the records of the Church of Scotland. In many parishes as many as 60% of church members were unemployed. The Church was particularly disturbed by the effects of unemployment and poverty on the urban population of Scotland (80% of the whole), and could see 'little hope of any speedy progress being made towards the solution.'[31] The Church saw no evidence of that heightening of the 'capacity and will for healthy living' reported by Cathcart. Cathcart had given a decline in alcoholism as evidence of an improvement in life-style. There was some statistical evidence that, at first sight, might seem to support this claim. Over the year 1931–32 the consumption of spirits in Scotland had decreased by 946,000 gallons and beer by 3,370,00 gallons and total spending on licensed alcohol sales by 10.5%. The Chief Constable of Glasgow reported to the General Assembly of the Church of Scotland that 'drunkenness *as ordinarily understood* showed a decided decrease' (my italics). However, 'the number of persons proceeded against for drunkenness produced by drinking methylated spirit has increased.' Methylated spirit could be bought surreptitiously from street vendors for a few pennies, and in the 1930s Scotland's Chief Constables had come to recognise 'meths' drinking as a serious menace.

In presenting a somewhat benign view of social conditions in Scotland the Cathcart Committee was being circumspect.[32] The picture painted by the Department of Health for Scotland, the Church of Scotland, Edwin Muir and Walter Elliot is more convincing and continues in the memories of many still alive. The continuing problems of poverty, poor diet and bad living conditions – the worst features of urbanisation – were all too evident in the 1930s and their legacy has not yet disappeared.

Urbanisation

The effects of urbanisation have been observed in different societies and cultures since the Bronze Age.[33] While the elite remains relatively unscathed, the poor become shorter, less heavily built and suffer an earlier death. The urbanisation that accompanied the Industrial Revolution in Britain produced people smaller than their grandparents and with an average lifespan shorter than in the first century BC.[34] In Scotland, where

---

31 *Reports to the General Assembly of the Church of Scotland*, xiv, 1934, p. 465.
32 All papers relating to the Cathcart Committee were destroyed during the Second World War and Professor Cathcart left no papers of his own. The comments on the considerations that shaped the Committees decisions can only be speculative.
33 W. J. MacLennan and W. I. Sellars, 'Ageing Through The Ages', *Proceedings of the Royal College of Physicians of Edinburgh*, xxix, 1999, p. 72.
34 A study in 1994 produced evidence that the median life span in the period 1850 to 1899 was shorter than in the first century BC. J. D. Montague, 'Length of Life in the Ancient World,' *Journal of the Royal Society of Medicine*, dxxxvii, 1994, p. 25.

urbanisation was 'abrupt and swift',[35] the effects had been particularly severe and reached a nadir in the first decades of the nineteenth century. The changes in physique that occurred over the following 100 years were therefore not 'improvements,' as described by Cathcart, but the restoration of normality.

The first phase of the Industrial Revolution in Scotland, the years from c1760 to c1830, formed a 'bridge between the Old World of rural Scotland and the urbanised society of the later nineteenth century.' By the 1840s, 40% of the Scottish population already lived in towns of over 5,000 inhabitants.[36] There were damaging consequences for the rural population. On average, agricultural wages had increased slightly but they had not always kept pace with the inflation of the last years of the eighteenth century and the first two decades of nineteenth century. When prices fell after 1820, agricultural prosperity suffered and the depression soon filtered through from the farmers to their labourers.[37] Real wages in the 1840s were therefore lower than they had been before the Napoleonic Wars and there was less opportunity to supplement low wages by earnings from outworking in textile production. Rural housing was primitive. The typical farm labourer's house of the period was described as.

> . . . about 12 feet by 14, and not so high in the wall as will allow a man to get in without stooping . . . without ceiling, or anything beneath the bare tiles of the roof; without a floor save the common clay; without a cupboard or recess of any kind; no grate but the iron bars which the tenants carried to it, built up and took away when they left it; with no partition of any kind save what the beds made; with no window save four small panes on one side.[38]

In the towns and cities living conditions were becoming even harsher. By 1850, as an urbanised society, Scotland was second only to England in Europe. The growth of the industrial centres across the central belt was fed by the migration of poor young adults from the rural Lowlands, with small numbers from the Highlands and a flood of both Protestant and Catholic immigrants from Ulster and southern Ireland.[39] As both a major port as well

---

35 T. M. Devine, 'Urbanisation,' in T. M. Devine and R. Mitchison (eds.), *People and Society in Scotland*, i (Edinburgh, 1988), p. 31.

36 Between 1831 and 1861 less than 40% of the population lived in settlements of more than 5,000. R. J. Morris, 'Urbanisation and Scotland,' in W. H. Fraser and R. J. Morris (eds.), *People and Society in Scotland*, ii (Edinburgh, 1995), p. 74.

37 E. Royle, *Modern Britain* (London, 1987), p. 157.

38 A. Somerville, *The Autobiography of a Working Man* (London, 1848), p. 10.

39 B. Collins, 'The Origins of the Irish Immigration to Scotland in the Nineteenth and Twentieth Centuries,' in T. M. Devine (ed.), *Irish Immigration and Scottish Society in the Nineteenth and Twentieth Centuries* (Edinburgh, 1991), p. 1.

as a major industrial centre, Glasgow experienced the effect in full. Thousands of power looms served a thriving textile industry. More than a hundred pig-iron furnaces produced hundreds of thousands of tons each year. Ships trading with North America and the West Indies were berthing in creasing numbers at the Broomielaw. Glasgow's first railway opened for traffic in 1831.[40] As industrial activity increased, the Clyde became an open sewer. Disposal of human and industrial waste was grossly defective; cattle were slaughtered in the street; the older parts of the city became increasingly filthy.[41]

'While the higher ranks in Glasgow were advancing in wealth and luxury, a large proportion of the lower rank were receding towards barbarism.'[42] Housing conditions were appalling. The crowded tenements in which the working classes lived were owned by a large number of the middling classes intent on making a profit from tenement properties in which, in many cases, they themselves lived. An uncontrolled building boom, beginning in 1831, continued well into the 1870s. Large houses were partitioned and subdivided and shoddy new dwellings sprang up in their backyards. New tenements were erected round squares which then became built up by the erection of further smaller squares to form a complicated arrangement referred to by Glasgow's Medical Officer of Health as 'Chinese puzzles.'[43] The dwellings were without drainage or ventilation. The central courts of the 'Chinese puzzles' became middens with dunghills reaching the height of the first floor.

The slum ghettos were persisting nests of typhus and their populations were victims of recurring epidemics of cholera. These were the conditions found by the Poor Law Commissioners visiting Scotland for the Sanitary Inquiry (Scotland) in 1842. Some of the most damning evidence of the appalling housing conditions in Scotland's cities was provided by doctors – Neil Beaton, Neil Arnott, Alexander Miller, W. P. Alison and Robert Cowan. These doctors could bear witness to the association between the housing conditions and the incidence of fevers and pestilential disease; the overcrowding and squalor the Commissioners could see for themselves.[44]

From the 1840s there was a second phase of industrialisation and the

40 The Glasgow and Garnkirk Railway.
41 Butchers were much to blame. In the previous century 'slaying and building the whole bestial they kill on the High Street in Trongait on baith sides of the gait, quhilk is very loathsome to beholders and also raises ane filthie and noysonme stink' – J. S. Clarke, *An Epic of Municioalisation* (Glasgow, 1928), p. 7. This had improved little by the early years of the nineteenth century.
42 Alison, *op. cit.*, p. 182.
43 E. Robertson, *Glasgow's Doctor: James Burn Russell* (East Linton, 1998), p. 98.
44 *Report on the Sanitary Condition of the Labouring Population of Scotland* (Edinburgh, 1842).

process of urbanisation accelerated, eventually shaping the Scotland of the 1930s. Textile manufacturing was surpassed by heavy industry. Glasgow and the western Lowlands became the Workshop of the World and, supported by a flourishing coal-mining industry, had come to dominate the production of ships, locomotives, heavy engineering and steel. Existing industrial cities and burghs expanded and new centres were created, often on greenfield sites and named after the nearest village. In 1831 Coatbridge had been a village of 107 houses on the Monkland Canal;[45] by 1931 it was a town with a population of over 40,000. Airdrie grew almost as rapidly and acquired 'the ramshackle and dangerous character of a frontier town.'[46] Although cotton spinning was in decline, the more specialised textile industries prospered – jute in Dundee, lace in the Irvine valley, canvas in Arbroath, and high-quality woolen goods in the Borders. Hawick soon became as overcrowded as Glasgow.

These upheavals created a new and multiplying urban poor who suffered as much in their diet as in their housing and working conditions. Traditionally the diet of the rural population was oats, barley, peas, potatoes and milk with meat only as an occasional luxury. The basic diet of the new urban poor differed little from that of the rural population but the same food was more expensive and less likely to be fresh. The family diet depended on income and families could only be fed and housed while the breadwinner remained healthy and in employment.

By the middle of the nineteenth century almost nothing had been done to relieve the living conditions of the urban poor. Tucked away in the most squalid parts of the towns and cities the poor, and the squalor in which they lived, were out of sight and the more prosperous citizens could remain oblivious to the conditions in the ghettos. There was little public pressure for improvement and central Government did not actively intervene in the interest of public health in Scotland until the Public Health Act of 1867. Even then the Board of Supervision[47] chose not to put pressure on the many local authorities that were reluctant to invest in public health measures. In 1869 the Board issued an 'Instructional Letter' to its officers: 'You will understand that the Board do not expect that the whole of the provisions of the Public Health Act can be immediately and simultaneously put in force in all places.'[48]

In the second half of the century Britain, and particularly England, had begun to enjoy a period of increasing prosperity. In 1851 the *Manchester Guardian* could claim that 'we have at least as much, if not more, substantial

45 A. Fullerton (ed.), *Gazetteer of Scotland* (Glasgow, 1842).
46 T. C. Smout, *A Century of the Scottish People* (London, 1986), p. 9.
47 'An absurd executive' according to Glasgow's MOH.
48 T. Ferguson, *Scottish Social Welfare* (Edinburgh, 1958), p. 11.

reason for contentment and thankfulness, than at the close of any past year in our history.'[49] Food was cheap and plentiful and 'clothing, fuel, shelter and transition from place to place within the reach of all, except those whom demerit, or extraordinary misfortune, has reduced to complete destitution.' Working people were beginning to enjoy the benefits as well as the squalor of the Industrial Revolution. Expanding industry provided employment and higher wages. The cotton industry produced cheap washable clothing and the chemical industry cheap soap; personal cleanliness was at least as important as a health benefit from the new water supplies as the safer drinking water. The new railways were more efficient in distributing the food produced by more modern farming to the towns. Protection of home markets had been abandoned, and improved transport within North America and across the Atlantic allowed the importation of cheap grain and lowered food prices. Those who suffered 'extraordinary misfortune' and even some of those destitute because of 'demerit' received support from an extraordinary expansion of philanthropic societies and the widening scope of middle-class good works. The process of urbanisation continued but the increasing prosperity and the gradual, even if uneven and haphazard, implementation of public health legislation prevented any further deterioration in the health and physical wellbeing of the people, certainly in England and Wales.

In Scotland conditions were much less satisfactory. Industrialisation, beginning later, had proceeded even faster than in England. Except in coalmining, even skilled employees in Scotland's industries earned substantially less than their opposite numbers in England.[50] The proportion of skilled workers was smaller than in England and wage differentials between the skilled and unskilled and between male and female workers were greater. Scotland had a low-wage economy and greater poverty, and support for the poor was slow in coming. The Poor Law (Scotland) Act of 1845 had transferred the responsibility for the poor of each parish from the Kirk Session to new parochial councils under the guidance of a Board of Supervision in Edinburgh. Each parish was directed to appoint an Inspector of the Poor to judge the merits of applications for relief. But there was still no provision for the able-bodied. The parochial councils were authorised to levy a compulsory rate for public health measures but it was several years before most parishes in Scotland took up this option. As a result parochial councils, in the great majority of cases, did not have the funds to make full use of their powers. Into the twentieth century

49 Quoted by A. Briggs, *Victorian People: A Reassessment of Persons and Themes* (Folio Society edition, London, 1996), p. 41.
50 W. W. Knox, *Industrial Nation: Work Culture and Society in Scotland, 1800 – Present* (Edinburgh, 1999), p. 90.

spending on the poor in Scotland was much more niggardly than in England.[51]

Without active central direction, it was left to local authorities to find their own solutions to their public health problems in local Police Acts. Local authorities varied in their enthusiasm for public health measures and in their financial resources to implement them. In Glasgow a succession of outstanding Medical Officers of Health, supported by sympathetic Health Committees, succeeded in setting up a Public Health service that was ahead of its time in Britain. But overall Public Health services remained patchy and uneven across Scotland until central Government, in the Public Health Act of 1897, began to make important public health legislation compulsory.

In these circumstances of poverty and overcrowding the uneven and uncertain public health measures of the second half of the century failed to prevent further deterioration in health standards as urbanisation continued. The death rates in Scotland which, in the middle years of the century, had compared favourably with those in England and Wales, began to deteriorate as the century advanced, and by the end of the century the deaths rates had deteriorated to match those south of the border.[52] Over the same period real wages improved by some 45%[53] and opportunities for regular employment in the industrial regions of Strathclyde and Lothian had more than doubled. Even so, the diet of the working classes in 1901 was still barely adequate[54] and living conditions were still squalid.

Improvement in the social conditions began to accelerate in the first years of the new century. Cathcart drew attention to the 'progress of the last forty years.' 'With the exception of a few backward areas, practically all populous centres have now more or less adequate services for water, drainage, sewerage, public cleansing and the other elements of sanitation, and, although much progress has still to be made, the housing conditions are greatly improved.' There had been satisfactory progress in the relief of poverty. Cathcart's buoyant assessment was not substantiated by published statistics. The *Annual Reports of the Registrar General for Scotland* and the *Annual Reports of the Registrar General for England and Wales* show that almost to the end of the nineteenth century the problems had hardly been contained at all. Real measurable improvement had begun only in the last few years of the nineteenth century and had then proceeded at a significantly slower rate in Scotland than in England and Wales.

---

51 M. A. Crowther, 'Poverty, Health and Welfare,' in Fraser and Morris, *op. cit.*, p. 269.
52 Appendix II.
53 E. Royale, *Modern Britain* (London, 1987). p. 168.
54 N. Paton, J. Dunlop and E. A. Inglis, *A Study of the Diet of the Labouring Classes in Edinburgh* (Edinburgh, 1901).

Table 4.1   **Scotland's Worst Mortality Rates, 1930–1933**

Large Towns		Small Burghs	
Glasgow	16.3	Johnstone	17.7
Coatbridge	16.1	Denny	16.9
Paisley	16.1	Lanark	16.2
Greenock	16.1	Hawick	15.5
Port Glasgow	15.9	Alloa	15.5
Falkirk	15.3	Lochgelly	15.3
Dumbarton	15.3	Kilwinning	15.3
United Kingdom	10		

Source: *Annual Reports of the Registrar General for Scotland 1930–33; Annual Report of the Registrar General for England and Wales 1930*

Scotland's poor showing was due to the greater disruption caused to a greater proportion of the Scottish population by the upheaval of the Industrial Revolution than had been the case in England and Wales. In the 1930s almost every part of Scotland was still suffering from its aftermath. In England and Wales the evil legacy of the Industrial Revolution was confined to certain definable areas of the north and of Wales. In Scotland damaging living conditions were widespread and worse even than in the most distressed areas of England and Wales. Using the general death rate as an index, Table 4.1 lists the large towns and small burghs which, in the four years up to and including 1933, suffered the worst of Scotland's living conditions. All had death rates more than 50% greater than the prevailing rate for the United Kingdom.

As these figures illustrate, the poor social conditions left in the wake of industrialisation were not confined to the large towns and cities but extended into almost every part of the Lowlands and Borders and were suffered by a majority of the population. The towns and burghs listed as black spots in Table 4.1 were home to no less than 30% of the population of Scotland, and their living conditions differed little from the average conditions suffered by Scotland's working population. In Scotland as a whole the death rate was over 30% greater than that of the United Kingdom.

In these, the most distressed towns and burghs in Scotland, the population had increased since 1800 (Table 4.2). In the first phase of Industrial Revolution, Glasgow, Paisley, Johnstone and Hawick and other textile towns increased well above the average rate in Scotland, as did the mining villages like Lochgelly. Steel towns like Coatbridge increased dramatically only in the second stage after 1831. Over the whole period from 1800, the increase in these towns and small burghs varied widely from over 5000% in some to no more than 97% in others, and not all had increased beyond the average for Scotland. It is also significant that for over a century the increase in population had been much greater in England and Wales (187.5%) than in Scotland (100.3%)[55] yet, as measured by death rates, social conditions in England and Wales had never been so badly affected. It becomes evident that increase in population does not, of itself, account for the relatively poor living conditions in Scotland.

Table 4.2 **Population Increases, Scottish Burghs, 1801–1931**

	Population		Percentage Increase	
Large Towns	1801	1801–31	1831–1931	1801–1931
Glasgow	83769	141	288	1199
Coatbridge	585	21	5711	7260
Paisley	31179	84	50	177
Greenock	17458	57	186	352
Port Glasgow	3865	34	277	406
Falkirk	8838	44	187	314
Dumbarton	2862	21	495	653
Small Burghs				
Johnstone	1434	292	129	795
Denny	2033	98	136	367
Lanark	4692	64	19	135
Hawick	2798	78	267	552
Alloa	5214	21	109	296
Lochgelly	620	21	1084	1400
Kilwinning	2700	40	41	97
Scotland	1.625m	46	104	199
Eng. & Wales	9.061m	54	128	253

Sources: *Census of Scotland*, 1931; *Gazetteer of Scotland*, 1842; *Abstract of Historical Statistics*

A more constant factor was the poor quality of the housing stock. Table 4.3 shows that, in almost all these distressed communities, the proportion of the local housing stock made up of houses of one or two rooms was higher than the average for Scotland and considerably higher than the average in England and Wales (much higher even than in Northumberland and Durham where in England, the proportion was highest).

The small houses in these distressed communities accommodated a proportion of dependant children higher than the average for Scotland and much higher than the proportion in England and Wales (Table 4.4).

These differences were a reflection of the changing birth rates. During the nineteenth century, until 1895, the birth rate had been lower in Scotland than in England and Wales. Thereafter the rate fell in both countries. By 1900, while the rate in Scotland had fallen only to 29.6, the rate in England and Wales had reached 28.7. Thereafter the gap between the countries widened progressively. In 1930 the rate in Scotland was 19.6, and 16.3 in England and Wales. The greater numbers of children combined with the

55 Calculated from N. L. Tranter, *British Population in the Twentieth Century* ((London, 1996), p. 3.

smallness of the houses to cause greater overcrowding in Scotland than in England and Wales. The effect of overcrowding is indicated by its particular severity in those Scottish communities that suffered Scotland's highest death rates.

Table 4.3 **High Mortality and Percentage of Small Houses, Scottish Burghs, 1931**

Rooms	1	2	1 & 2		1	2	1 & 2
Large Towns				**Small Burghs**			
Glasgow	14.5	43.6	58.1	Johnstone	13.2	46	59.2
Coatbridge	23	50.9	73.9	Denny	4.1	40.7	41.5
Paisley	14.9	50.3	65.2	Lanark	8.8	32.7	41.5
Greenock	10.2	44.8	55	Hawick	9	36.2	45.2
Port Glasgow	8	59.5	67.5	Alloa	8.4	32.9	41.3
Falkirk	7.2	46	53.2	Lochgelly	5.2	55.2	60.4
Dumbarton	5.4	42.7	48.1	Kilwinning	15.2	35.4	50.6
Scotland	9.5	36.9	46.4	Eng. & Wales	0.4	4	4.4
				N & Durham	0.7	3.4	4.1

Sources: *Census of Scotland*, 1931; *Census of England and Wales*, 1931

Inadequate housing, large numbers of dependant children and overcrowding were all factors in making living in Scotland's black spots dangerous, but none of these variable factors operated consistently in every one of these communities. In each community their effects were cumulative and all were fundamentally expressions of poverty. Scotland's bad housing was essentially attributable to poverty.[56] The continuing high birth rate and the resulting large numbers of dependant children were also functions of poverty.[57] There were no relevant official surveys of nutrition in Scotland in the nineteenth century but there were a number of later studies from that by Paton and his colleagues in 1901 (above) to that by John Boyd Orr in 1935,[58] all of which demonstrated that the diet of the masses in Scotland was unsatisfactory and that this too was related to poverty.

This poverty was longstanding. The poverty caused by the unemployment during the Depression of the 1930s, most severe in the shipbuilding areas of the Clyde (Clydebank, Port Glasgow and Dumbarton[59]) but experienced across Scotland, was no more than an exacerbation of an existing problem. For centuries Scotland, when compared with England, had been a poor country. The years of its Economic Miracle had been too insecurely based[60] and too short-lived to correct that relative poverty. The upheaval of the Industrial Revolution had affected a greater proportion of

56 T. M. Devine, *The Scottish Nation, op. cit.*, p. 341.
57 J. Caldwell, 'Paths to Lower Fertility,' *BMJ*, cccix, 1999, p. 985.
58 J. Boyd Orr, *Food Health and Income* (London, 1936).
59 *Annual Report of the Department of Health for Scotland*, 1932, Cmd. 4338, p. 182.
60 R. H. Campbell, *The Rise and Fall of Scottish Industry, 1707–1939* (Edinburgh, 1980).

the population of Scotland and its effects had been more severe even than in the worst-affected industrial communities in the south. In the 1930s Scotland, unlike England, had become a proletarian nation with an established culture of poverty.[61]

Table 4.4 **High Mortality, Percentage of Population under 14yrs, Persons/Room (P/R), Scottish Burghs, 1931**

Large Towns	%Population 14 yrs or less	P/R	Small Burghs	%Population 14 yrs. or less	P/R
Glasgow	27.3	1.54	Johnstone	30	1.67
Coatbridge	32.4	2.03	Denny	28.9	1.55
Paisley	46.9	1.62	Lanark	25	1.16
Greenock	30.6	1.61	Hawick	21.1	1.21
Port Glasgow	33	1.93	Alloa	27.7	1.29
Falkirk	26.8	1.49	Lochgelly	32.5	1.77
Dumbarton	29.5	1.48	Kilwinning	30	1.53
Scotland	26.9	1.27	Eng. & Wales	23.8	0.83

Sources: *Census of Scotland*, 1931; *Census of England and Wales*, 1931

Health

In the 1930s little was known about the extent of life-threatening disease in the population of Britain and nothing whatever about the amount of minor illness and disability that disturbed the day-to-day activities of the people. Although records were available from 1855, when registration of death became compulsory in Scotland, Cathcart made use of death rates only from 1870 when they had already begun to fall. Over this period,[62] the general death rate had fallen steadily from 22.3 per thousand to 13.4. Over the same period the death rates in the major cities had shown greater improvement than the rate for the country as a whole (Edinburgh from 25.9 to 13.4; Glasgow from 30.4 to 14.3; Dundee from 27.5 to 14.3; Aberdeen from 22.8 to 13.4). Cathcart quoted these figures as evidence that health in Scotland had improved significantly over this period and that while health in great cities had been worse than in the rest of the country in 1870, the gap had narrowed by 1930.

The Cathcart Committee could only attempt a 'general view of the extent and nature of the ill-health' in Scotland. Even when suitable corrections were made to the figures to make allowance for changes in the age and sex structure of the population, a decline in the overall death rate did not immediately reveal much that was useful; it did not show which

61 J. Foster, 'A Proletarian Nation? Occupation and Class since 1914,' in A. Dickson and J. H. Treble (eds.), *People and Society in Scotland*, iii (Edinburgh, 1992), p. 201.
62 Appendices II and III.

sections of the population were surviving in greater numbers and therefore gave no indication of which causes of death were being contained or diminished. A method of presentation of the death statistics was devised by Cathcart's statisticians[63] that made it possible to draw a few but important conclusions. Figures were derived for ten separate age groups, giving the percentage reduction in death rates in each group between 1870–72 and 1930–32. This showed that while every age group had experienced a fall in death rate, infant mortality had fallen less than the death rate of any age group under 45 years of age. This was taken to disprove a theory that was prevalent at the time[64] that efforts to reduce infant mortality were counter-productive since they had the undesirable effect of prolonging the survival of weaklings. It was also noted that the greatest saving in life was among children between the ages of one and five years, the age group most vulnerable to infectious disease. Based on these and all the other figures, Cathcart ventured the hypothesis that 'the death rates of the adolescent and the adult depend on the constitution acquired during the first fifteen years or so of life and that the latter had undergone a very substantial improvement, presumably as a result of the general rising of the standard of life and the amelioration of social conditions.'

The statistics showed very clearly that since 1870 many more people, especially women, were surviving into old age. That the improvement in survival had been greater in Glasgow than in Scotland generally was offered as evidence that, over a period of 70 years, the threats to life in Scotland's industrial centres were being rapidly overcome while recovery was less rapid where the pressures of urbanisation had been less.

The Causes of Death

The causes of death, as recorded on death certificates, were much less certain than the fact of death itself. In the nineteenth century many deaths went uncertified because no doctor had been consulted about the terminal illness. In Glasgow in 1874 over a third of children dying in the first years of life had not been seen by a doctor; for those between 1 and 5 years the proportion was over a quarter and of those over that age almost 15%.[65] In some Highland parishes no cause was established in 75% of all deaths.[66] Not

---

63 Dr McKinlay of the Department of Health for Scotland and Drs McKendrick and Kermack of the Research Laboratory of the Royal College of Physicians of Edinburgh.
64 Professor Cathcart had himself expressed this fear in his address at Anderson College in 1933. *Glasgow Medical Journal*, i, 1933, p. 185.
65 J. B. Russell, *Report on Uncertified Deaths in Glasgow* (Glasgow, 1876).
66 Ferguson, *op. cit.*, p. 32.

until the early years of the twentieth century did this cease to be a significant problem.[67]

There were other difficulties. In many cases where the death had been certified, the diagnosis was grossly inaccurate. For much of the nineteenth century and into the twentieth, it was often impossible to make a reliable diagnosis in the dark overcrowded homes of the poor and, in many cases, the difficulty was made worse by personal filth. 'The skin is to such people virtually a lost organ, coated with the accumulated excretion of years.'[68] Infectious diseases such as typhus were impossible to diagnose until the body had been thoroughly washed to expose the skin rash. The medical examination of the body before certification was often cursory in the extreme and the diagnosis of acute deaths little more than guesswork.

Even when a diagnosis was attempted, the classification of disease used by the Registrar General was imprecise and unhelpful. A death classified as due to heart disease could have been due to the recent onset of degenerative disease or equally could have been the late effect of rheumatism or syphilis contracted early in life. Other broad diagnoses – 'nervous disorders' or 'kidney disease' – were equally uninformative. The changing age and sex structure of the population added to the difficulties in trying to detect a pattern of change over the years.

Cathcart's statisticians attempted a full analysis of the causes of death only for the short period after 1891 and then only in relation to a 'relatively small number of causes of death.' The crude death rates indicated that deaths from cerebral haemorrhage in 1932 had increased by 42% since 1910, but when this figure was corrected for age it was shown that the incidence had actually declined. Similarly it was shown that an apparent increase of 42% in deaths from cancer was in fact a real increase of only 9%. On the advice of their statisticians, the Cathcart Committee concluded that, from the records of the causes of death as they were presented in 1936, 'detailed comparisons with past experience are not possible.'

Sickness and Defect

Until the end of the nineteenth century the records of the incidence of disease (as opposed to deaths from disease) were totally unreliable. The Infectious Disease (Notification) Act, applying to the whole of Scotland, was not passed until 1889. It was then only adoptive and applied only to smallpox, cholera, diphtheria, erysipelas, scarlet fever and the 'fevers known by any of the following names – typhus, typhoid enteric, relapsing,

67 In 1901 the percentage of death in Scotland going uncertified had fallen to 1.7.
68 J. B. Russell, MOH of Glasgow, quoted by Robertson, *op. cit*, p. 52.

continued or puerperal.'[69] Notification of infectious disease (now including all forms of tuberculosis) became compulsory in 1897 but even then it was far from being an exact science. During the period from 1891 reviewed for the Cathcart Report, the statistics could only be used to indicate some general trends. By 1891 smallpox and typhus had disappeared completely and there were marked reductions in deaths from all the common infectious diseases – abdominal tuberculosis by 71%, pulmonary tuberculosis by 65%, scarlet fever by 63%, diphtheria by 66%, measles by 68% and whooping cough by 59%, erysipelas by 39%. There had also been significant reductions in 'dysentery and diarrhoea' (listed together without mention of typhoid) and in 'infectious and other parasitic diseases.'

Without meaningful statistics, the Cathcart Committee was unable to draw any useful conclusion about the cause or causes of these trends and could report only the theories put forward by medical witnesses. The marked decline in deaths from enteric fevers and the diarrhoeal illnesses of children was attributed to the introduction of pure water supplies, the diminution of the fly menace and the increase in communal and domestic cleanliness; the fall in mortality from scarlet fever was attributed to a (speculative) lessening in the virulence of the infecting organism; the lessened death rate from diphtheria could possibly be attributed in small part to the very recent introduction of serum treatment;[70] the incidence and severity of measles and whooping cough had perhaps declined as the result of improvement in nutrition and overcrowding. However, none of these explanations was entirely convincing; nor was the suggestion that the decrease in the severity of the infectious diseases of children might be associated with the decline in the incidence of rickets in Scotland's cities.

Cathcart concluded that any 'deductions relating to the future incidence and severity of infectious disease should be made with caution.'

Other than on notifiable infectious disease, there was almost no hard information about the prevalence of disease in the general population. The ill-defined disorder of rheumatism had apparently declined by 40% and bronchitis and pneumonia by 44%. It was tentatively suggested that these improvements might be the late effects of the diminution of infectious disease earlier in life. Other disorders had been increasingly recorded as the cause of death – Bright's disease (nephritis) by 46%, suicide by 41%, diseases of the nervous system by 25%, violence by 16% and diseases of the circulatory system by 5%. These increases might possibly be related to the ageing of the population rather than to a true increase in incidence.

69 Quoted from the Act by Ferguson, *op. cit.*, p. 405.
70 Serum treatment had been possible since 1891 but its use met with resistance and introduction into practice had been slow.

However, the explanations for the changes in the pattern of disease remained obscure.

The School Medical Service provided little information on what was an important sample of the population. As will be discussed in a later chapter, school medical inspections gathered more information on the physical appearance of the children than on their state of health. Information on the adult population was no better. Since 1930 the Morbidity Statistics Scheme, set up by the Department of Health for Scotland to record incapacitating illness in the insured population, had provided information on a large sample of the adult population. But only disorders causing absence from work were recorded. The scheme therefore did not reveal the incidence of the common chronic disorders – hernias, migraine, haemorrhoids, chronic bronchitis, carbuncles – that made up such a large proportion of the medical problems of the mass of the working population.

From the very little reliable information available Cathcart could only conclude that the amount of sickness in the population was very great and that 'there was ample scope for reduction.'

Anthropometric Data

There was even less information about the growth and physical development of the people. In 1903 the Royal Commission on Physical Training had deplored the lack of anthropometric data, and the Inter-Departmental Committee that followed in 1904 had recommended that an anthropometric survey should be established. This had not been done and by 1936 the only data available were from Glasgow and derived entirely from children attending school. (Crucially, disabled children, children with chronic illnesses and children who were absent from school because of illness were therefore excluded.) Measurements made at the age of five years and again at nine years and at 13 years showed that, over the period from 1910 to 1933, there had been significant increases in both height and in weight. The increases in boys ranged from 0.7 ins. and 0.9 lb. in five-year-olds to increases of 1.5 ins. and 5.5 lb. at 13 years; in girls from 0.8 ins. and 0.1 lb. at 5 years to 1.3 ins. and 2.8 lb. at 13 years. It was shown that these increases were shared by children of all classes.[71] Sir Leslie Mackenzie of the Scotch Education Department and other experts accepted that the data were sufficient to establish that Scottish children in 1933 were 'better physically' than their predecessors. Cathcart was more cautious; height and weight were measures of growth and by themselves were of little significance as indicators of health or nutrition of individual children. (It would later be

71 Indicated by the number of rooms in the family home.

claimed that the cause was, at least in part, genetic.) Although measurement of comparable groups of children at different times and under different circumstances had been used by many investigators as indications of improved nutrition, Cathcart was unwilling to accept such conclusions in the absence of other supportive evidence.

While the Cathcart Committee considered that no matter what interpretation was put on the improvement in height and weights of a small sample of Scottish children, it certainly could not be taken to signify an improvement in the nutrition or a relative absence of disease in the general population.

Observations and Impressions of Medical and Other Witnesses

Without satisfactory statistics on which to base a sound assessment of health trends in Scotland, Cathcart recorded anecdotal evidence. A number of medical witnesses attested to a striking decline in rickets, especially in its more severe forms. Medical witnesses from the larger towns reported that, although rickets was still not uncommon, it was now in much milder form than formerly.

On blindness, it was suggested that ophthalmia of the newborn had become rare and that the infectious diseases of childhood were less frequently followed by loss of vision. But nothing at all was known of the trend in blindness due to congenital causes, injuries or the affections incidental to old age

The incidence of deaf mutism among Scottish schoolchildren was thought to be decreasing since, between 1891 and 1931, there had been a definite decrease in the number of children attending schools for the deaf and, of these children, the proportion with acquired deafness had fallen from 50% to 27.8%.

A number of witnesses suggested that venereal diseases had become less common but the statistics on the venereal diseases were considered to be too recent to allow a categorical statement to be made.

Only on pernicious anaemia and diabetes was there reliable evidence of an improvement, if not in the incidence of disease, at least an improvement in management. The *Annual Report of the Registrar General for Scotland* for 1931 had shown that the mortality from pernicious anaemia had fallen by a half since liver extract was introduced over the period 1921–1926. There had been a similar improvement in the survival of young adults suffering from diabetes following the introduction of insulin treatment.

On mental disorders the evidence submitted to the Cathcart Committee was as uncertain as that relating to physical disease. The Committee found that 'it is not possible to say by reference to any body of statistics whether or not mental disease and psychoneurotic conditions are increasing.' The number of certified lunatics had increased from 205 per 100,000 of the population in 1861 to 392 per 100,000 in 1931, but to what extent this represented a true increase was uncertain. One authority stated that it was 'very largely due to different diagnosis. Forty years ago almost half the cases that are now being certified as mentally defective would not have been so certified.' There was greater confidence among the expert witnesses that psychoneurotic illnesses had increased. The Industrial Health Research Board had reported that 'not less than 10–20% of time loss through sickness by employed persons should be debited to the so-called psychoneuroses or minor psychoses.' There was also a growing body of opinion that the psychological determinants of ill health had been underestimated and that organic disease was often intensified by accompanying psychoneuroses. A leading authority attributed the apparent increase in psychoneurosis to 'the change in ethical and moral standards that has taken place.' In the absence of hard information Cathcart accepted the opinion of the acknowledged experts of the time that the incidence of mental deficiency had probably remained constant while there had probably been a true increase in psychoneurosis.[72]

The Cathcart Committee was satisfied that it had been clearly established that, over the period of its review, there had been a significant prolongation of life at all ages. However, in the absence of proof, it could only be assumed that the reduction in death had been accompanied by greater freedom from sickness, ill health and physical defects and had not merely extended the duration of disability. 'It would be impossible for us to present anything like a complete picture of the present state of the people.' Everyday experience indicated there was still 'a large mass of sickness and defects.' But since much of the country's disease and disability never came 'within the purview of the local authorities', the true extent of the burden of illness could not be known. Cathcart could only speculate.

There had been a great reduction in the number of deaths from infectious disease but there had been no proportionate decline in the incidence of infectious disease. While the incidence remained high, especially among children, and recovery was often incomplete, it must be assumed that the volume of chronic disorders in the adult population was increasing.

The Cathcart Committee was confident that, in the 1930s, the greater

72 'The stress and anxieties of present-day living have been potent agents in the production of the neuroses, while a widespread pursuit of pleasure and excitement with a corresponding lack of balance among the post war generation is to be regarded with some anxiety.' Memorandum from the Royal College of Physicians of Edinburgh.

rates of survival into middle and old age had caused an important change in the general pattern of disease. The incidence of the conditions associated with ageing – cancer, chronic bronchitis, and degenerative circulatory and mental conditions – were already increasing and the increase could be expected to continue.

Although it seemed certain that chronic illness and degenerative disease of old age would increase, Cathcart forecast that they would continue to be vastly outnumbered by the minor disorders which did not threaten life or lead to long-lasting disability but caused temporary disruption of employment or other normal activities and comfort. The Morbidity Statistics Scheme, initiated in 1930, had already brought to light the great volume of these disorders – 'common colds, influenza, catarrhal affections of the throat and nose, and tonsillitis, gastritis, the various manifestations of rheumatism, inflammations of skin and septic conditions, and by a vague and ill defined group of affections of the heart and nervous system into which a psycho-neurotic element enters or in which mental symptoms predominate.' Cathcart suggested that it was these complaints that would make up the chief burden to be taken on by a comprehensive medical service.

The Cathcart Committee's predictions of the changing pattern of disease were logical. They correctly forecast the general shape of the health problem that would be faced in the future. However, the best efforts of the Committee failed to provide sufficient warning of the sheer volume of sickness and disability that would suddenly confront the NHS in 1948. When the White Paper on the NHS was drawn up in 1944, the Cathcart Report was the most thorough and most up-to-date review available.[73] However, it failed to provide the depth of intelligence and analysis necessary for the rational planning of a comprehensive health service, even for Scotland. In part this was unavoidable; the necessary information on the incidence of disease and disability was not available. However, for reasons of polity, the Cathcart Committee avoided making a full declaration of the social conditions that lay behind the country's diseases and disabilities, even when the relevant information was available in the records of the Registrar General for Scotland and the Department of Health for Scotland. This was unfortunate for Scotland, and since no study comparable to the Cathcart Report had been attempted for England and Wales, it was also unfortunate for Britain. A few years later the planners of the NHS were working in the dark.

---

73 More limited surveys had been carried out in England, notably *The Social Survey of Merseyside in 1928* and the *New Survey of London Life and Labour* in 1933.

5

The Promotion of Health

In a new policy for health, the Cathcart Committee proposed that the state should no longer be essentially defensive, intervening only to protect the population by public health measures, and providing personal health services only as additional support for certain particularly vulnerable groups. The state was to adopt a more positive approach. Personal medical services would be made comprehensive in scope and available to all. But, while corrective and restorative services would continue to be essential and a responsibility of the state, they would play a secondary role in the state's positive campaign to promote health. The individual citizen was to be encouraged to take responsibility in promoting and maintaining his own health; the state's primary role was to attend to those factors which made a healthy life possible and which could be influenced positively by government action – heredity, nutrition, housing, the environment and education. In the 1930s each of these matters presented its own particular set of difficulties for the Cathcart Committee.

Heredity

In reviewing the health of the people of Scotland the Cathcart Committee had made no mention of heredity. But in considering the part the state might play in promoting the health of the people, in the 1930s it would have been quite impossible to neglect the disputed potential of eugenics. Eugenic programmes had been introduced in almost every country in Western Europe and North America except Britain, and many in Britain had come to believe that only eugenics could 'save the world.'[1]

In 1888, it had been feared that 'the great cities are the graves of our race.'[2] It seemed then that working-class families, in London and the other great cities, could survive beyond the third generation only with 'a steady influx of sound, energetic, physically strong recruits from the salubrious countryside.'[3] By 1903, even that mechanism for survival seemed to be failing. 'The people residing in urban districts already number four fifths of the population and the proportion is rising, while the country bred who in

1 C. W. Saleeby, *Parenthood and Race Cultures* (London, 1909), p. 182.
2 F. Farrar, *The Fortnightly Review*, 4 March 1888.
3 R. Soloway, *Demography and Degeneration* (North Carolina, 1990), p. 39.

the past recruited the weakened blood of the cities are either stationary or actually decreasing.'[4] In Parliament, Lord Meath set out the problem as it appeared at that time. The size of the population, then accepted as a sure measure of the strength of the nation, was clearly in decline; the decline was greater among the more prosperous and the better educated; the poor and less successful were reproducing at a greater rate than their betters; the poor, deteriorating in the urban conditions in which they lived, were passing on their acquired defects to their over-numerous offspring, producing a race of deteriorating quality.[5]

In the aftermath of the Boer War the quality of the people had become a cause of acute concern. The disappointing performance of the British forces had given rise to a drive for 'National Efficiency.'[6] Proclaimed by Lord Rosebery in his Rectorial Address at Glasgow University in 1900, National Efficiency was for a time an attractive and adaptable, even if very uncertain, ideology which grouped together all manner of projects intended to rescue the nation from decline. In most fields of national activity the drive for Efficiency soon died, but the promotion of National Efficiency by improving the quality of the people attracted much more lasting attention. The idea of eugenics had obvious attractions although its acceptability, morally and ethically, was uncertain. Nevertheless, for some influential enthusiasts, eugenics came to transcend politics, ethics or any other system for the improvement of the condition of man.[7]

Francis Galton had first introduced the concept of eugenics in his *Inheritance of Human Faculties* in 1883, several years before the emergence of the science of genetics. For centuries farmers and others had improved the quality of their stock artificially, and in a very few generations, by selective breeding. Galton proposed that the race of men could be similarly improved artificially by using two complementary approaches – by getting rid of the 'undesirables' and multiplying the 'desirables.'[8] However, any scheme, like that of the farmers, had to be based on the simple observation that like seems to breed like. Without a fuller understanding of the mechanisms of inheritance Galton's eugenics was no more than a hopeful idea.

In 1900 eugenics began to find a more secure scientific basis. Following his rediscovery of Mendel's studies of the inheritance of characteristics,

4 *Ibid.*
5 The Earl of Meath, *Hansard*, cxxiv, HC 6 July 1903, col. 1324.
6 P. Addison, 'Churchill and Social Reform', in R. Blake and W. R. Louis (eds.), *Churchill* (Oxford, 1996), p. 59.
7 Saleeby, *op. cit*, p. viii.
8 D. L. Kelves, 'From Eugenics to genetic Manipulation', in J. Krige and D. Pestre (eds.), *Science in the Twentieth Century* (Amsterdam, 1997), p. 301.

published in an obscure journal in 1865, Hugo de Vries developed a new Mendelian hypothesis of inheritance. This was taken up at Cambridge as the basis of a new academic discipline of genetics and, although understanding of inheritance was still at a primitive stage, its scientific basis uncertain and disputed, enthusiasm for eugenics increased.

However, even the most enthusiastic eugenists accepted that they could not run too far ahead of public opinion. This was a difficulty that had to be overcome by the 'education of the democracy' before legislation for eugenic measures could become a political possibility.[9] 'About two hundred people of influence'[10] came together to form the Eugenics Education Society (EES) to provide that education and to encourage public support. The EES was promoted by the Fabian Society, and many of those who were to become influential between the wars – including J.M. Keynes, Harold Laski, J.B.S Haldane, H.G. Wells, G.B. Shaw – became members. Eugenics gained wide support in the universities, especially among biologists and sociologists. (Many politicians were eugenists but, with Balfour as the only notable exception, they were reluctant to declare their position by joining the EES.) Eugenists looked to the potential of both positive and negative eugenics. Positive eugenics presented the attractive prospect of improving the race by promoting breeding from the best stock. The Fabian Society hoped to correct the differential birth rate by a system of family allowances for the more able sections of society ('Endowment of Motherhood'). More active programmes of selective breeding were clearly impossible; apart from the immediate practical and ethical difficulties, there was no clear definition of the desirable human qualities that should be encouraged. The promotion of negative eugenics was more feasible. While some of the same ethical and practical problems would have to be overcome, the undesirable qualities that a programme of negative genetics might eliminate were more easily identified. The attentions of the EES and eugenists therefore tended to focus principally on preventing the reproduction of the 'unfit' and particularly the mentally 'unfit.'

The eugenics lobby had a degree of success in influencing the Royal Commission into the Care and Control of the Feeble Minded in 1904. This investigation had been set up by Government in response to the concern of prison and poor law authorities about the rising cost of maintaining large numbers of the feeble-minded in custody. The Commission was persuaded by leading eugenists that feeble-mindedness was a hereditary condition and that the feeble-minded, as a class, had a fertility well above the average. The

9 A. F. Tredgold, 'Heredity and Environment in Regard to Social Reform', *Quarterly Review*, ccxix, 1913, p. 382.
10 Searle, *op. cit.*, p. 10.

Commission therefore recommended that the feeble-minded should be segregated, not only from the general community, partly in the interest of the majority and partly for their own protection, but also by sex to prevent their procreation. This proposal was endorsed by both the Majority and the Minority Poor Law Commissioners but no immediate effective Government action followed. The EES and other interested groups continued their pressure and a new Bill was drafted. Some sponsors of the Bill wished to make it an offence to marry a defective; others proposed to sterilise all defectives. The Mental Deficiency Act of 1913[11] was less radical. No provision was made for sterilisation but four groups were to be compulsorily institutionalised and segregated – idiots, imbeciles, the feeble-minded, and moral imbeciles.[12] These groups consisted mainly of defectives who had come to the attention of the authorities because they were already in prisons, lunatic asylums or workhouses, or had been picked up in the street without visible means of support, or as habitual drunkards. Those women in receipt of public relief during pregnancy or at the time of giving birth to an illegitimate child were also to be compulsorily institutionalised. This last group was to be particularly targeted since it was believed that the number of such feeble-minded young women was on the increase. The Government hoped to solve what was thought to be an increasing problem of lax morality and feeble-mindedness among women.

The Mental Deficiency Act came into effect in April 1914 but its implementation was inhibited by the First World War, and by the early 1920s little had been done to implement the Act of 1913.[13] The necessary institutions had not been built; parents had proved reluctant to agree to the certification of their children as mentally abnormal; doctors had been unwilling to certify patients against the wishes of their families. Even more important, social attitudes had changed and there was no longer general support for either the purpose or the provisions of the Act. Scientific opinion had also turned against eugenics 'because of the scientific shoddiness that coloured its theories of human heredity.' Eugenic science was also suspect 'for its racial and class bias' and for its disregard for the effects of social and cultural environment.[14]

However, Britain's fiscal difficulties began to revive the anxieties of those who had to find the cost of institutionalising the mentally defective and the criminal. In February 1929 the Minister of Health, Neville Chamberlain, received a petition, once again urging the sterilisation of criminals and

11 In Scotland the Mental Deficiency and Lunacy (Scotland) Act, 1913.
12 A classification that was ill-defined at that time and is now unrecognisable.
13 The membership of the EES had dispersed during the war and its provincial branches had been disbanded.
14 Kelves, *op. cit.*, p. 310.

mental defectives. Chamberlain set up a Joint Committee of the Board of Education and the Board of Control on Mental Deficiency to inquire 'into the possibility and advisability of legalising sterilisation under proper safeguards and in certain cases.'[15] The Joint Committee took account of experience in other countries. Since the early years of the century sterilisation laws had been passed in more than twenty American states and in Canada, Sweden and Switzerland. However, public opinion in most countries and states had remained effectively opposed to sterilisation on humanitarian grounds.[16] In America the laws had only been enforced on any considerable scale in two states. The results of the programme in California, where sterilisation legislation had been in operation since 1909, had been published and a review published in London in 1929.[17] The reports on the Californian programme claimed, in the light of their experience, that if mental defectives in the school system were sterilised, the number of mentally defective persons in the community could be reduced by as much as half in three or four generations.[18] From a smaller series in Switzerland it was reported that after castration a number of patients formerly unable to live in the community were able to go back to a normal social life.[19]

In the first part of its report the Joint Committee[20] concluded that if mental defectives in the current population were sterilised only after they had been certified, this would have little effect in reducing the incidence of mental deficiency in the next generation. The Joint Committee was persuaded that mental disease was a genetic as well as a social problem and that 'if we are to prevent the racial disaster of mental deficiency we must deal not merely with mentally defective persons but with the whole subgroup from which the majority of them come.'[21] In the second part of its report the Joint Committee looked at possible social benefits, suggesting that by sterilising some groups of certified mental defectives it would be possible to return them safely to the community, thus reducing the financial burden on the state of their maintenance in institutions.

The *BMJ* was horrified. Dismissing the American trials as biased and unscientific, it went on to state that if 'nothing short of the sterilisation of one-tenth of the whole population can be an effective preventive measure along such lines, the question whether systematic sterilisation should be

15 *BMJ*, i, 1929, p. 481.
16 *Lancet*, ii, 1929, p. 143.
17 E. S. Gosney and P. Popenoe, *Sterilisation for Human Betterment* (London, 1929).
18 *Ibid.*
19 *BMJ*, ii, 1929, p. 1070.
20 *Report of the Joint Committee of the Board of Education and the Board of Control on Mental Deficiency*, HMSO, 1929.
21 *BMJ*, ii, 1929, p. 108.

resorted to has only to be asked to be dismissed.' In a leading article the *BMJ* also dismissed as a crank W.M. Gallichan who, in a book published in 1929,[22] had claimed that 'the alarm now shown by an increasing number of responsible citizens in the United Kingdom lest the unfit may soon vastly out number the fit is almost of the nature of a panic.' The book was condemned as misleading and hysterical, 'illustrating the kind of propaganda to which the population is being subjected on the subject of sterilisation.' The *BMJ* was convinced that 'all compulsory measures are beyond practical possibility.' It conceded only that any measure that might result in the safe return to the community of a somewhat larger number of defectives than would otherwise be possible merited further investigation.

The *Lancet* was even more restrained. It published a summary of the report of the Joint Committee on Mental Deficiency without comment but later reviewed an article by K. B. Aikman in the *Edinburgh Review* in which the author attacked the doctrine of the equality of man and deplored the 'suicide of the middle classes.'[23] Dr Aikman argued that rather than attempting to influence the breeding of those few at the extremes – the frankly mentally defective and the 'highly superior' – much more would be gained by using economic inducements to increase the family size of the mass of people just above the mean and to reduce the numbers just below the mean. The *Lancet* claimed that economic measures had been tried before and had always failed. It also doubted that the necessary efficient 'selection of individual beneficiaries by bureaucrats' could be expected. The *Lancet* insisted that no measure should be introduced that might interfere with the liberty of the subject and drew attention to useful reforms that could be achieved easily and without reasonable objection. For example, there was no law in Britain requiring that persons discharged from mental hospitals should be warned that their weakness might be transmissible. The *Lancet* particularly deplored the common practice by which magistrates discharged mentally defective girls from asylums only on condition that they married.

In December 1933 the *BMJ*, still resolutely opposed to compulsory sterilisation, reprinted in full a lecture on 'Eugenics and the Doctor'[24] given by Lord Horder, not only a leading member of the medical profession in London, as has been described, but also a prominent eugenist.[25] Horder accepted that eugenics must 'seek only to operate by voluntary measures,

22 W. M. Gallichan, *Sterilisation of the Unfit* (London, 1929).
23 *Lancet*, ii, 1929, p. 142.
24 Lord Horder, '**Eugenics and the Doctor**'. Lecture to the Hampstead Hospital Postgraduate Session and published in December 1933. *BMJ*, ii, 1933, p.1057.
25 Lord Horder, physician to King George V and senior physician at St. Bartholomew's Hospital.

thus doing nothing by which the liberty of the individual may be in-fringed.'[26] However, he suggested that local authorities should be empow-ered to provide instruction on contraceptive methods for married women on economic and eugenic grounds, in addition to the gynaecological and medical grounds which were already allowed. Horder believed that birth control, as then practised, was acting dysgenically; while practised by the educated sections of society, it was not practised by the less well endowed 'from want of adequate knowledge.' Not only did this virtual 'veto put upon the spread of contraceptive methods' enhance differential fertility, it also encouraged the dangerous practice of abortion.

Horder believed that while compulsory sterilisation was legally en-forced in some countries, in Britain even voluntary sterilisation, sanc-tioned by the patient and his responsible relatives, was still an actionable offence. He recommended that in the case of mental defectives and mental convalescents voluntary sterilisation should be made legal as an alter-native to segregation. He accepted that there were difficulties to be overcome before such a scheme could be introduced. First there was the attitude of the public. For the great majority, 'either from sheer exigency, or from fundamental inability to think clearly, there is a dull acceptance of things as they are.' But there was a minority able 'to project the problem outside themselves.' Of these, one section believed that, as this was the best of all possible worlds, any attempt to exercise biological control over heredity was meddlesome interference. Another section he believed to be persuaded principally by their religious beliefs in actively opposing all eugenic measures; this section of the population was en-couraged by the church to regard the arrival of each new individual as a direct act of providence. He quoted the Bishop of Exeter – 'If the Lambeth conference should approve birth control then there will be a new breach in the growing unity of Christendom.'

Lord Horder urged that the public should be persuaded to think of their responsibility to future generations. Voluntary schemes of eugenics were clearly necessary, but impossible until the public was convinced of their benefits and their morality. It would also be essential for the medical profession to be better informed[27] since the informed general practitioner would be vital, 'for without him this newest and most hopeful of the humane sciences must inevitably stand still.'

As a result of the country's financial problems in the 1930s, there was further pressure from the local authorities. The segregation required by the existing legislation was proving difficult; the number of institutional beds in

26 *BMJ*, ii, 1929, p. 1058.
27 Genetics was not taught formally at any British medical school at that time.

place was far short of the estimated requirement. In June 1932, following a deputation from the County Councils Association, the Association of Municipal Corporations and the Mental Hospitals Association, the government appointed a Departmental Committee under the chairmanship of Sir Lawrence Brock, the Chairman of the Board of Control:

> To examine and report on the information already available regarding the hereditary transmission and other causes of mental disorder and deficiency; to consider the value of sterilisation as a preventive measure having regard to its physical, psychological and social effects and to the legislation in other countries permitting it; and to suggest what further inquiries might usefully be undertaken in this connexion.[28]

By 1932 the science of genetics had moved on. Biologists had come to see that biometrics and the Mendelian genetics were entirely compatible. The differences that had caused acrimonious disputes at the beginning of the century were finally resolved by the publication of *The Genetic Theory of Natural Selection* by R. A. Fisher in 1930. By then even the initially sceptical T. H. Morgan and his group at Columbia University in New York had not only accepted the Mendelian model and the existence of discrete genes, but had gone on to demonstrate that genes, the messengers of inheritance, were carried in chromosomes lying in pairs in most cells and singly in the germ cells. The scientific community had come to some elementary understanding of the mechanisms of inheritance. After almost two years of deliberation the Departmental Committee (Brock Committee), of which R. A. Fisher was a member, completely rejected compulsory sterilisation. The Committee was unimpressed by experience in other countries. The practice in Denmark, where compulsory sterilisation was included in the penal code, was particularly deprecated. In California the scheme seemed to have been pointless; over 16,000 sterilisations had been carried out but only one in five had been on mental defectives. Elsewhere in the United States, 27 schemes had not been followed through, partly from lack of resources but mainly because of 'a lack of support for laws promoted by groups of enthusiasts not backed by public opinion',[29] and the schemes had not resulted in the discharge of any significant numbers of patients from institutions. In Switzerland, where the laws had been interpreted very liberally, many operations had been carried out, but as there had been no follow-up studies it was impossible to draw any useful conclusions. Quite

---

28 *Report of the Departmental Committee on Sterilisation*, Cmd. 4485, 1933/34; reported in *BMJ*, i, 1934, p. 161.
29 *Report of the Departmental Committee on Sterilisation*, op.cit.

apart from the discouraging experience in other countries, the Brock Committee found that their chief objection to compulsory sterilisation was the uncertainty of diagnosis. The part played by heredity in causing mental deficiency was also uncertain; only two causes of mental deficiency – mongolism and amaurotic family idiocy – could be accurately diagnosed and were known with certainty to be genetically transmitted.

The Brock Committee concluded that 'if the test is to be the certainty with which the results of procreation can be predicted in individual cases, the case for compulsion cannot be established.' However, it did consider that there might be a case for voluntary sterilisation for:

a) A person who is mentally defective or who suffers from mental disorder.

b) A person who suffers from or is believed to be a carrier of a gross physical disability which has been shown to be transmissible.

c) A person who is believed to be likely to transmit mental disorder or defect.

But these suggestions were made in principle only. The Committee believed that it was possible that the incidence of mental defects was indeed rising, but clearly it was not rising at a rapid rate; there could be no case for immediate legislation. Research on a number of key questions would be required before any programme of sterilisation could be carried out with any degree of confidence. The Government, less influenced by the lack of research than by the uncertainty of public opinion, agreed. In the Commons the Parliamentary Secretary to the Minister of Health said: 'I wish an occasion would arise when birth control and the sterilisation of the unfit were more ventilated. We want guidance of public opinion on the sterilisation of the unfit.'[30]

Meanwhile the Government remained cautious, even on birth control. The policy of the Ministry of Health would continue to be 'that it is wrong for a maternity and child welfare centre or a clinic paid for out of public funds to be used for giving contraception advice except where further pregnancy would be injurious to health.'

In 1936, the Cathcart Committee was therefore under no pressure to differ from Government policy. The studies recommended by the Brock Committee were still to be carried out and in Scotland eugenics and birth control were not, at that time, matters of public debate. The subject did not occupy the press. The Church of Scotland, in its various committees and at

30 *Hansard*, ccciv, HC 17 July 1935, col. 1171.

its General Assembly (a useful indicator of public opinion), discussed all the social problems of importance in the 1930s – unemployment, poverty, housing, immigration, emigration, malnutrition, physical and metal health – but the issues of eugenics and the sterilisation of the unfit were not raised.[31] The Cathcart Committee was content to accept the recommendations of the Departmental Committee on Sterilisation, and eugenics did not feature in its health programme for Scotland.

Nutrition

In 1936 the Cathcart Committee reported that even after years of industrial depression there was no evidence of widespread malnutrition in Scotland.[32] This echoed the Ministry of Health Report in 1933 that claimed that in England and Wales, 'though specially sought for, of evidence of widespread malnutrition there is none.'[33] However, the Cathcart Committee carefully included the *caveat* that 'the fact that there is no evidence of widespread and gross malnutrition does not imply that there may not be a considerable amount of under or wrong feeding that does not manifest itself in specific disease or in other recognisable ways.' 'It is impossible to put on record . . . the state of nutrition at one examination.' This was one of the questions facing the Cathcart Committee in attempting to secure the proper nutrition of the people of Scotland; how was proper nutrition to be assessed? The second question was whether a family's failure to secure an adequate diet was due to poverty or to ignorance.

In England and Wales, in 1933, the BMA had appointed a Committee to determine 'the weekly minimum expenditure on foodstuffs which must be incurred by families of varying sizes if health and working capacity are to be maintained, and to construct specimen diets.'[34] For the purpose of the survey, it was assumed that a family apparently healthy, working and functioning normally must be consuming a normal and healthy diet. As expected, there were regional variations both in the cost of food and in dietary preferences but the Committee concluded that 'the minimum cost of feeding the average adult male a reasonably varied diet sufficient to maintain health and working capacity was 5s 11d. per week.' The BMA calculated that for a family of five this minimum diet would cost 23s 2d. Theoretically for such a family on benefit this would leave only 6s 1d for all other needs. On the basis that such an allocation of financial resources was

31 *Reports to the General Assembly of the Church of Scotland.*
32 Cathcart Report, p. 95.
33 *Annual Report of the Chief Medical Officer*, 1932, p. 41.
34 P. Bartrip, *Themselves Writ Large; the British Medical Association 1832–1966* (London, 1996), p. 203.

impossible it was calculated that the diets of some eight million people in the United Kingdom must necessarily fail to reach the BMA's recommended minimum.[35] The BMA published these findings as a pamphlet which sold thousands of copies within a few days. There was considerable coverage in the press and the BBC made the BMA's statement the subject of a radio programme. Under this increasing pressure, in 1935 the Minister of Health appointed a special Advisory Committee

> . . . to inquire into the facts, quantitative and qualitative, in relation to the diet of the people, and to report as to any changes therein which appear desirable in the light of modern advances in the knowledge of nutrition.

In Scotland the problems of inadequate diet had been studied since the beginning of the century and different methods of investigation had been developed. By 1900 it was already clear that children were growing up smaller than their grandparents, and it was widely accepted that this was a consequence of poverty and urbanisation.[36] In Edinburgh, which suffered less from the effects of industrial urbanisation than many other communities in Scotland, it was observed that:

> Everyone who is accustomed to pass through the slums of our city must have been struck by the large proportion of puny children and of poorly-developed, undersized adults, and the question doubtless presents itself: 'How far are these conditions due to insufficient food supply and how far to general unhygienic surroundings.'[37]

These were the opening sentences of a study of the diet of the poor of Edinburgh by Noel Paton and his colleagues in 1901. At the time vitamins were unknown and the importance of these and other essential elements in the diet had yet to be recognised. Scientific assessment of the diet was limited to the measurement of its caloric value. Although the authors of the study had no knowledge of vitamins or the importance of minerals, in general terms they recognised the relationship between the content and quality of the diet and morbidity.[38] Even in the light of the limited knowledge of nutrition at that time, the quality of the diet of the poorest sections of Scottish society was unsatisfactory. The diet histories taken for the survey showed an over-dependence on potatoes, bread and jam and an

35 *BMJ*, ii, 1933, p. 1098.
36 A. H. Kitchin and R. Passmore, *The Scotsman's Food* (Edinburgh, 1949), p. 52.
37 D. Noel Paton, J. Dunlop and E. Inglis, *A Study of the Diet of the Labouring Classes in Edinburgh* (Edinburgh, 1901), p. 1.
38 All physicians at this time included advice on diet when prescribing for their patients.

almost total lack of fresh food and uncooked vegetables. Noel Paton did not attribute the poor quality of the diet directly to the prohibitive cost of a better one but believed that the poor quality could be overcome by better education and training.[39] Nevertheless, he found that in 1900 nutrition was a major problem in Scotland. After investigation of diets in England, Germany, Sweden, Russia and America, Paton found that, even in caloric value, 'the food supply of our poorer working classes compares unfavourably ... with the diets of inmates of poor houses, prisons and pauper lunatic asylums, with the single exception of the diet allowed to the working inmates of the Scottish poor houses.'[40]

Conditions for the working classes in Scotland eased to some extent in the years before the First World War. The shipbuilding, engineering and steelmaking industries prospered. Employment also increased in mining and the service industries from 1914. But in Scotland wages continued at least 10% lower than in England while food and fuel prices were higher in Scotland than elsewhere in Britain.[41] The working class in Scotland was therefore at a disadvantage when dietary habits in the more prosperous part of the United Kingdom began to benefit from the revolution in food production at the end of the nineteenth century and from the marketing skills of the new multiple grocers. In Scotland the typical diet of much of the working class continued to be made up of white bread, margarine, tea, sugar, jam, and sausages often of poor quality.[42]

Wheat was plentiful and imported at low cost from North America; the introduction of roller milling[43] and improved food technology in Britain contributed to the reduction in cost. Bread could now be made as white as fashion demanded without adulteration with alum or copper sulphate. But in the new processes of milling, the wheat germ was removed from the flour and along with it all the minerals, vitamins and much of the protein. The bread on which the poor depended so heavily had become cheaper but of less nutritional value.[44] Margarine had been produced in quantity in Britain from 1889. It had originally made from beef fat, but by the end of the century beef fat had been replaced by vegetable oils. While the new margarine looked better and tasted somewhat better, the vitamins of beef fat margarine were almost completely absent from new vegetable-oil

39 Cookery and household management had been introduced as 'domestic science' into the Scottish school curriculum in 1897.
40 Paton *et al, op. cit.*
41 O. Checkland and S. Checkland, *Industry and Ethos: Scotland 1832–1914* (Edinburgh, 1989), p. 175.
42 Kitchin and Passmore, *op. cit.*, p. 37.
43 The first roller miller in the UK was set up in Glasgow about 1872.
44 The price of a 4lb loaf in 1832 was $10\frac{1}{2}$ d. In 1913 it was $5\frac{3}{4}$ d.

margarine produced by Van den Burgh. Meat became more affordable in Britain with the introduction of refrigerated ships after 1880; cheap beef was imported from Argentina, lamb from New Zealand and pork from America; meat became affordable, at least on occasion, for most people. But for the poor, meat could only be bought in its cheapest forms, as sausages or mince – both open to adulteration and 'expansion' to increase profit margins. Carbohydrate made up a large part of the diet. From about 1900 mechanisation, and the better understanding of the biochemistry of the processes involved, had made jam-making into a large and profitable industry. Manufacturers were able to take advantage of the surplus production of the English fruit growers, and sales of jam became enormous, especially in the industrial areas where a sweet, highly flavoured spread was cheaper than butter and made margarine more palatable. The poor could also usually afford tea; for much of the nineteenth century tea had been an expensive luxury often adulterated by the addition of leaves from British hedges. The introduction of lead-lined packets reduced the risk of adulteration but tea remained expensive until its marketing was taken up by the new multiple grocers. Lipton began trading tea in Glasgow in 1889, cutting the prevailing price of 2s 6d to 1s 7d.[45] The poor could buy even cheaper brands at Co-operative Stores, and with tea went sugar. For the poor, sugar in its various forms provided calories and some comfort but it was of little nutritional worth.

The constituents of the less than ideal diet in Scotland – white bread, margarine, tea, sugar, jam and sausages – were not only what was cheap; they were also what was made available. Much of the food of Scotland's working class was bought at Co-operative Stores. There were 130 Co-operative Societies in Scotland, mostly in weaving and mining communities, when the Scottish Co-operative Wholesale Society (SCWS) was founded in Glasgow in 1860.[46] By 1914 the SCWS had 16 factories and 4000 employees and had become Scotland's largest food wholesaler. Retail societies, concentrated in the central belt, had a membership 470,000.[47] Customers looked to these stores for low prices (cash only) and the additional benefit of the 'dividend' which could be as much as 2s 6d in the pound and for many families was the only method of saving for major purchases of any kind. The Co-operative Stores acquired a virtual monopoly in the sale of provisions to the poorer sections of society and greatly influenced the shopping habits of working-class families. Unfortunately, their sales of fish, fruit and green

45 J. Burnett, *Plenty and Want: A Social History of Diet in England from 1815 to the Present Day* (London, 1966), p. 107.
46 J. Kinloch and J. Butt, *History of the Scottish Co-operative Wholesale Society Ltd* (Manchester, 1981).
47 T. Johnston, *The History of the Scottish Working Classes* (Glasgow, 1929), p. 386.

vegetables were 'negligible.' The Co-operatives supplied food cheaply but did little to encourage good dietary habits.[48]

The First World War brought opportunities for improvement in the nutrition of the working classes throughout the United Kingdom.[49] A Food Department at the Board of Trade was created in August 1916 and the Ministry of Food four months later. Rationing and direction of food supply were introduced from 1 January 1918. Full employment meant that the working population was able to afford all the food allowed by rationing.[50]

In *The Great War and the British People*,[51] Winter has claimed, not only that by the end of the War the people had healthier diets than ever before, but that the wartime diet had provided the poorer section of the population with reserves that allowed them to withstand the deprivations of the Depression. This interpretation is in line with the reassurances given by the Ministry of Health in 1932 but was disputed at the time[52] and has been disputed by historians since.[53]

Whether or not there was real hunger in the 1930s is an English question. In Scotland, there was never any doubt. The evidence of subnutrition[54] was as obvious in the 1930s as it had been to Noel Paton in 1901. (John Maclean famously said that if people could not afford the food they needed, they should take it. He was jailed for sedition.) The Ministry of Food had been abolished in 1921. The many wartime government-funded organisations throughout the country, including the canteens that had ensured that workers were properly fed, no longer operated. Unemployment had increased from 2% in 1913 to over 15% throughout the 1920s. Although the collapse of agricultural prices after 1921 had lowered the cost of food, the families of the unemployed or those on short-time working were unable to afford an adequate diet.[55] Almost as its last act the Ministry of Food doubled the price of milk. In the poorer areas of Glasgow milk consumption fell by a third in spite of a surplus of

48 As the Co-operative movement was closely associated with the temperance lobby, no alcohol was sold in the stores.
49 J. Burnett, 'A Context for Boyd Orr: Glasgow Corporation and the Food of the Poor, 1918–1924', unpublished paper delivered at the International Committee for Research into European Food History, Aberdeen, September, 1997.
50 Burnett, 1966, *op. cit*, p. 218.
51 J. M. Winter, *The Great War and the British People* (London, 1986).
52 H. Pollitt, in A. Hutt, *The Condition of the Working Class* (London, 1933), p. xii.
53 C. Webster, 'Health, Welfare and Unemployment During the Depression', *Past and Present*, cix, 1985, p. 205.
54 Subnutrition is distinguished from clinical malnutrition with manifest deficiency disease. 'The signs of under-nourishment in children take time to develop and are not always easily recognised though they leave scars in the constitution that last for life.' Edwin Muir, *Scottish Journey* (Edinburgh, 1935), p. 135.
55 J. Burnett, 1967, *op. cit.*

milk in the city.[56] It was reported that 'the very poor here never use milk as they should, but give the infants tea with toast soaked in it.' Porridge made with milk and milk puddings were given up. Nursing mothers continued to breast-feed for as long as possible. While the great influenza epidemic was raging, the Independent Labour Party campaigned under banners reading '1914 – Fighting; 1920 – Starving.'[57] In Glasgow, while the typical artisan living in a room and kitchen, a member of a trade union and a provident society, and with some savings, could finance an adequate diet for his family, the very poor were close to famine. A study of the families of the unemployed and those on short working showed that over a period of two years from 1920 the caloric intake of the men had fallen from 2500 calories to 2200 calories and the weight of boys and girls had fallen by 7.5% and 7% respectively.[58] In 1920, A. K. Chalmers, the Medical Officer of Health for Glasgow, made it clear that poverty and the lack of proper food was already leading to ill-health.[59] In 1921 the miners' strike made matters worse. The Scottish Board of Health reported:

> The stoppage in the coal-mining industry in the spring of 1921 was responsible for great destitution in the areas affected, and the local authorities of these areas found themselves faced with the necessity of exercising their powers on a scale that had never been contemplated. Emergency arrangements for supplying food to mothers and children were rapidly made with our full concurrence.[60]

In 1920 Noel Paton still argued in the *Glasgow Medical Journal*[61] that the main problem was not poverty itself but the fecklessness of the poor. But evidence to the contrary was growing stronger. In 1923 the Scottish Board of Health, in reporting that death rates of children were higher than in England, attributed the difference in part to climate and housing conditions but also to poor feeding.[62] In 1926 the Empire Marketing Board made a grant to John Boyd Orr at the Rowett Institute to demonstrate the nutritive value of milk.[63] A committee was formed, under the chairmanship of Sir

56 Webster, 'Health, welfare and Unemployment During the Depression', *op.cit.*
57 G. Aldred, *John Maclean* (Glasgow, 1940), p. 47.
58 A. Tully, 'A Study of the Diet and Economic Conditions of Artisan Families in Glasgow', *Glasgow Medical Journal*, ci, 1924, p. 1.
59 A. K. Chalmers, 'A Complete Health Service'. Unpublished lecture given in 1920, quoted by Burnet, *op. cit.*
60 *Annual Report of the Scottish Board of Health*, Cmd. 1697, 1921, p. 47.
61 D. M. Paton, 'Physiology: The Institutes of Medicine', *Glasgow Medical Journal*, xii, 1920, p. 321.
62 *Annual Report of the Scottish Board of Health*, Cmd. 2156, 1923, p. 50.
63 J. Boyd Orr, *As I Recall* (London, 1966), p. 110.

Leslie Mackenzie, to supervise the scheme for the Scottish Board of Health.[64]

This was a clinical trial in which, as in all Boyd Orr's investigations, sound nutrition was defined as 'the state of well-being such that no improvement can be effected by change in the diet.'[65] The results of the trial demonstrated that the children who were given free milk 'showed a marked improvement, in weight and height, and by better general condition.'[66,67] The Ministry of Health was sceptical, claiming that the benefit to the children came from the supervision and general regulation of their lives during the period of the trial and not from the nutritional supplement. However, in 1931, Tom Johnston, the Under-Secretary for Scotland in the Labour Government, arranged for a further trial in Lanarkshire to meet this objection.[68] On the evidence of these trials, Walter Elliot, the Conservative Minister of Agriculture in the National Government, successfully introduced a Bill in 1934 to allow local authorities in Scotland to provide cheap milk for all schoolchildren.

In 1934 the Rowett Institute received a grant from the Carnegie Trust 'to estimate the diets of different classes, including the whole population, according to family income.'[69] The survey was promoted by Walter Elliot, supported by the Agricultural Board and the Linlithgow Committee on the Import of Food[70] and carried out by John Boyd Orr[71] in centres in England as well as Scotland. The survey showed that, by Boyd Orr's standard, an adequate level of nutrition was not being reached by families in which the income per week was less than 20s – families that made up 47.1% of the population of Scotland. 'Complete adequacy' was 'almost reached' by the families – 25.3% of the population – with a weekly income between 20s and 30s. For more affluent families 'the diet has a surplus of all the constituents considered.'

This report was rejected by Kingsley Wood, the Minister of Health, who continued to insist that such defective nutrition as existed could not be attributed to poverty since poverty had been effectively abolished by the existing state welfare schemes. Official support was withdrawn from the Rowett Institute. It was even suggested that the medical members of the

64 *Ibid.*, p. 114.
65 Boyd Orr, '*Food, Health and Income*,' (London, 1937), p. 11.
66 *Lancet*, i, 1929, p. 41
67 *BMJ*, i, 1929, p. 23.
68 Boyd Orr, *As I Recall, op. cit.*
69 Boyd Orr, *Food, Health and Income, op. cit.*
70 Boyd Orr, *As I Recall, op. cit.*, p. 115.
71 Professor Cathcart collaborated in this trial. J. Brotherston, 'The Development of Public Medical Care', in G. McLachlan (ed.), *Improving the Common Weal*, Edinburgh, 1987), p. 82.

research team might be reported to the General Medical Council and removed from the Medical Register for unethical conduct in publishing work that had been unfairly represented for political ends. Because of this threat, co-authors withdrew and the results were issued under Boyd Orr's name alone and published by Harold Macmillan, not only chairman of Macmillan and Company but also MP for Stockton who was greatly concerned about the plight of the poor in his own constituency. *Food, Health and Income* went through three editions and attracted international interest.

Although rejected by the Ministry of Health, Boyd Orr's findings were accepted by the Department of Health for Scotland[72] and by the Cathcart Committee. However, the Committee's comments on the nutritional problems in Scotland were careful and non-committal. There remained the 'major issue of controversy on this subject of nutrition' – whether improvement was to be brought about 'by economic changes or by education.'[73] The Cathcart Committee 'was of the opinion that one of the most valuable means of making good the deficiencies of home feeding was the provision of free or cheap milk and meals to school children.' But at the same time the Committee claimed that 'there is abundant room for practical education of the people on the purchase and preparation of food.'

The Cathcart Committee did not set out a plan to overcome the acknowledged deficiencies in the diet of the mass of the people in Scotland. It decided that it should be left to the Advisory Committee on Nutrition, of which Professor Cathcart was a member, to decide whether 'any considerable departure from national health policy would be justified.'

In this as in other matters, the Cathcart Committee wished to avoid unnecessary conflict with central government in devising what was intended as a policy for the whole of Britain. The Report did emphasise that 'an adequate supply of food in the form of a well-balanced mixed diet is the most important single factor in the maintenance of health', and by including a section on nutrition in its Report the Cathcart Committee ensured that, in future, problems of nutrition would be kept under review and would feature in all subsequent reviews of health and health policy. However, it is undeniable that the Cathcart Report missed the opportunity to draw attention to the particular and persisting problems in Scotland. Poverty, high food prices, hidebound marketing practices, long-established habits and housing with inadequate equipment and services for the preparation of meals[74] were all factors which continued to prejudice the diet of the

72 *Annual Report of the Department of Health for Scotland*, 1937, Cmd. 5713, p. 52.
73 Cathcart Report, p. 97.
74 Domestic services such a kitchen stoves and sinks were not fully surveyed until the census of 1951.

majority of the Scottish people in 1936 and for many years after the introduction of the National Health Service.

Health Education

It was central to Cathcart's plan for the future that every member of society should be able to play a full part in maintaining his or her own health. In the 1930s it was

> ... generally agreed that public ignorance regarding matters of health, especially in regard to dietetics, child welfare and nursing, is a serious obstacle to the efficient functioning of the medical services.[75]

Cathcart believed that considerable improvement in public understanding of health had already been achieved. The sanitary measures introduced in the previous century had created a much more enlightened 'outlook' among the people:

> The introduction of a public water supply may have effects on the population concerned far beyond its results in an adequate provision for the purposes of drinking and personal cleanliness. In such matters it is not possible to become accustomed to decency in one aspect of life without attaining to a wider sense of personal and communal responsibility.

The Cathcart Committee was confident that over the previous hundred years 'the habits and outlook of the people' had been changed by their experience of improved sanitation and their increasing familiarity with a higher standard of living, supplemented by practical guidance from the better-informed – including doctors, welfare services, voluntary organisations ('boy scouts, girl guides, youth hostels and folk dancing'). The effect of this experience and the example had been cumulative. Cathcart now recommended that health education should continue on the same principles. There was still a frustrating gap between what was known and what was practised – in nutrition, dress, recreation, the management of the home and the parental care of children.

In 1911 the National Insurance Act had empowered Insurance Committees to spend money on health education; a few of these bodies had organised public lectures and issued pamphlets to the public but the majority had not. In England in 1927, the Society of Medical Officers of Health, funded by a number of voluntary bodies and by local authorities, set

---

75 Evidence to the Cathcart Committee by the Scottish Branch of the Society of Medical Officers of Health (Scottish Branch).

up the Central Council for Health Education. Its aims were to promote research in the 'science and art of healthy living' and to promote the prevention and cure of disease by 'health education and propaganda.'[76] The Central Council organised health weeks and propaganda campaigns in England but most doctors and teachers remained unconvinced that they served any useful purpose. In 1927 the British Broadcasting Corporation made a brief contribution to health education. A series of lectures on 'Health in the Home' was broadcast in March and April and published, first in the *Listener* and later as a pamphlet.[77]

Cathcart rejected these methods:

Health education is frequently taken to mean propaganda by lecture, leaflets and the like. These methods have their place, but, at present, they seldom reach the section of the population that has the most need of instruction . . . Unless they fit into a larger scheme, they may do harm. Health propaganda tends frequently to concentrate on disease rather than on health. While propaganda against particular diseases (e.g. venereal diseases and tuberculosis) has achieved excellent results, it may have had the effect of creating unnecessary fears.

Cathcart stressed that health education should not be prescriptive but should aim at stressing the advantages of healthy living. 'Health is not a negative state, it involves more than the mere absence of disease . . . It is obvious that there are many people who, despite the absence of any signs of disease, nevertheless fail to reach a satisfactory standard of health and usefulness or to enjoy the sense of well being that might be reasonably expected.' In its evidence to the Cathcart Committee, the Scottish Committee of the BMA also stressed the importance of this sense of wellbeing. It drew particular attention to the part that education could play in meeting the new problems of leisure, not only the increased leisure which came with the reduction in the working week to 48 hours, but 'especially when leisure is enforced by lack of employment and carries with it the special strains caused by economic anxiety:'

Leisure is an evil for those who have no capacity for using it, and though the questions relating to leisure are not entirely medical, the doctor best knows the evil influence upon health, especially mental health, of the excess of leisure in unemployment and also the lack of tastes that make leisure healthful.

Cathcart proposed that the leisure time of young people could best be taken up in athletic and other physical activities. For older adults the educational

76 I. Sutherland (ed.), *Health Education* (London, 1979), p. 3.
77 M. C. Green, *Health in the Home* (London, 1927).

system should provide instruction in handicrafts and gardening. Since these activities would not usually fill all leisure time, the educational system should also foster the taste for new interests – literary, musical, dramatic and artistic. Cathcart suggested that it was the lack of such cultural interests that, in the past, had 'favoured the more anti-social alleviation of leisure – intoxication and methods of extraneous stimulation.'

The Cathcart Committee recommended that, while both general practitioners and the Department of Health clearly had some part to play, there was general agreement that the overall responsibility for health education should lie with the Department of Education and instruction on health related subjects should be included in the school curriculum. It set out a very detailed scheme. It was particularly important that the school environment should be improved and more facilities should be provided for exercise, sport and the development of ideas and skills that might later be useful for adult leisure. As organised games provided a valuable form of physical and social training, they should be compulsory. In schools where children did not go home at midday a hot meal should be provided 'in seemly and comfortable conditions.' For children who lived at some distance from school there should be a properly staffed and equipped hostel.

Instruction on healthy living should begin in infancy with informal day-to-day guidance to develop good healthy habits. Until the age of 12 'formal health lesson are unnecessary; the lessons should be incidental to other school subjects.' After the age of 12, incorporated in the teaching of biology there should be systematic instruction to provide 'a sufficient knowledge of the working of the human body to enable them to realise the value of health.'[78] In the senior classes every girl was to be given 'some practical instruction in plain household cookery, food values and economic buying' and, since in the interval between school and marriage many would have forgotten what they had been taught, local authorities should provide courses for women on cookery and in baby and child management.

The Cathcart Committee proposed that health education should be continued into adult life as a joint responsibility of the Department of Health, the Department of Education and the Local Authorities. Valuable work was already being done in health education in Scotland through a number of special agencies, such as the National Association for the Prevention of Tuberculosis. In England the work of all such organisations was co-ordinated by the Central Council for Health Education; a similar body was proposed for Scotland.

The Committee also recommended that the teacher training colleges and Scottish universities should play their part. Teacher training should be

78 Ibid.

revised to include more instruction in biology, physiology and hygiene and more opportunity for the practice of physical education and hygiene. At the universities, every student should be medically examined on entry and should be expected to take part in some form of physical training as a normal part of the curriculum. 'We consider this necessary for the proper mental and physical development of all students, who in after life may become leaders in the community.'

The Cathcart Committee had in mind that health education should have more ambitious objectives than the correction of the 'ignorance and fecklessness' of the poor:

> The aim of health education should be to train each individual to adopt such a way of living as will enable him to derive full enjoyment from the exercise of his faculties not solely for his own benefit, but also for the benefit of the community. There is an essential unity of life, and the physical should be interpreted in association with the intellectual and emotional; but the physical aspect is fundamental.

Health education was to be a cornerstone of the health policy advocated by the Cathcart Committee. The ideas behind Cathcart's proposals were not new. There were distinct echoes of Juvenal – *orandum eat ut sit mens sana in corpore sano*. Cathcart's originality was in attempting to bring health education to the forefront of national health policy and to contend that the necessary education should be by precept and practice and not by exhortation and propaganda.

In the 1930s Cathcart's proposals were not well received. It has been claimed that Whitehall found the emphasis on physical activities and training in Cathcart's scheme too close to the fascist methods then practised in Germany and therefore inappropriate for Britain.[79] Government preferred to rely on exhortation and propaganda. In 1937 Neville Chamberlain, recently Minister of Health and now Prime Minister, launched the first national health education campaign. This was carried out by the distribution of leaflets, by posters and by lectures, exhibitions and film shows.

The Environment

The Cathcart Committee was satisfied that, since the middle years of the nineteenth century, great improvements had been made in the general sanitary condition in Scotland. As public health arrangements had been reviewed by the Department of Health for Scotland in 1929, the Cathcart

---

79 M. Grant, 'The National Health Campaigns of 1937–8', in D. Fraser (ed.), *Cities, Class and Communication: Essays in Honour of Asa Briggs* (London, 1990), p. 217.

Committee considered it 'unnecessary to attempt anything approaching a sanitary survey of Scotland.' During the years of financial stringency since 1929, improvements had continued with support from the Unemployment Grants Committee.

The aim of the reforms proposed by Cathcart was to remove, as far as possible, the sources of friction between local authorities. The burghs and county councils were to remain the responsible authorities but their areas of responsibility were to be more clearly defined. The Special Districts for drainage and water supply that had been set up since 1889 to serve ill-defined rural areas, usually centred on large villages, were to be abolished. Central supervision by the Department of Health was to be increased, to control levels of expenditure, to promote co-operation between local authorities and to ensure a more even provision of services across the country.

The Committee recommended that greater attention should be given to atmospheric pollution. New legislation on smoke abatement was needed, applicable to counties as well as burghs. Cathcart also drew attention to a new problem. Since the war, the building of electricity power stations had resulted in the release of great quantities of sulphur gases that must be assumed to be harmful to health.

Housing

Scotland's housing was a longstanding problem and recognised as a major cause of illness and poor health. In the nineteenth century the state had accepted some responsibility for the elimination of unfit dwellings but had done little to ensure that the poorer members of society would be properly housed. From the First World War, a new housing policy had emerged and the Cathcart Committee was confident that the housing programmes already in place by the 1930s were already raising the standard of living of a large part of the population and making a substantial contribution to their wellbeing. Cathcart made no new proposals but the 'magnitude of the problem' that remained in Scotland had to be kept in mind.

Although, in the first years of the century, Government had been principally concerned with the removal of pestilential slums and the improvement of sanitation, the Housing and Town Planning Act of 1909 had given local authorities optional powers to set down plans for new developments, to design street layouts, to restrict building densities and to acquire and set aside land for development. However, the construction of new houses was left almost entirely in the hands of private enterprise. The Act placed some obligation on local authorities to provide houses for those displaced in the destruction of slums but most local authorities were dilatory and few development schemes were submitted for Government approval before the First World War. In 1914 a memorandum of the Local Government Board for Scotland recognised that there was not only an increasing need for more houses but also that the existing slum clearance programmes would fail 'unless there is other proper accommodation for the persons displaced.'[80] The local authorities in Scotland had again failed to respond.[81]

The issue was forced by the military requirements of the war. Houses were required for the large number of munitions workers and other civilians needed for war work. At Rosyth, the Admiralty sponsored a public utility society, the National Housing Company, to house 'in a manner that shall secure to the future community, at reasonable rentals, a model standard of health and comfort.'[82] This wartime initiative proved to be a watershed. Local authorities now showed how quickly houses could be built and the high standards that could be achieved. The shift towards local authority housing received further impetus in 1915. In response to the serious and potentially dangerous unrest in Glasgow provoked by wartime inflation in rents, the Increase of Rent and Mortgage Interest Act limited rents to the levels which had prevailed at the outbreak of the war. Rent control continued after the war[83] and proved to be an effective disincentive to private-sector house building. The building of houses for the working class in Scotland became almost exclusively the province of the state.

In July 1917 a committee, established jointly by the President of the Board of Trade and the Secretary for Scotland, laid down levels of construction and design that became the accepted standards between the wars. From 1917 Lloyd George's government also addressed the problems of working-class housing. The Ministry of Reconstruction planned that, after the war, a housing drive would be organised and funded by the state. The Ministry favoured direct action by central Government, but the Treasury insisted that local authorities should be responsible, supported by Treasury funds only when the need could be proved. The Treasury view prevailed; thereafter the building of working-class housing of a national standard became the responsibility of local government. A Royal Commission in 1917 showed how much had to be done.[84] There were too few houses and much of the stock was of very

---

80 T. Begg, *Housing Policy in Scotland* (Edinburgh, 1996), p. 15.
81 In 1914 Dundee refused to re-house those displaced by the clearing of Greenmarket and Overgate.
82 Begg, *op. cit.*, p. 16.
83 Rent control was first partially removed in 1957.
84 Royal Commission on the Housing of the Industrial Population of Scotland, Rural and Urban.

poor quality and too small – 53.2% of Scotland's houses were of only one or two rooms.

The House and Town Planning (Scotland) Act of 1919 required local authorities to review their housing stock and to submit schemes for housing the working class. In addition to borrowing, local authorities were given permission to raise rates (by four-fifths of a penny). The difference between the expected income from rates and rents and the cost of borrowing was to be borne by the Treasury.

Progress was slow. Then in 1921 the financial climate changed for the worse. The Chancellor feared that when the scheme became fully operative, the cost would be insupportable; the scheme was abandoned. In Scotland only 25,129 houses had been built. In 1923 the Chancellor attempted to shift the responsibility back to the private sector, with the state providing a subsidy of £6 for each house built. While in England and Wales these subsidies led to the building of 438,000 houses, in Scotland there was no such response and public-sector house completions in 1924 and 1925 fell back to what proved to be the lowest levels of the inter-war years.

Scotland's building programme revived following the Wheatley Act of 1924.[85] Local authorities received a subsidy of £9 per house (£12 10s in rural areas) for forty years. Rents could be raised to cover costs in excess of the rate contribution of £4 10s per house. Building increased steadily over the following years and by 1933 over 100,000 council houses had been completed.

In the economic crisis of the Depression the Wheatley Act was repealed. It was replaced by the Housing Act of 1933 that focused only on the clearing and the replacement of slums. The Act did not work well in England where there was disagreement about the definition of a slum. In Scotland there were easily recognisable slums in abundance; under the new Act a record number of 18,814 council houses were completed in 1935.

In 1936, Cathcart was 'gratified to record' that almost all local authorities in Scotland had performed well. Between 1919 and 1935 over 200,0000 new houses had been built for the working classes in Scotland under state-aided schemes. However, overcrowding remained a serious problem and there were still many slums to be cleared although 'the numbers of new houses required will not be known with anything approaching precision until the surveys that are now being carried out under the recent Housing Act are completed.' It was already known that apart from an inadequate number of houses, there were in Scotland over 300,000 houses with water closets common to two or more houses, some 30,000 without any water closet and many without running water. Cathcart was confident that housing pro-

---

85 Housing (Financial Provisions) Act, 1924.

grammes under way throughout the country were already 'raising the standard of living of a large part of the population.'

Cathcart was being circumspect. Overcrowding in Scotland was still severe. While Census figures showed that between 1881 and 1931 the average number of persons per house had fallen from 5.06 to 4.08 and the number of persons per room had fallen from 1.59 to 1.27, this could be attributed to the falling birth rate and the reduction in family size. Even if this trend continued, it would only have a marginal effect on the problem. There was still a serious absolute shortage of houses of an acceptable standard. In 1925, local authorities had been required to inspect the houses in their areas and report their findings. Local authorities were slow to respond[86] but gradually the full picture began to emerge. The housing problem did not, as previously assumed, exist only in the towns and cities. In the rural areas up to 75% of the working-class houses were found to be unfit for human habitation.[87]

The local authority surveys were completed in 1936, after the Cathcart Report had been published. They showed that of 259,194 houses built in Scotland since 1919, 83% were built under state-aided schemes, and a record number of contracts had been approved for 1936. However, the number of houses actually completed was beginning to fall because of a general shortage of building workers, particularly bricklayers.

The surveys provided new information on overcrowding. The percentage of houses in Scotland found to be overcrowded was 22.6% compared with 3.8% in England. The worst overcrowding was found, not in the cities, but in the industrial towns in the West of Scotland – Clydebank 44.9%, Coatbridge 44.8%, Port Glasgow 42.1%, Motherwell 40.5%. Overcrowding was almost as bad in the mining areas and there was no evidence of improvement since the Royal Commission on Housing reported in 1917 – in Fife (Cowdenbeath 39.9%, Lochgelly 35%), in landward Lanarkshire 36.9% and landward West Lothian 34.1%.

While there could be no doubt that a very large proportion of Scotland's overcrowded houses were in the large cities, in percentage terms their number was obscured by the houses of a large middle class. The percentage of overcrowded houses was therefore lower than in less prosperous small towns but still dreadful – Glasgow 29.1, Dundee 23.9, Aberdeen 22.1% and Edinburgh 17.2%. Of comparable cities in England only Sunderland (20.6) had overcrowding of this degree. In other great cities in England – for example, Liverpool (7.4), Bristol (2.1) and Plymouth (6) – overcrowding was of a different order.

86 *Hansard*, cccxxiv, 24 June 1937, col. 1462.
87 *Ibid.*, col. 1463.

In 1936 the Department of Health estimated that 161,749 additional houses would be required to put an end to overcrowding. The situation was complicated by the continuing process of slum clearance. Since 1931, 241,243 people had already been displaced by the demolition of their slums and had been re-housed. Many more would need to be re-housed in the future. 'The Department's own inspectors continue to disclose housing conditions which are almost beyond belief.' How many new houses would be required could only be guessed at.

The Cathcart Report gave evidence of the deleterious effect of bad housing, citing deaths from measles and tuberculosis, childhood deaths, and overall death rates. In Glasgow, where 55% of houses were of one or two rooms, deaths from measles were three times higher than in Birmingham where only 4% of houses were of equal size. Again in Glasgow, a study in 1932 had shown a clear association between the number of rooms and both the case rate and the death rate from tuberculosis. The same relationship between the number of rooms and the death rates of children under five and the general death rates had been shown in studies in Glasgow by Dr. A.K. Chalmers in 1911.

These relationships were no longer controversial and were a strong argument for re-housing much of the urban population. However, 'It has been suggested in some quarters that tenants transferred from slum areas to re-housing schemes have to forego necessary food in order to pay the higher rents.' Cathcart accepted that this would be serious if it were true. However, the Committee was 'of the opinion that there is no first hand data to justify a definite conclusion on this point.'

In 1936, McGonigle and Kirby, in *Poverty and Public Health*, were to claim that in England, where the housing problem was less extreme, re-housed tenants found themselves unable to pay for an adequate diet.[88] In Scotland this question was discussed at the General Assembly of the Church of Scotland. It was described as 'the most important problem of all'[89] in schemes for slum clearance:

> The people have been compulsorily removed from their old envir-onments into houses where rents are higher than those to which they are accustomed. It is no longer possible for them to live on the few shillings on which formerly they were able to make ends meet. Many, even of the most careful, become involved in debt, and with debt comes discouragement. The size of the slum clearance house, too, presents its own difficulties. Many of the families arrive at their new homes pushing all their worldly goods in front of them in a wheel-

88 G. M. C. McGonigle and J. Kirby, *Poverty and Public Health* (London, 1936).
89 *Minutes of the General Assembly of the Church of Scotland*, 1935, p. 389.

barrow. They cannot afford to furnish the extra rooms with which they have been provided, but these empty rooms mean constant calls from hire-purchase canvassers and it is difficult to refuse the 'easy' terms which they offer. Soon, for many, the burden of debt is overwhelming.[90]

In 1936, slum clearance programmes had become controversial. They were slowing because of an increasing shortage of skilled labour and rising cost of building. There was growing competition for local authority and other state funding. It could be argued that the Cathcart Committee did not reveal the true severity of the deficiencies in the 1930s and the extent of the difficulties to be overcome and its confidence was misplaced.

Nevertheless, the Cathcart Report was the first statement of policy for health in Britain in the twentieth century to give housing first place in the improvement of the environment of the population.

90 *Ibid.*

6

The State Medical Services

It was the Cathcart Committee's criticism of the state medical services that they had not come together to form a coherent organisation or to embody any coherent national policy. Mindful of the need to retain the good will of all those who would be essential to future health services, the Committee tempered the very substantial evidence that the existing medical services had failed to achieve the objectives for which they had been set up.

The Poor Law Medical Service

The reform of its Poor Laws in 1845 gave Scotland its first rudimentary national medical service. In the early years of the nineteenth century the case for some new provision for the poor had become compelling in every part of Britain. The remorseless industrialisation of Britain had created a new underclass – the overworked, badly paid and badly housed urban industrial workforce. In the years of economic depression that followed the Napoleonic Wars, the poverty and discontent of this ever-growing proportion of the population deepened even further. There seemed a real possibility of some catastrophic social upheaval. 'Something ought to be done.'[1]

In 1834, a Poor Law (Amendment) Act was passed for England and Wales, based on Utilitarian principles. The greatest good of the greatest number was to be achieved by reducing the threat that pauperism and its attendant evils presented to the general public and by containing the financial burden that increasing numbers consigned to pauperism were forcing on the self-supporting majority.

The Act, drawn up by Edwin Chadwick, encouraged the many small local Poor Law authorities to come together in Unions to build larger and more economically efficient workhouses. Chadwick was also confident that pauperism could be reduced by removing what he saw as its principal cause, the diseases of the working poor that caused the decline of so many of their number into destitution. Like many in England at that time, he was persuaded that the chief source of the diseases of the urban poor was miasma, the noxious effluvium from urban filth. He was confident that

1 T. Carlyle, *Chartism* (Boston, 1840), p. 1.

eliminating miasma from the country's towns and cities by a programme of sewerage and drainage would remove the chief cause of pauperism. Not only would pauperism be reduced, but the slums which harboured the urban poor would no longer be the breeding grounds of diseases that constantly threatened to spread to the community at large.

Chadwick made no specific provision for the medical care of the poor. Their diseases were to be prevented, not cured. He was confident that, as a result of his projected sanitary measures, doctors would soon become redundant; doctors were 'necessary evils not likely to last.'[2] It was not until 1842 that the Poor Law Commissioners established an official medical service under the English Poor Law to be staffed by medical officers holding English licences to practice. (Scottish graduates were excluded.)

It had been the Government's intention in 1934 that the provision of the Poor Law (Amendment) Act should be extended to Scotland. However, this was resisted by those then pressing for reform in Scotland. They were not persuaded by Utilitarian ideology and they discounted miasma as a cause of pauperism. Physicians in Scotland had long held that poverty – through poor diet, inadequate clothing and shelter, overwork and overcrowding – led to 'debility.' Since the eighteenth century, medical students at Glasgow and Edinburgh were taught that it was the 'debility' of poverty that was at the root of the health problems of the urban working class.[3] In the 1830s and 1840s, W. P. Alison, the most eminent advocate of social reform at that time, argued that any new Poor Law for Scotland must include support for the able-bodied poor so that, when deprived of employment for whatever reason, they and their families would not be reduced to debility, depression, disease and pauperism.[4] He also insisted that appropriate support for the able-bodied poor must include medical aid. Equally, those who had become paupers because of ill health must have access to the medical treatment that might allow them to return to work. More workhouses must be built large enough to included hospital wards.[5] (Scotland had only four such work-houses, three in Edinburgh and one in Paisley.)

Alison and his fellow-reformers were only partially successful in influ-encing the provisions of the Poor Law (Amendment) Act of 1845. The Act transferred to the state the responsibility for the administration of the Poor Law that, for three centuries, had been devolved to the Kirk. Parochial

2 R. Hodgekinson, *The Origins of the National Health Service* (London, 1967), p. 639.
3 Robert Cowan, Professor of Medical Jurisprudence and Police, Glasgow University; W. P. Alison, Professor of Medical Jurisprudence and Professor of Medicine, Edinburgh University.
4 W. P. Alison, *Observations on the Management of the Poor in Scotland* (Edinburgh, 1840).
5 W. P. Alison, *Remarks on the Report of Her Majesties Commissioners on the Poor Laws of Scotland Presented to Parliament in 1844* (Edinburgh, 1844).

Boards were set up to 'have and exercise all the Powers and Authority hitherto exercised by the Heritors and the Kirk Sessions.' However, the administration of the new Poor Law was not to have the strong central control that Alison had advocated; the new Board of Supervision in Edinburgh was created only as an advisory body and given no powers of direction.[6] The Parochial Boards, although obliged to raise funds to provide for the poor, were required to impose 'assessments' for this purpose only as they thought fit. There was no provision in the Act that might have led to the building of the Poor Law hospital accommodation that Alison thought so necessary.

Since the sixteenth century, the Poor Law in Scotland had not required parish authorities to provide for the able-bodied, and that ancient principle was continued under the new Poor Law. However, it did offer those pauperised by ill health some assistance to recover their ability to work. Parish Boards were to be obliged 'to provide for Medicines, Medical Attendance, nutritious diet, Cordials and Clothing for such poor and in such a manner and to such an extent as seem equitable and expedient.'

In the House of Commons, Scottish members objected that this did not go far enough. They demanded that the Poor Law must ensure that every parish had the services of a resident medical officer and that, to provide the necessary funds, assessment should be made compulsory. The Home Secretary, Sir James Graham, agreed that 'general assessment must be desirable but considering the difference of opinion he thought it infinitely more wise to leave the public of Scotland, by a voluntary act, to adopt assessment themselves rather than by an enactment to make it compulsory.'[7] The Prime Minister, Sir Robert Peel, considered that the provision of a paid medical officer in every parish was impractical and that Scottish members were being over-ambitious.

Nevertheless, Scottish pressure continued and in 1848 the government offered a compromise. An annual grant of £10,000[8] was made to the Board of Supervision to provide a financial supplement for every parish ready to raise an equivalent sum to employ its own medical officer. Sir John McNeil, the Chairman of the Board, was confident that, with this inducement, a full

6 Technically the Board was a sub-department of the Home Office. The Chairman was Sir John McNeil, a Tory, but the Board was not intended to reflect general opinion in Scotland. Three sheriffs (Ross, Perth and Renfrew) represented the counties. The Lord Provosts of Edinburgh and Glasgow represented the towns. The Scottish legal system was represented by the Solicitor-General. There were two further Crown appointments; McNeil insisted that one should be a Whig. I. Levitt, *Government and Social Conditions in Scotland 1845–1919* (Edinburgh, 1988).

7 *Hansard*, lxxxi, HC 12 June 1845, col. 425.

8 Increased to £20,000 in 1882.

complement of parish medical officers would be recruited in every parish in Scotland.[9]

From the beginning the rudimentary medical service that emerged was unsatisfactory. In rural areas, even in the largest parishes, the number of parishioners able to contribute to parish funds was often too small to provide the financial contribution that would have attracted a grant from central funds. Parishes that were able to accept the subsidy often used their funds unwisely and unfairly, and many of the medical officers they employed proved unsatisfactory. Most rural parishes could afford only a few pounds as a 'salary' or subsidy for a medical officer; the doctors engaged continued to be essentially dependent on private practice and based themselves in the centres where they were most likely to earn a living. As a result the distributions of Poor Law medical officers had little relation to the parish structure of the counties. In the rapidly growing industrial centres the problems were even more overwhelming. The old parish structure could not support the vastly increasing numbers of their new poor.[10] With or without a Treasury grant, parishes could not afford to appoint a sufficient number of medical officers. In Scotland there were no Unions, and individual parishes proved unwilling to join forces to build poorhouses. Only in very exceptional circumstances could individual parishes build poorhouses with hospital accommodation.[11] When pauperism in Scotland reach a record level in 1869 (41 per thousand of the population), only 6.7% were lodged in Scotland's poorhouses and, of these, only a minority had hospital accommodation.

While in the middle years of the century the number on parish Poor Rolls increased, the number of the destitute able-bodied increased even faster. As the extent of local poverty became more compelling, parochial boards became more liberal in the interpretation of 'able-bodied' and more and more parochial boards were at last forced to impose assessments on their parishes.[12]

---

9 Sir John McNeil, letter to the Royal College of Physicians. Quoted in the report of a Committee of the College, 3 February 1852. RCPE Archive.

10 Thomas Chalmers' parish, St John's in Glasgow, was an outstanding exception. S. J. Brown, *Thomas Chalmers and the Godly Commonwealth* (Oxford, 1982), p. 153; Cave, *op. cit.*, p. 143.

11 In 1865 the St Cuthbert's Parochial Board in Edinburgh was able to sell its poorhouse in Lothian Road to the Caledonian Railway Company which required the site for its Edinburgh terminal. The sale price of £115,000 allowed the parochial Board to build a new poorhouse to a high standard at Craigleith. In Glasgow in 1889 the City and Barony parishes took the most unusual decision to combine forces; the site of the old City Poorhouse was sold to the railway company providing funds sufficient to build small hospitals at Duke Street and Oakbank and a hospital for the chronic sick at Stobhill.

12 All Scotland's parishes were eventually assessed by 1909.

In 1894 the responsibilities of the Board of Supervisors were taken over by a Local Government Board. Parochial boards were replaced by elected parish councils to be responsible for both the administration of the Poor Law and the Public Health. In this new organisation, the services provided under the Poor Law remained much as before and the proportion of the population entitled to Poor Law medical relief remained almost constant for some years at approximately 22 per thousand.

Poor Law Services in the 1930s

Real change came with the introduction of Old Age pensions in 1908. Those over 70 and now supported by a pension were removed from the Poor Rolls; by 1910 the numbers entitled to medical care under the Poor Law had fallen dramatically. During the First World War there was a further sharp fall and many of Scotland's small poorhouses were made over to the armed forces. By 1919, the number of poor accommodated in poorhouses was little more than half what it had been in 1914. At the end of the war, of the poorhouses no longer required by the armed forces, several were renovated to provide accommodation for infectious disease, mental deficiency or convalescence and others were sold off. From a total of 65 (all but three without hospital accommodation) at the turn of the century, there were only 18 in 1919. In the more optimistic and more enlightened climate of the years immediately after the war, it became usual to drop the name 'poorhouse' in favour of 'house,' and in three cases, 'hospital.'

Sir George McCrae, the Chairman of the new Board of Health, felt that in 1920 parochial councils could afford to 'adopt a broad view'[13] in providing outdoor support for the unemployed. However, rising unemployment and a miners' strike in 1921 created an unforeseen crisis. The case for providing for the able-bodied unemployed became overwhelming and was at last officially accepted in the Poor Law Emergency Provision (Scotland) Act of 1921.[14] In 1921, outdoor aid was given to 1,478 able-bodied unemployed and their dependants. By 1922 that number had risen dramatically to 147,420, outnumbering the 100,981 officially recognised 'ordinary poor.' The numbers on the Poor Roll still continued to rise. Then in 1930 one of the effects of the Unemployed Insurance Act was to reduce the number of able-bodied unemployed recorded on the Roll by almost a half; after 1932 lunatics and mental defectives (at that time 4.1 per thousand of the population) were also excluded from the Poor Law statistics. In spite of

13 I. Levitt, *Government and Social Conditions in Scotland 1845–1919, op. cit.,* p. 106.
14 The provisions for the unemployed in this Act were renewed annually by Expiring Laws Continuation Acts until established by the Poor Law (Scotland) Act of 1934.

this statistical redistribution of those in need of relief, the proportion of the population recorded as being entitled to Poor Law relief, reached 82 per thousand in 1934.[15]

The Local Government (Scotland) Act of 1929 had transferred the administration of the Poor Laws from parish councils to county councils and the town councils of large burghs. In 1932 the Department of Health for Scotland complained that, although the old parish councils had made valiant efforts to meet the needs of the poor, they had been 'armed with a defective instrument.' The Department, in its turn, had inherited a 'machine' that was still defective. The resources and organisation of the Poor Law medical services were clearly inadequate to cope with the increasing numbers in need of support and the problems caused by a new wave of ill health. Medical care was being provided but at a very low standard. There was an acute shortage of hospital accommodation. All institutions were over-crowded and 'it was not uncommon to find in one institution the acutely sick, the chronic invalid, the senile poor, young children, able bodied, vagrants, mental defectives and lunatics.'[16] Since no proper medical records were kept, the effectiveness or otherwise of their medical care could only be guessed at.

In 1935, the Department of Health set up a committee, chaired by James Keith K.C, 'to examine the existing statutory provisions relating to the relief of the poor in Scotland.'[17] Its findings were anticipated by the damning conclusion of the Cathcart Report:

> The poor law medical service is generally regarded as unsatisfactory, and efforts at improvement cannot overcome the difficulties inherent in the maintenance of a separate service for persons only when they are destitute. The legislature has already recognised that a separate hospital service for the sick poor is undesirable; a separate domiciliary medical service for the sick poor is no less undesirable.

Cathcart was confident that the Keith Committee would recommend that, where necessary, medical treatment should be available to all without any distinction between the general public and the poor.

Other Local Authority Medical Services

The key figures in the promotion and organisation of local authority medical services were the Medical Officers of Health. In 1847 a Public

15 *Annual Report of the Department of Health for Scotland*, 1930, Cmd. 3860, p. 155.
16 *Annual Report of the Department of Health for Scotland*, 1929, Cmd. 3529, p. 167.
17 *Annual Report of the Department of Health for Scotland*, 1935, Cmd. 5123, p. 148.

Health (Scotland) Bill would have allowed the appointment of Medical Officers of Health across Scotland. However, the Bill proved to be controversial and was lost. It was not until 30 September 1862 that, on the uncertain basis of a Police and Improvement Act of August 1862, the Town Council of Edinburgh agreed to appoint Henry Littlejohn as Scotland's first Medical Officer of Health. In 1863, a local Police Act allowed the appointment of William Gairdner in Glasgow. Other towns followed, and in 1867 the appointment of Medical Officers in all burghs became obligatory under the Public Health Act.

The appointment of this first generation of Medical Officers of Health proved highly successful, and they and their successors won the active support of the Town Council Committees (later the Public Health Committees)[18] to which they were answerable. It was this combination of reforming Medical Officers of Health and their supportive Public Health Committees that developed the municipal services that served a large section of the Scottish population until the establishment of the NHS.

Infectious Diseases

Until the first half of the nineteenth century Scotland had no permanent system for the management of infectious disease. At the approach of epidemics, in the larger towns at least, special temporary shelters were set up to accommodate those who could not be managed at home. Houses of quarantine were designated as places of refuge for the healthy hoping to escape infection. Dispensaries were established to issue medicines, and a list of doctors willing to give their services was drawn up. As each crisis passed, these arrangements were abandoned.

Lister's success with antiseptic surgery in Glasgow, and later in Edinburgh, and the work of Pasteur in France inspired a new interest in the possibility of controlling infectious disease. An essential first step was the notification of infections. It was first suggested (in Greenock in 1877) that the patient should be responsible for notifying his own illness. In Edinburgh a Municipal and Police Act of 1879 made notification obligatory and placed the obligation on the diagnosing doctor. This, the first programme for the notification of infectious disease in the United Kingdom, was gradually adopted by other authorities and became compulsory in Scotland in 1889.

By then the arrangements for the care of patients with 'fevers' had changed radically. In Glasgow, during a typhus epidemic in 1864–5, the Poor Law authorities gave notice that they would no longer admit 'fever'

---

18 The appointment of Public Health Committees followed the Public Health (Scotland) Act of 1867 but in many cases they were not inaugurated for some years. J. A. Gray, *Edinburgh City Hospital* (East Linton, 1999), p. 30.

patients other than paupers to hospital accommodation under their con-trol.[19] William Gairdner, the Medical Officer of Health, then successfully argued for the establishment of a permanent fever hospital. Scotland's first fever hospital was opened at Parliamentary Road in 1865. In 1866 when a cholera epidemic threatened in Edinburgh, the Royal Infirmary gave notice that it would not admit infectious cases to its small unit for 'fevers.' The Medical Officer of Health persuaded the Corporation to set aside part of the City Poorhouse Hospital for acute infectious disease. When this proved inadequate, the Corporation agreed to buy and convert the Canongate's Poor House as the first of Edinburgh's succession of City Hospitals for infectious disease.[20] Similar provisions were made across Scotland and in 1897 all local authorities were required to provide infectious disease hospitals according to a formula that recommended one bed for every 1000 of the population in urban areas and one bed per 1500 in rural areas.[21]

In 1929, when the Department of Health for Scotland became the responsible authority, it found that there were 179 hospitals and 18,670 beds almost entirely for the treatment of infectious disease. By then, as a result of the improvement in social conditions and the success of immu-nisation schemes, the incidence of infectious disease had declined. The space no longer required for infectious disease was often taken up for the treatment of pneumonia and other non-notifiable diseases. There was also a trend for infectious disease hospitals to become centres for treatment rather than for isolation. This was possible in the large city hospitals, with appropriate accommodation and adequate medical staff. But most Scottish 'fever' hospitals remained, as they had been for many years, small, with poorly trained nursing staff and with medical direction in the hands of the local Medical Officer of Health as a part-time responsibility.[22]

In 1936, Cathcart concluded that, although local authority infectious disease services were still passively accepted by the public, they had not been developed to an acceptable standard. Not only was there a great lack of modern accommodation but the medical and nursing care provided in the patient's home was clearly inadequate. It was anticipated that the proposed extension of the general practitioner service would ensure earlier diagnosis and more effective treatment at home. However, infectious disease hospitals should no longer be seen merely as places for isolation but as centres for modern treatment. For this purpose the existing small hospitals were clearly unsuitable and must be replaced.

19 A. K. Chalmers, *The Health of Glasgow 1818–1925* (Glasgow, 1930), p. 277.
20 Gray, *op. cit.*, p. 48.
21 Public Health (Scotland) Act, 1897.
22 T. S. Wilson, 'The Public Health Services', in G. McLachlan (ed.), *Improving the Common Weal* (Edinburgh, 1987), p. 229.

Tuberculosis Services

The wasting condition of *phthysis* (consumption) had been seen in Europe since the sixth millennium BC. In the eighteenth century it was identified with pulmonary tuberculosis. In the seventeenth century, *phthisis* become 'The Captain of the Men of Death'[23] in Britain's growing urban populations. Consumption, as it was commonly known, again became a major problem as the population became more intensely urbanised in the Industrial Revolution, and by the middle of the nineteenth century it had become the commonest cause of death among young adults. It was clearly associated with poverty; in Edinburgh in the 1860s deaths (3 per 1000) were most frequent in the slums of Canongate and St Giles. Later in the century it was shown in Glasgow that the mortality rate for pulmonary tuberculosis for families living in one room was almost twice that for families in two rooms and more than three times that of families living in all other houses.[24] The disease also affected particular groups identified by 'the special duties and indoor nature of their duties' – seamstresses, tailors, indoor servants and unmarried women living at home[25] but, above all, young married women caring for young families in conditions of overcrowding.

In 1882, Robert Koch proved that pulmonary tuberculosis was caused by an airborne infection. Nevertheless, it remained a common perception, shared by many in the medical profession, that tuberculosis, so often seen to affect every member of a family, was essentially an inherited defect. The belief that the disease was a hereditary 'taint', and inevitably fatal, discouraged attempts to find a scheme of rational management.[26] In 1868, Herman Weber publicised the notion that exposure to high mountain air could, at least, arrest progress.[27] The wealthy were drawn to the mountain resorts of Switzerland but for the less wealthy, who made up the vast majority of sufferers, treatment, if any, could only be palliative.[28]

Although the death rate from tuberculosis had been falling for over 30 years, in 1898 increasing public interest in the health of the race led to the formation of the National Association for the Prevention of Consumption and other Forms of Tuberculosis. By 1904 over 70 sanatoriums had been established in the United Kingdom, almost all for private patients following

23 J. Bunyan, *The Life and Death of Mister Badman.*
24 Chalmers, *op. cit.*, p. 96.
25 *BMJ*, i, 1892, p. 150.
26 A. G. Leitch, 'Two Men and a Bug: One Hundred Years of Tuberculosis in Edinburgh', *Proceedings of the Royal College of Physicians of Edinburgh*, xxvi, 1996, p. 296.
27 This notion persisted and influenced sanatorium treatment in the United Kingdom until after the Second World War.
28 Malt to counter debility, a mixture of opium, extract of senega and ammonium bicarbonate to control the cough.

the regime advocated by Weber. Treatment was still that advocated by Weber: rest, a sound diet and the supposed benefits of exposure to fresh air. The cure rates in these private institutions are unknown but there is nothing to suggest that they were better than those in the few charity sanatoriums where the cure rate was known to be 4%.[29]

In Edinburgh, R. W. Philip had already introduced a new system of management in 1887 devised not for the wealthy few but for the general public. Anyone thought to be suffering from tuberculosis could be seen at a public dispensary for diagnosis and assessment; if found to have active disease, their families, and as far as possible their contacts, were also assessed. Those found to be at an early stage of the disease were isolated as in-patients in a 'sanatorium' to prevent the spread of disease; those who improved were later transferred to a 'colony' for gradual return towards normal activities under supervision. Those who seemed unlikely to recover were admitted to a 'tuberculosis hospital' for terminal care.

However, many of those diagnosed at the dispensary refused admission. Although aware of the potential benefits, men were reluctant to give up work, particularly in times of relatively high wages. Mothers were reluctant to leave their families. The proportion accepting admission could be as low as 50% and many of those admitted could not tolerate the regime and discharged themselves.

For some years Philip's system was regarded as a 'visionary concept.'[30] Then, in 1911, a Departmental Committee reviewing the administration of the Sanatorium Benefit of the new National Health Insurance Scheme advised that his system should be adopted nationally. The National Insurance Act of 1911 allowed responsibility for tuberculosis schemes to be assumed by large burghs and counties in preference to the many small rural local authorities. However, the powers of the small local authorities were not repealed. To add to the confusion, the administration of the financial Sanatorium Benefit remained the responsibility of the Insurance Committees.

The First World War brought a sudden and alarming increase in the incidence of the disease and a large number of deaths. The problem was seen to be beyond the disparate capabilities of the 309 Public Health Local Authorities (serving populations that ranged from 300 to 1,000,000), all of which had some responsibility for tuberculosis and some of which had used the lack of clarity in the legislation to avoid providing any service.

The scheme for the management of tuberculosis was not rationalised

---

29 F. Smith, *The People's Health 1830–1910* (London, 1990), p. 291.
30 C. I. Holmes, 'Trial by TB', *Proceeding of the Royal College of Physicians of Edinburgh*, xxvii, 1997, p. 15.

until the 1920s. The Scottish Health Board placed entire responsibility for the scheme clearly on the counties and large burghs. In 1929, when the Scottish Board of Health was replaced by the Department of Health for Scotland, there were 39 dispensaries and a total of 119 hospitals and sanatoriums, 50 with fewer than 50 beds. By 1936, the number of dispensaries had increased to 42 while the total number of beds had remained for some years at a little over 5000.

The system introduced by Philip had demonstrated that the spread of the disease could be confined by isolation of the victims and by accepting that the unit for management was not the patient alone, but his family and contacts. In other respects success was limited. Although the incidence of tuberculosis continued to fall after the First World War, the mortality of those discovered to have active tuberculosis continued to be over 50%. Not all patients could be admitted for treatment and 60% of the women and 50% of the men who died of tuberculosis died at home.

In the 1930s, pulmonary tuberculosis was still the commonest single cause of death of young adults. The overall death rate in Scotland had fallen from almost 170 per thousand at the end of the nineteenth century to 78 per thousand in 1933, but in the distress of the Depression, the disease had begun to increase once more. Because of the considerable social stigma still associated with the disease the diagnosis was often denied until the disease had reach 'a stage when response to treatment is slow or negligible.'[31] The true incidence of the infection was unknown but there could be no doubt that pulmonary tuberculosis was a major and uncontrolled problem.

Cathcart called for new legislation that would put greater emphasis on support for the patients and families at home. Domiciliary services were to be made more effective by ensuring co-operation between local authority tuberculosis officers and the patient's general practitioner. (In Cathcart's proposed scheme for general practice everyone would have a general practitioner.) The outpatient tuberculosis services were to continue on Philip's model but the dispensary component was to be sited with other specialist services in local authority medical centres. The existing number of beds available for in-patient treatment was satisfactory, but many of the institutions were 'not always adequate in quality.' It was recommended that the existing institutional accommodation should be overhauled and that specialist skills and equipment should be concentrated in regional referral centres.

---

31 *Annual Report of the Department of Health for Scotland*, 1935, p. 84.

The School Medical Service

The School Medical Service had its origins in the findings of a Royal Commission on Physical Training.[32] The inquiry was set up by the Secretary of State for Scotland to

> ... enquire into the opportunities for physical training now available in the state aided schools and education institutes of Scotland and to suggest means by which training may be made to conduce to the welfare of the pupils.[33]

The Royal Commission did find a place for physical training but, as the Secretary for Scotland later explained to Parliament, its most important findings had come 'in a more or less accidental way.'[34] The Commission had chosen to assess the 'the general physical condition of the youth of the country.' It found that:

> There exists in Scotland an undeniable degeneration of individuals of the classes where food and environment are defective which calls for amelioration ... School Boards should have command of medical advice and assistance in the supervision of schools; a systematic record of physical and health statistics should be kept. They should provide facilities for the provision of suitable food by voluntary agencies without cost to public funds. If this proves inadequate power should be given to provide a meal and to demand from the parents a payment to meet the cost.[35]

The Conservative government of the time took no action on the recommendations of this Report, or the support that followed in 1904 in Reports from the Scottish Royal Medical Corporations[36] and an Interdepartmental Committee.[37]

However, after the election of 1906, which introduced the period of New Liberalism and its social reforms, the poor physical condition of schoolchildren was taken up by the Scottish member, Arthur Henderson. In the

---

32 During the Boer War, the army had been particularly disappointed by the quality of recruits form Scotland, usually the source of its best physically developed men.
33 *Report of the Royal Commission on Physical Training (Scotland), op. cit.*
34 *Hansard*, cxxiv, HC 6 July 1903, col. 1353.
35 *Report of the Royal Commission on Physical Training (Scotland)*, 1903, Cd. 1507, p. 5.
36 *Report on Health Conditions of School Children of Scotland.* The Scottish Royal Corporations proposed that accurate data should be collected to determine whether or not degeneration of the race was taking place. It urged the examination of children to the highest attainable standards of accuracy including anthropomorphic measurements. This was communicated to the Scottish Secretary without effect. *Minute of the Royal College of Physicians of Edinburgh*, 8 March 1904.
37 *Report of the Interdepartmental Committee on Physical Deterioration*, 1904, Cd. 2175.

Commons, he recalled the findings of the reports of 1903 and 1904 and their evidence of a need for 'the proper and sufficient feeding of children.'[38] He quoted from the 1903 *Report* that 'in the slums of Edinburgh a large proportion of the children were half starved and that to subject half starved children to the routine of school would be the height of cruelty and that the results of education would be poor.'[39]

A private member's Bill was passed without difficulty as the Education (Provision of Meals) Act, 1906. The Act encouraged local authorities to introduce school meals and allowed the cost to become a charge on the rates. In most local authority areas schemes were organised by voluntary committees with financial support from the local education authority.[40]

In 1907 Robert Morant, then Permanent Secretary to the Board of Education, contrived the inclusion in the Educational (Amendments) Bill of a clause 'to provide for the medical inspection of children immediately before . . . their admission to a public school and on such other occasion as the Board of Education direct, and the power to make such arrangement as may be sanctioned by the Board of Education for attending to the health and physical condition of children in Public Elementary Schools.'[41] This legislation for England and Wales slipped through almost unnoticed.[42] The equivalent legislation for Scotland came later in the Education (Scotland) Act, 1908, again without significant opposition. The School Medical Service had been created.

Across Britain, local education authorities viewed their new responsibilities with varying degrees of enthusiasm and there was vigorous opposition from parents. Many regarded the examination of their children as an intrusion on liberty.[43] In 1909, an Amendment Act established that parents could not be compelled to accept either examination or treatment of their children and that 'there must be reasonable regard for the susceptibilities of parents and child. There must be no attempt to introduce controversial issues such as the pros and cons of vaccination, particular medical theories or fanciful investigations or minute anthropometric measurements.'[44] 'The examination should not take more than a few minutes.'[45]

The medical examinations were therefore never carried out as recom-

---

38 *Hansard*, clii, HC 2 March 1906, col. 1394.
39 *Ibid.*
40 Voluntary bodies, such as the Poor Children's Dinner Table in Glasgow, had been providing meals since 1868.
41 Education (Administrative Provisions) Act, 1907, Clause 10 (section 131(b)).
42 B. M. Allen, *Sir Robert Morant: A Great Civil Servant* (London, 1934), p. 231; *Hansard*, clxxix, HC 31 July 1907, col. 1097.
43 A group of irate mothers in Glasgow smashed the windows of the Education offices in Glasgow (A. Macgregor, *Public Health in Glasgow* (Edinburgh, 1967), p. 82).
44 Sir G. Newman, *The Building of a Nation's Health* (London, 1939), p. 202.
45 *Report of the Board of Education*, 1909, Cmd. 4566.

mended in 1903. Instead a quick inspection was designed to answer eight simple questions:

1. Has the child had any illness in the past which would be likely to affect his physical future?
2. What is the present condition of his body as regards cleanliness and nutrition?
3. Are his senses normal – hearing, touch, smell, taste?
4. Has he sound or decayed teeth?
5. Are his throat and tonsils normal and healthy?
6. Is he normal and sound of mind?
7. Does he show any signs of disease or deformity (rickets, tubercle, rheumatism, rupture, glandular disease, ringworm, anaemia, epilepsy, psychoneurosis)?
8. Has he any weakness or defect unfitting him from ordinary school life and physical exercise, or requiring any exemption from any branch or form of instruction?[46]

The School Medical Service was crippled from the beginning by the restrictions on its powers and capabilities.

In 1904, the Interdepartmental Committee on Physical Deterioration had commented that the period of school life offered the only opportunity to 'take stock' of the nation and monitor changes in physical development. The School Medical Service was prevented from fulfilling that function. No anthropomorphic measurements could be made and no attempt was made to derive any useful statistics from the cursory inspections.[47] 'Variation in the methods of tabulating the results made effective collation of statistics impossible.'[48]

The brief medical inspections carried out did prove useful in recognising the blind, deaf and otherwise severely disabled children who could not usefully be accommodated in the normal school system and for whom special provision had to be made. However, the great majority of the defects that could be discovered in a few minutes of superficial inspection were relatively trivial. In 1929 the new Department of Health reported that school medical inspections had revealed nothing that had not already been documented in greater detail in the *Report of the Royal Commission on Physical Training* in 1903.

Statistics for the whole of Scotland first appeared in 1929. In that year 33.3% of Scottish school children were inspected.[49] The scope of the

---

46 Newman, *op. cit.*, p. 199.
47 The School Medical Service in Scotland did not have an effective record system until 1938. H. P. Tait, 'Maternity and Child Welfare', in McLachlan, *op. cit.*, p. 428.
48 *Annual Report of the Scottish Board of Health*, 1924, Cmd. 2416, p. 105.
49 Based on my own many years' experience of Scottish children, I find these figures almost incredible. I would have found them surprisingly good even 30 years later.

inspections and the small number of defects discovered are listed in Table 6.1.

Table 6.1   **School Medical Examinations, Scotland, 1929**

Poor Nutrition	6.1%	Dental decay	74%
Overt Tuberculosis	0.1%	Hearing Loss	1%
Head Lice	1.8%	Enlarged adenoids	3.9%
Other Vermin	0.8%	Discharging ears	2.4%
Poor Sight	5.8%	Heart disorders	1.9%
Skin diseases	3.7%	Rickets	1.6%

Source: *Annual Report, Department of Health for Scotland*

Throughout the 1930s annual reports showed no significant change.[50]

When school medical inspection was first introduced in Scotland in 1909, it was assumed that it would only be necessary to draw the presence of defects to the attention of parents for appropriate treatment to be arranged by them. However, many parents remained unconvinced that treatment was necessary, and even more could not afford the expense involved. Local authorities were allowed to make grants for medical treatment from 1912, and in 1918 it was made a statutory duty for local education authorities to provide some limited forms of treatment.

Visual defects were identified and spectacles provided; hearing defects were recognised and, where relevant, referred for specialist treatment; cases of heart disease, tuberculosis and rickets were referred to hospital. Treatment carried out at the school clinics was usually only for skin and other minor disorders although the extent of the service offered varied widely from authority to authority; the dental service was perhaps the most effective and the most widely available.[51] How much was achieved by treatment cannot be accurately known since no records were kept. The Department of Health for Scotland found that services were provided unevenly across the country and that there remained a large body of children with remediable defects 'whose ranks were proving difficult to reduce from year to year.'[52]

The chief difficulty was that the service was administered and financed at local level. This limited the resources of the School Medical Service and prejudiced the quality of the medical staff recruited. Local authorities were known as poor and uncertain employers. By 1938, of medical staff of the School Medical Service, only 18% held full-time appointments. For most the School Medical Service was a fringe activity taken up only to supple-

50 Appendices VI (i) and (ii); Appendix VII.
51 Appendix VII.
52 *Annual Report of the Department of Health for Scotland*, 1930, Cmd.3860, p. 70.

ment income from other preferred forms of medical practice. There was little opportunity to develop professional skills in the care of children and there was no proper career structure. As a result the quality of the medical staff remained unimpressive.[53]

By the late 1930s the School Medical Service employed 233 doctors, 97 dentists, 140 nurses, 20 dental dressers and 10 masseuses providing a service to 3,344 schools and 795,079 pupils. A doctor who had been in the service from the beginning recorded after 40 years that 'I have long been impressed with the wastage of manpower and money.'[54] The inadequacy of the cursory inspections was revealed by their failure to detect the appallingly high incidence of rickets[55] found by a special survey carried out by the Scottish Board of Health in 1925 and by the unexpected severity of sub-nutrition found by John Boyd Orr in 1928.[56]

The School Medical Service did not, at that time, take part in prevention schemes. Vaccination against smallpox was never included in the programme, and when immunisation against diphtheria became available, it was not provided. The School Medical Service made no significant contribution to the dramatic fall in childhood deaths from infectious disease in the first half of the century.

Cathcart concluded that the School Medical Service had been 'prevented by legal, and other restrictions from achieving its full potential.' In future the task of the School Medical Service should continue to be to monitor the state of health of children but its main task should be to advise on the curriculum 'so as to strike a sound balance between physical welfare and book work,' and on school life generally – assisting in the siting, planning and construction of new schools, on the provision of playing fields and other facilities for recreation, on physical training and on health education. Medical services for children of school age should become the responsibility of the local authority clinics 'in wide terms, similar to those for maternity and child welfare.'

Maternity and Child Welfare

Scotland's Maternity and Child Welfare Services were introduced early in the century to meet what were then perceived to be two major, distinct but related, threats to the nation – the loss of a great part of its population in the first year of life and the disruption of a great many families caused by the deaths of young mothers.

53 'I do not believe that our ablest men and women will look for a career in the School Medical Service.' Sir Charles McNeil, *BMJ*, 28 October 1950, p. 1170.
54 *BMJ*, ii, 1950, p. 1001.
55 In one community in central Scotland the incidence was over 70%.
56 J. Boyd Orr, *Lancet*, i, 1928, p. 871.

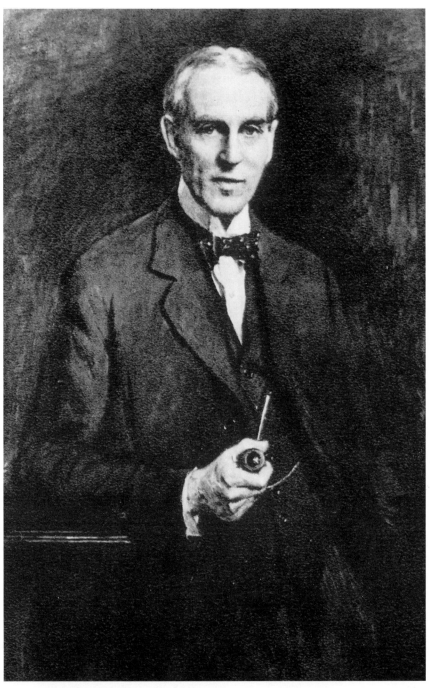

1. Sir Godfrey Collins, Secretary of State for Scotland, 1932 – 1936
(Scottish National Portrait Gallery)

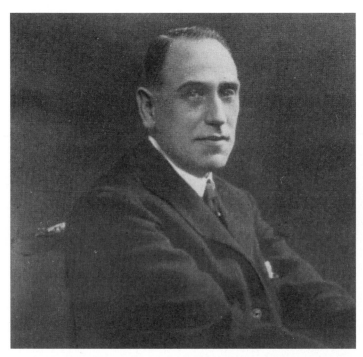

2. Professor Edward Cathcart *(Scottish National Portrait Gallery)*

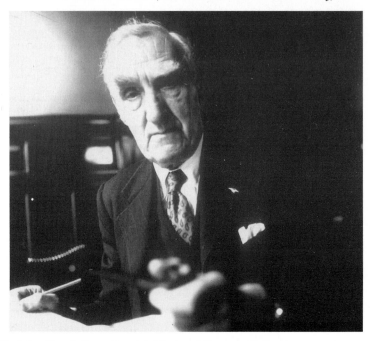

3. Sir John Boyd Orr *(Scottish National Portrait Gallery)*

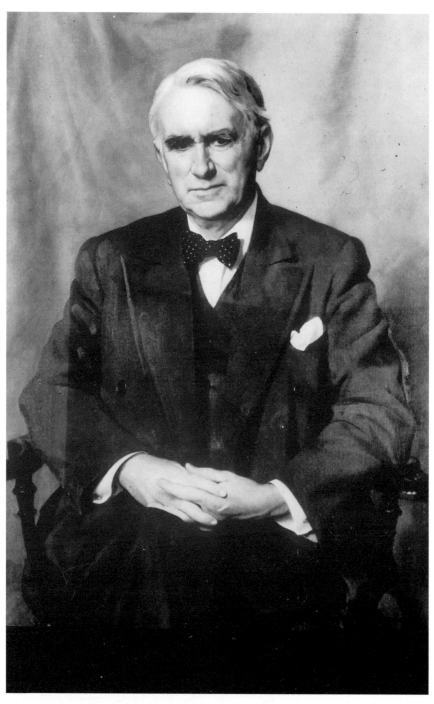

4. Tom Johnston *(Scottish National Portrait Gallery)*

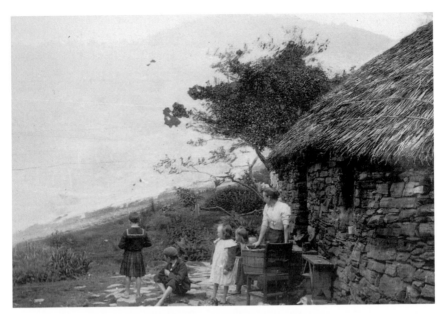

5. Crofter's house and healthy family, Morar 1905. The cottage had two rooms with a bed in each. The father and two sons slept in one; in the other the grandmother, mother and three daughters
(Scottish Life Archive, National Museums of Scotland)

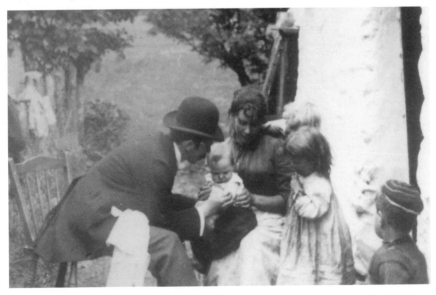

6. General Practitioner, Highlands and Islands Medical Service, 1930. Examining the patient in the daylight rather than in the interior gloom of a blackhouse *(Scottish Life Archive)*

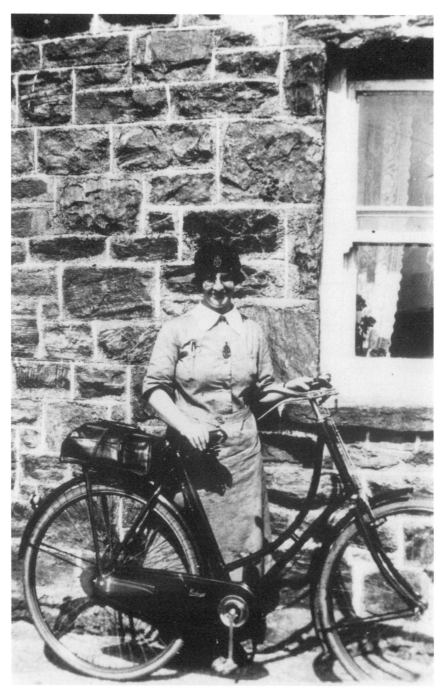

7. Nurse a'Bhugalair (District Nurse), Highlands and Islands Medical Service, Lewis, 1930 *(Scottish Life Archive)*

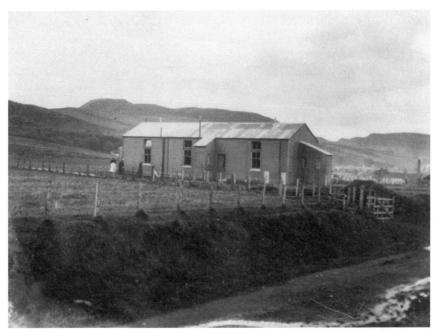

8. Isolation Fever Hospital, Campbeltown, 1910 *(Scottish Life Archive)*

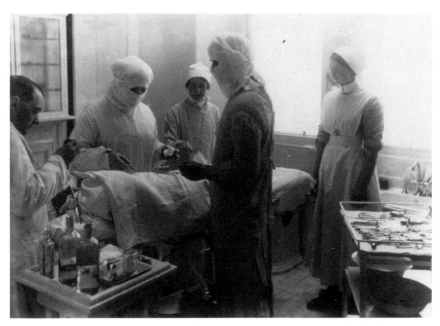

9. Gilbert Bain Hospital (Highlands and Islands Medical Service), Lerwick, 1929 *(Scottish Life Archive)*

the Miners' Strike, 1921. They fought bravely for four months...

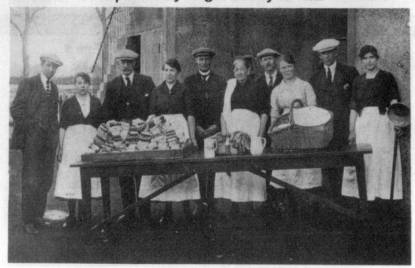

10. Soup kitchen, Fife, 1921 *(Scottish Life Archive)*

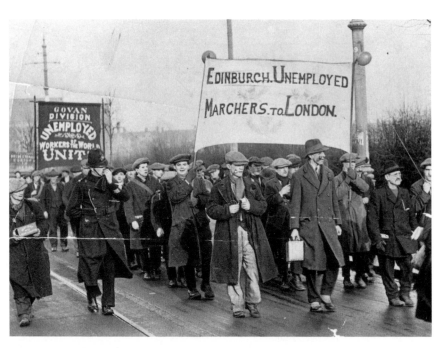

11. Hunger March, Edinburgh, 1932 *(Scottish Life Archive)*

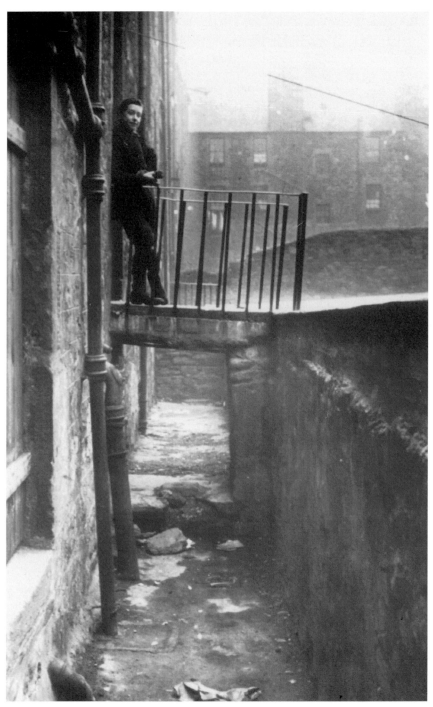

12. City life, Edinburgh, 1910 *(Scottish Life Archive)*

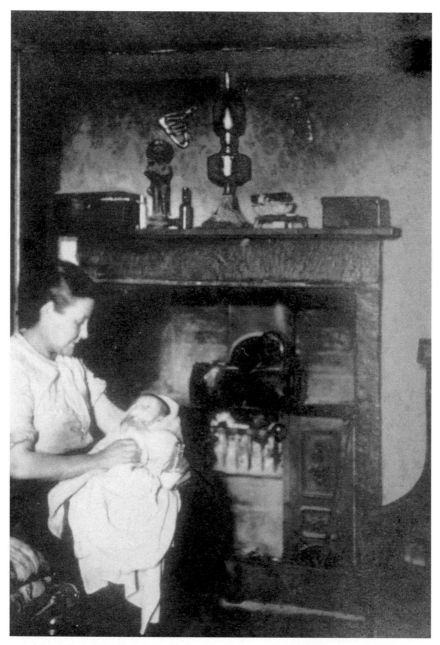

13. Interior, Edinburgh Old Town, 1905. Grandmother and infant at home in a one-room flat. Total contents of the single room listed as: 'a chair, a bed covered with old coats, a box for a second seat, a table, a lamp, a pot and kettle, a strip of old carpet, a few dishes and a few ornaments' *(Scottish Life Archive)*

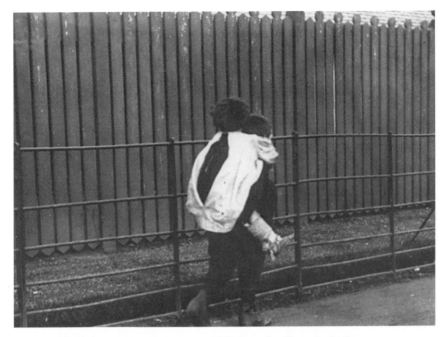

14. Taking young sister to Edinburgh Royal Infirmary, 1929
(Lothian Health Board Archive)

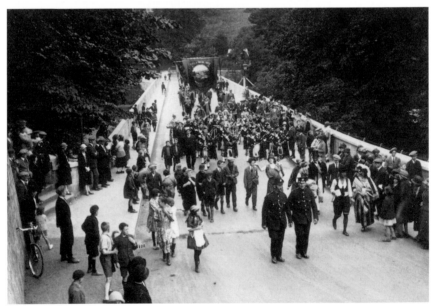

15. Fund-raising for Edinburgh Royal Infirmary, 1935
(Scottish Life Archive)

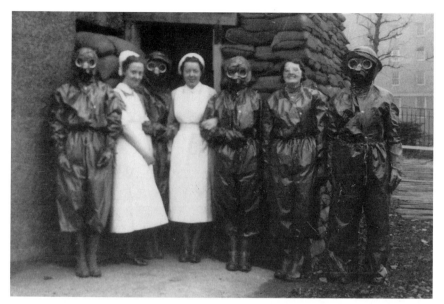

16. Preparing for war, Western General Hospital, Edinburgh (*Miss Christine Orr (centre)*)

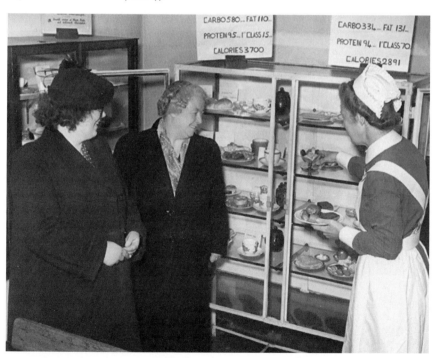

17. Nutrition in wartime: advice on making the best of the rations (*Scottish Life Archive*)

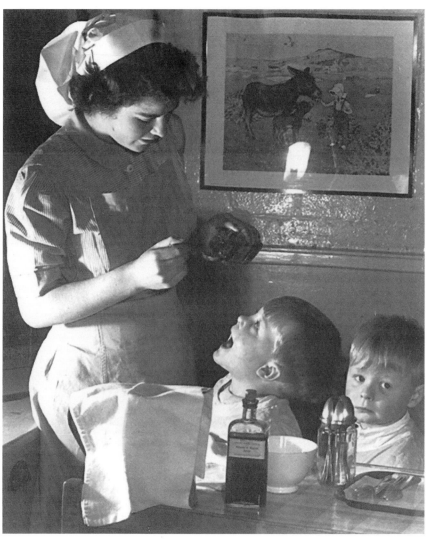

18. Management of nutrition in wartime: cod-liver oil and fruit syrups
(Scottish Life Archive)

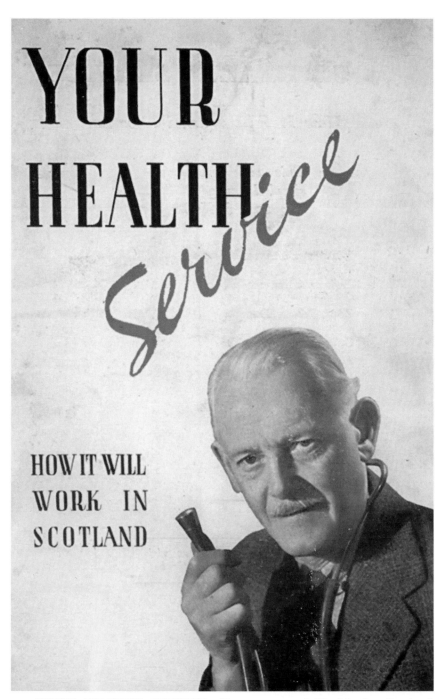

19. YOUR HEALTH SERVICE, Department of Health for Scotland pamphlet *(Lothian Health Board Archive)*

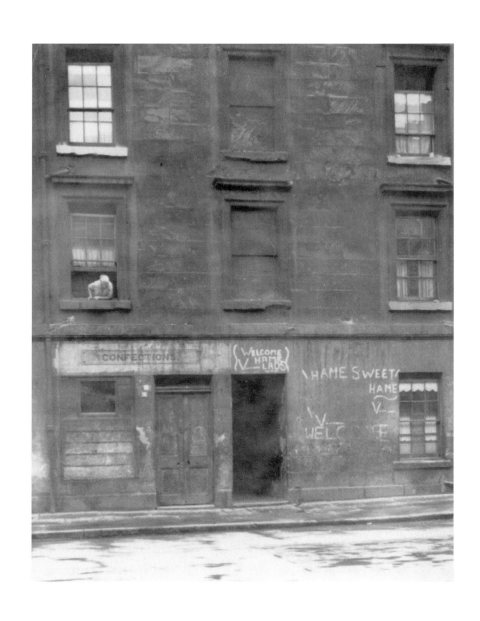

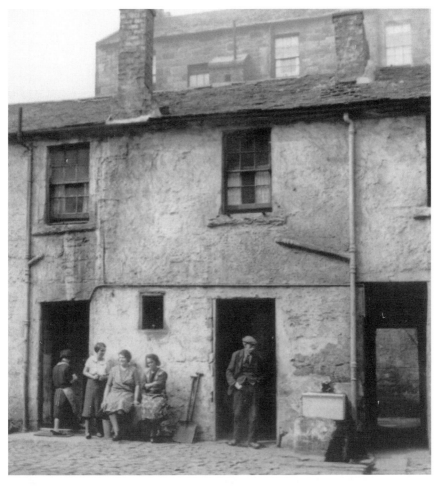

20. Post-war tenement, Glasgow, 1945 (left) *(Mitchell Library, Glasgow)*

21. Behind the tenement, 1945 (above) *(Mitchell Library, Glasgow)*

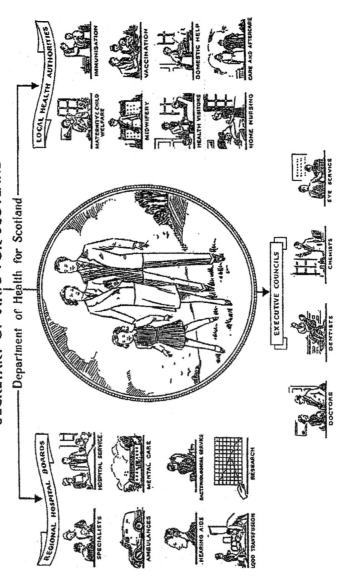

22. Pictorial plan of the National Health Service in Scotland, from Department of Health for Scotland pamphlet (*Lothian Health Board Archive*)

a) Infant Mortality

The high infant mortality that accompanied the industrialisation of the country reached its peak in the 1870s. In Scotland, the Infant Mortality Rate (IMR),[57] even at worst, as in Dundee and Glasgow, was never as high as it was in England at that time. In the last decades the IMR declined, rapidly in England, more slowly in Scotland. By 1910 the rate was equal in the two countries. But that rate was still enormous at approximately 110 per thousand live births.[58]

For the greater part of the nineteenth century this loss of life was accepted with some equanimity. But towards the end of the century, as the birth rate began to fall, there were fears that a reduction in population must inevitably reduce the strength of the nation. The high IMR now attracted more anxious attention. The association of a high infant mortality with poor living conditions was well known.[59] It was a contemporary view that the cause of so many infant deaths was 'in two words, poverty and ignorance.'[60] Voluntary bodies were set up in Scotland, supported in a number of cases by a grant from the local authority, to offer support to young mothers in need. It became clear that, against this background of poor social conditions, the greatest immediate cause of death of infants was the summer plague of infective diarrhoea. A new generation of Medical Officers of Health with training in the new discipline of bacteriology focused their attention on the control of this recurring epidemic. In 1901 William Robertson, the Medical Officer of Health of Leith, persuaded his committee to follow the example of the scheme in Fécamp in France, where free 'clean' milk was supplied and the health of the children carefully monitored.[61] The first Milk Depot in Scotland was opened in Leith in 1903,[62] followed by others in Glasgow and Dundee in 1904. These Milk Depot schemes were again dependent on voluntary workers.[63] Their success in preventing deaths was not measured.

Useful statistics on the survival of infants only became available a few years later. For many years it had been known that many infant deaths,

---

57 The number of deaths under one year per thousand live births.

58 *Annual Abstract of Statistics.*

59 In Edinburgh at the beginning of the century the IMR was 38 in Morningside, 54 in Newington, 102 in Haymarket and 344 in the Cowgate. A. D. Fordyce, *The Care of Infants and Young Children* (Edinburgh, 1911), p. 62.

60 *Ibid.*, p. 57.

61 W. S. Craig, *Child and Adolescent Life in Health and Disease* (Edinburgh, 1946), p. 158.

62 The first in the UK was at St Helens in 1899.

63 O. Checkland and M. Lamb (eds.), *Health Care as Social History: The Glasgow Case* (Aberdeen, 1982), p. 123.

especially among the illegitimate and those that had fallen victim to baby farming,[64] went unrecorded. A. K. Chalmers, Medical Officer of Health in Glasgow, led a campaign that led to the Notification of Births Act of 1907. This new evidence prompted Edinburgh to appoint its first official health visitor, and by 1910 this single official was assisted by 300 volunteers.[65] To varying degrees other local authorities in Scotland followed this lead.

In the early years of the First World War many young mothers found employment in industry. The IMR rose to 125.5, reversing the earlier trend:

> The overcrowding of houses, the urgency of labour demand, the stresses of the labour required, the ill organised food supplies, the sporadic provision for sickness or injury or temporary unfitness – these and the multitude of derivative effects tend, in the aggregate, to destroy the life of the child and to make the life of the mother superlatively difficult.[66]

In 1915 the Notification of Births (Extension) Act made the notification of births compulsory. It also offered by a 50% grant from central funds to support Milk Depots and all other voluntary feeding schemes approved by the local authority. Local authorities were empowered to 'make such arrangements as they think fit and as may be sanctioned by us, for the attending to the health of expectant mothers and nursing mothers and of children under the age of five years.' Local authorities differed widely in their willingness to devote scarce financial resources to this new enterprise and a number of local schemes had again to rely on voluntary support.[67] At the end of the war this growing service was put on a more professional footing. Numbers of well-trained nurses, released from war service, found an opportunity to continue their nursing careers as health visitors.

In 1920 the new Scottish Board of Health laid down guidelines for a more uniform Maternal and Child Welfare service. Local authorities were encouraged to develop domiciliary services for expectant and nursing mothers and children up to the age of five, based on Maternity and Child Welfare Centres. Some medical treatment and milk and food for mother and child were to be available but the emphasis was to be on instruction in the general hygiene of maternity and childhood and given in the home. Midwifery and a medical service for disorders of pregnancy and the newborn were to be set up where they were not already provided by

---

64 Parents of illegitimate infants could pay up to £20 to a 'baby minder' to assume total responsibility for the child.

65 H. P. Tait, *A Doctor and two Policemen: The History of the Edinburgh Public Health Department* (Edinburgh, 1997), p. 83.

66 W. L. Mackenzie, *Scottish Mothers and Children* (Dunfermline, 1917), p. 17.

67 The last voluntary health visitors retired in 1948.

other agencies. Wherever possible, local authorities were to provide day nurseries, play centres and children's gardens.

The Act stated frankly that 'all local authorities can not be expected to make provision of all these services.' By the end of 1920 there were 165 child welfare centres and 1,162 health visitors; maternity and child welfare schemes had been set up in the districts of local authorities representing 83% of the population. However, in 1932 not all schemes were complete and further progress had been halted. The Scottish Health Board reported that 'owing to the national financial situation' it had been forced 'to discourage local authorities from entering into new commitments for extending maternity and child welfare services.'[68] By 1936 the number of health visitors (now including school nurses) had fallen to 1085, of whom only 462 were full-time. Of the 254 Maternity and Child Welfare Centres, 14 were entirely voluntary bodies and many others were still dependent on voluntary assistance. A number of unsatisfactory health centres had been closed and no new centres were planned. What remained in 1936 was a small and poorly resourced scheme unable to provide an adequate service for Scotland's 410,095 children under five. It was also unevenly distributed. In Glasgow local authority services for infants and young children were well organised, adequately funded and fully professional.[69] But, except in a few of the large local authority areas, much of the service in Scotland remained part-time, amateurish and rudimentary.

Nevertheless, as Cathcart reported, the death rate of children under five had almost halved over the previous 15 years; the IMR had fallen from 110 at the end of the war to 77. The improvement was attributed, to an extent, to the control of infections but undoubtedly the major factor had been the improvement in living conditions. In Scotland, the worst infant mortality rates were not in the great cities but in the industrialised counties (Renfrew IMR, 85) and in the industrial burghs (Coatbridge IMR, 94). It is possible that the lower mortality achieved in the large towns should be attributed to their more effectively organised and financed Maternity and Child Welfare Services.

In 1936 the Cathcart Committee found that, overall, the domiciliary nursing and medical services for infants were inadequate. There were also many 'serious gaps' in the clinic arrangements for children under five. It recommended that out-patient clinic arrangements for children under five should be combined with those for schoolchildren in a single local authority service for children of every age.

68 *Annual Report of the Board of Health for Scotland*, 1923, Cmd. 2156, p. 52.
69 Checkland and Lamb, *op. cit.*, p. 131.

b) Maternity Services

In the mid-1930s the loss of young mothers from the disorders of childbirth had become a scandal.[70] The Maternal Mortality Rate (MMR)[71] hardly reflected the extent of the problem; it did not reveal the volume of persisting disability and ill health that often followed delivery or the devastation of the families when the mother died.[72] In 1880 maternal mortality had been high in all social classes and particularly high in the lying-in hospitals where the death rate could be up to ten times that for deliveries at home. The introduction of first, antiseptic techniques and then asepsis brought a general reduction in deaths from puerperal sepsis and a spectacular reduction in maternal deaths in hospital practice. By 1900 the risk of puerperal sepsis was, for the first time, less in hospitals than in home deliveries. It was assumed that maternal mortality could be further reduced by more rigorous and more general application of best hospital practices. The Midwives Act of 1902 was intended to ensure that hospital trained midwives would be more generally available for deliveries at home.

Contrary to expectation, the Maternal Mortality Rate began to increase. In Scotland the MMR in the first decade of the century had averaged 5.6; by 1918 it had risen to 7 and continued in the next decade. The mortality figures for England were also alarming; in 1908 the overall MMR was 5.02 rising to 7.6 in 1918. In 1928 the British College of Obstetricians and Gynaecologists[73] was founded with a view to improving the standard of obstetric care. However, more intensive management of the delivery did not prove to be the answer. In 1933 a scheme in Rhondda that increased the part played by doctors in the management of the delivery conspicuously failed to improve the MMR. In 1935 the *Report on Maternal Morbidity and Mortality in Scotland* made the disconcerting judgements that: 'the general level of ante-natal care is unsatisfactory' and 'there is no doubt that one of the most disquieting features of present-day obstetrics is hurried and unnecessarily meddlesome midwifery.'[74]

From 1918 the MMR in Scotland continued to rise while in England it remained more or less stationary. In retrospect it is possible to offer a partial explanation of the greater problem in Scotland in the 1930s. In Scotland

70 I. Loudon, 'Some International Features of Maternal Mortality', in V. Fildes, L. Marks and H. Marland (eds.), *Women and Children First* (London, 1992), p. 10.
71 The number of deaths in pregnancy, delivery and the postnatal period per 1,000 births.
72 The problems were not unique to Britain The scandal affected most of Western Europe and the United States.
73 The predecessor of the Royal College of Obstetricians and Gynaecologists, founded in 1938.
74 *Report on Maternal Morbidity and Mortality in Scotland, op. cit.,* p. 16.

there was a higher proportion of 'at risk' pregnancies. The risks of pregnancy increase with maternal age and with the number of previous pregnancies, and both these factors were greater in Scotland at this time. (Birth rates for mothers aged 30–34 were 98.2 in Scotland compared with 81.4 for England and 60.42 between the ages of 35–39 in Scotland compared with 46.6 for England.) From the late 1930s the proportion of 'high risk' pregnancies in Scotland became smaller as the average family size became smaller and the average age of mothers became less. There was a corresponding fall in the MMR.

Nevertheless the MMR was still unacceptably high. Poverty, poor social conditions and inadequate antenatal care were the major factors. In the early years of the century the importance of a proper diet for the mother during her pregnancy had been described in Edinburgh and in Glasgow.[75] An experiment in Rhondda in 1935 again showed that the distribution of food to the women attending antenatal clinics could cause a dramatic fall in the MMR.

In part the high MMR in the 1930s was attributed to poverty and poor nutrition. It had also become evident that the meddlesome midwifery practised by general practitioners was less safe than management by a trained midwife. It had been found that in industrial areas general practitioners, in their daily practice, frequently dressed wounds infected by the streptococcus and carried the infection to their obstetric patients.[76]

When Cathcart reported, Scotland's MMR was still high at 6.2. In 1935 the Ministry of Health was satisfied with the overall rate for England and Wales (MMR 4) but launched investigations of the relatively poor rates in Lancashire and West Yorkshire and the burghs of Halifax and Rochdale. In Scotland, the worst rates were in the county of Renfrew (MMR 8.5) and in the burgh of Coatbridge (MMR 12).

Without a clear and full understanding of the problem Cathcart advocated the creation of a new comprehensive maternity service. In face of considerable evidence, it was recommended that the general practitioners should be central to the scheme, giving continuous supervision throughout pregnancy, delivery and puerperium and acting in co-operation with local authority clinics staffed by fully trained midwives and at which consultant advice and diagnostic services would be available. Hospital facilities were also to be improved with all obstetric units large enough to justify the employment of a resident medical officer. Since particular reliance was to be

75 J. W. Ballantyne, *Manual of Antenatal Pathology and Hygiene* (Edinburgh, 1904) and A. K. Chalmers, *Proceedings of the National Conference on Infant Mortality* (Liverpool, 1914).
76 G. Geddes, *Statistics of Puerperal Sepsis and Allied Infectious Diseases* (Bristol, 1912).

placed on midwives, it was recommended that their remuneration, conditions of service and status should be improved.

Cathcart also made the somewhat controversial recommendation that the local authority maternity service should include advice on contraception.

National Health Insurance

The National Health Insurance scheme came as a sudden and unexpected diversion from what was then thought to be a promising movement towards the development of state medical services. The Royal Commission on the Poor Laws and the Relief of Distress, set up in 1905, was intended to meet rising public concern over the increasing burden of pauperism by strengthening the existing provision for its management under the Poor Law. When the Commission reported in 1909, the Majority Report was in line with this intention. A Minority Report, however, called for the abolition of the Poor Law and all its services. It proposed the creation of a new state medical service that would serve a very much greater section of society.[77] This proposal had powerful support from the government's chief medical advisers, George Newman, Chief Medical Officer of the Board of Education, Robert Morant, its Secretary, and Arthur Newsholme, the recently appointed Chief Medical Officer of the Local Health Board.[78]

The Minority Report was welcomed in Scotland. *The Edinburgh Medical Journal* argued in its support:

> Of the fourteen Commissioners who signed the Majority Report five signed it with not unimportant reservations . . . The Minority Report is signed by four unanimous Commissioners. Counting heads is not a final test of authority. In two recent Royal Commissions within the last twelve years Minority Reports became the accepted reports of the general public and if unity of purpose and closeness of analysis are to count for anything, the Minority Report has all these.[79]

The *Edinburgh Medical Journal* went on to set out a plan for a National Medical Service 'analogous to State Education or the National Post Office.'

In England the response was slower. The *British Medical Journal* delayed its response until July 1909. It then supported the Majority Report for its own particular reasons. The *British Medical Journal* was a respected scientific journal but in its political sections it was the creature of the officers of the BMA who, in 1909, were struggling to become the accepted voice of the

---

77 At that time the Poor Law served only 2% of the Scottish population.
78 Sir A. MacNulty, *The History of State Medicine in England* (London, 1948), p. 71.
79 *Edinburgh Medical Journal*, ii, 1909, p. 209.

medical profession.[80] The Majority Report offered them an opportunity for power as the medical representatives on the proposed Medical Assistance Boards. But, as was to be the case on many occasions, the hierarchy of the BMA did not have the support of the profession or even of the majority of their own members. At the Annual Representative Meeting of the BMA in 1910, the officers were instructed to take the more progressive line of the Minority Report.[81] By 1911 the officers of the BMA reluctantly responded to these instructions and began to prepare 'for legislation along the lines of the Webb [Minority] report.'[82]

Then, suddenly, the full content of Lloyd George's National Insurance Bill became known at its first reading on 4 May 1911. Even to Sir George Newman, the Bill came 'out of the blue.'[83] The proposed National Health Insurance Scheme cut across the planning within the medical profession. The profession was already looking for a comprehensive reform of the country's system of health care that would address the great health problems of the country as a whole.[84] Lloyd George was coming from a different direction.

Lloyd George had been in consultation with the Friendly Societies and the commercial insurance interests since 1908.[85] His aim was the relief of poverty. He had studied the situation in Germany where Bismarck's legislation between 1880 and 1884 had introduced compulsory insurance of industrial workers against sickness, employers' liability in accidents and old age pensions. Lloyd George began work on a similar scheme of his own.

Lloyd George's Bill was complex and touched on many interests. Negotiation and consultations continued beyond the Second Reading at the end of May. As has been described in Chapter 1, following a last-minute amendment to the Bill, a separate National Insurance Fund and a separate Commission were established for Scotland.

From 1 January 1912, the Act brought in an insurance scheme, compulsory for persons employed under a contract of service in manual labour and open, on a voluntary basis, to non-manual workers whose annual remuneration did not exceed £160 a year.[86] In addition to a cash benefit (sickness or disablement) during periods of incapacity for work and a maternity benefit of £2 to be paid on the confinement of an insured woman or the wife of an insured man, every insured person was entitled to medical treatment

80 Appendix I.
81 *BMJ*, i, 1910, p. 273.
82 A. Cox, *Among the Doctors* (London, 1950), p. 85.
83 Newman, *op. cit*, p. 390.
84 *Edinburgh Medical Journal*, vii, 1912, p. 1.
85 B. Gilbert, *The Evolution of National Health Insurance in Great Britain* (London, 1966), p. 314.
86 Raised to £250 by the time of the Cathcart Report

by a general practitioner.[87] The doctor was required to provide 'all proper and necessary medical services other than those involving the application of special skill and experience of a kind which general practitioners as a class cannot reasonably be expected to possess.'

The cash benefits were administered by Approved Societies – usually Friendly Societies, Trade Unions or industrial insurance companies, often 'international' bodies managed from England. Each Approved Society was a separate financial unit, which, if found to have a surplus at each quinquennial valuation, could provide additional benefits either as increased cash payment or as additional medical services such as dentistry, ophthalmic services or additional medical support.[88] The statutory medical services were administered in Scotland initially by 39 local insurance committees (54 by the time of the Cathcart Report) under the supervision of the Scottish Insurance Commission. Every qualified medical practitioner in Scotland had the right to be included in the panel of insurance medical practitioners and to accept up to 2,500 insured persons on his list;[89] for each person on his list he received a capitation fee of 9s.

In Scotland the National Insurance scheme was generally welcomed although employers had some early reservations:

> The Chancellor of the Exchequer's great scheme of State insurance has had a very remarkable reception, which divides itself into two moods following a very unusual line of cleavage. On the one hand we have the politicians of all parties, the newspapers of almost all categories, and representatives of the working classes of all trades and grades, welcoming it effusively. There are, of course, the inevitable and altogether proper reserves. Details must be examined with critical care, actuarial wisdom must be consulted and deferred to, machinery must be closely scanned. But as regards the thing aimed at, the classes referred to are almost of one mind. On the other hand stand the businessmen. They cannot as a class be described as hostile, but their attitude is distinctly that of disturbance.[90]

There can be no doubt that the National Insurance scheme accomplished Lloyd George's immediate aim. It helped towards limiting poverty in the

---

87 There was also an ill-defined tuberculosis benefit that offered no more than was already generally available in Scotland. Braithwaite suggests that Lloyd George's concern about tuberculosis was the result of his own fear of the disease. W. Braithwaite, *Lloyd George's Ambulance Wagon* (London, 1957), p. 71.

88 The Post Office scheme did not accumulate such funds.

89 Few Scottish practices had lists of over 500. In 1913 the largest list, in Dundee, was 1,638.

90 *Dundee Advertiser*, 6 May 1911.

years of economic depression and unemployment in the '20s and '30s.[91] But the contribution of the National Health Insurance Scheme to the health of the nation or even of the working population was negligible. The scheme came quickly into operation in Scotland. With the exception of Edinburgh and four areas in the Highlands, panels of general practitioners had been set up across Scotland in time for the launch of the medical part of the scheme on 1 January 1913. There were already 102 Approved Societies in place and recognised by the Insurance Commission; 51 of these were new creations founded specifically to take part in the scheme. Further development was inhibited by the First World War. By 1919 the number of Approved Societies had been rationalised and reduced to 75. Some 21% of the population of Scotland were then contributing members of the scheme; of these contributors, 49% were members of Friendly Societies, 38% of Industrial or Colliery schemes and 12% of Trade Union schemes.[92] There were 17,340 deposit contributors. Over the years the number of Approved Societies was further reduced to 69. The total membership increased to 45% of the population of Scotland; the proportional distribution of members across the Friendly Societies, industrial insurance schemes and Trade Union schemes remained almost unchanged while the number of deposit contributors fell below 16,000.

By late 1930s the National Health Insurance scheme had extended to provide a service to a very large section of Scottish society. But that service was very limited and for many families the National Health Insurance Scheme had resulted in a reduction of medical care. Before 1913, many workmen, by a weekly deduction from their wages, had contributed to a works or other medical scheme that provided medical services for themselves and their families. Such schemes were displaced by National Health Insurance. Families now went without medical provision unless a second subscription was made to an appropriate special scheme provided by a trade union or other body or to a club organised by a general practitioner.

The service provided by the general practitioner for the insured workmen was limited by the Medical Benefit Regulations of 1920 which laid down that no insurance practitioner would receive payment in respect of any procedure that was held to be 'beyond the competence of a general practitioner of ordinary professional competence and skill.'[93] In a succession of rulings it was established that such emergency procedures such as appendicectomy, tonsillectomy, excision of tuberculous glands and other everyday surgery were considered to be beyond the ordinary competence

91 Gilbert, *op. cit.*, p. 452.
92 T. Johnston, *The History of the Working Classes in Scotland.*
93 *Annual Report of the Scottish Board of Health*, 1921, Cmd.1697, p. 153.

and skill of a general practitioner. For many practitioners in Scotland whose patients did not have ready access to hospital, these had always been regarded as domiciliary procedures. Since they were not financed by the NHI Scheme, the subscriber and his family still had to pay for such procedures carried out at home unless the doctor provided his services free.

A small proportion of the population of Scotland (4.4% by 1929) were entitled to hospital treatment as an additional benefit of membership of an Approved Society with actuarial surpluses. This very limited provision was thought to be tolerable since 'the great majority of insured persons in need of hospital treatment are accommodated in the large voluntary hospitals and are treated free of charge.'[94] However, for patients living at any distance from the main centres of population, treatment in a voluntary hospital was not readily available. For them, the restrictions on the services to be provided by general practitioners under the Medical Benefit Regulations resulted in a poorer service and many of their non-emergency surgical conditions went untreated.[95]

The insured population could have dental treatment, ophthalmic services and could receive appliances such as trusses, elastic stockings and other supports as additional benefits from their Approved Societies. The range of these additional services increased very little following their introduction after the war. The Approved Societies had been advised against using surplus funds to extend their services in 1913 and again in 1921.[96] In 1922 the need for further economies in public spending increased the pressure on the funds of the Approved Societies and prevented expansion of their medical benefits:

> The need for economy in the national expenditure was a special feature of the year common to all public services and led to an intensive scaling down of the whole field of National Health Insurance administration. Approved societies have accepted a full share of responsibility by shouldering till the end of 1923 the portion of the cost of medical benefit and related services formerly borne by special Exchequer grants.[97]

By the end of the 1930s, only 24.8% of the insured population were entitled to dental treatment, 25% to ophthalmic services, and 21.8% could have free appliances.

94 *Annual Report of the Department of Health for Scotland*, 1929, Cmd. 3529, p. 154.
95 Families were also liable for a fee when a doctor was required at maternity cases. The fee was usually greater than the Maternity Benefit from NHI and, in the working-class culture of the time, it was invariably paid.
96 *Annual Report of the Scottish Board of Health*, 1921, Cmd. 1697, p. 153.
97 *Annual Report of the Scottish Board of Health*, 1922, Cmd. 1887, p. 56.

The effect on the health of the insured population was also limited. In 1927, the Department of Health recorded an increase in sickness and disablement 'so continuous and of such magnitude as to cause concern among all engaged in the administration of these benefits.' The rising trend in reported sickness reached a peak in 1929 but accurate statistical accounting of the morbidity of the insured population did not begin until 1930 and useful reviews were first published in 1934. Reliable Department of Health statistics in 1936 showed that the total amount of sickness in the insured population had risen to the equivalent of 11 days for every insured person. The complaints being treated under the National Health Insurance scheme were 'not, in the main, those that were serious or life-threatening, but influenza, digestive disorders, rheumatism and skin conditions:'

> Much sickness is attributable directly or indirectly to general factors – housing, defective diet, poverty in the wide sense and the deleterious effects of occupational environment. Personal factors such as unhygienic habits, occupational misfits and maladjustments are not less important. Part of the high level of sickness can be attributed to the effects of unemployment which each act adversely though in totally different directions; unemployment when prolonged, leading to disabilities often of a psychoneurotic kind, re-employment producing such sequelae as accidents, myalgias and superficial sepsis.[98]

The increase in trauma (much of it associated with the increase in ownership of motor cars) was also presenting problems:

> The task of providing adequate treatment facilities for persons accidentally injured is rapidly becoming a serious problem. Violence accounts for approximately 10% of the certified causes of incapacitating sickness. This increasing accident incidence raises problems regarding provision for adequate, sometimes highly expert, treatment of the injured and the effect of the pressure of accident cases on available hospital accommodation.

In the 1920s and 1930s the Department of Health statistics showed no evidence of an improvement in the nation's health. In 1926 The Royal Commission on National Health Insurance[99] had recommended 'urgently desirable' extensions of the statutory medical benefits. In the prevailing financial climate these recommendations came to nothing. In 1936 the Cathcart Committee was more radical. In its view, the most urgent need in Scotland, both in the interest of the health of the people and as a matter of

98 *Annual Report of the Department of Health for Scotland*, 1936, Cmd. 5407, p. 15.
99 *Report of the Royal Commission on National Health Insurance*, 1926, Cmd. 2596.

administrative expediency, was that the services of the National Health Insurance Scheme should be extended 'to all classes in need,' on the same model, retaining the panel system, capitation fees and the part-time engagement of general practitioners, but administered by the state through the local authorities. It was hoped that this arrangement would be of mutual benefit to general practitioners and local authorities and perhaps improve relations between the two.

The National Health Insurance Scheme had not improved the health of the nation. That had not been the scheme's primary objective. Improvement in the nation's health could only have been hoped for, if at all, as an ultimate and long-term benefit. In the 1930s, the National Health Insurance scheme was barely able to fulfil the very modest role it had been given, to safeguard the workman's fitness to work and lessen the chance of his family falling into poverty.

However, the effect of the National Health Insurance scheme on the organisation of personal health care had been considerable. It had advanced the development of medical services in the United Kingdom. It had been administered separately in Scotland and had therefore been crucial in the separation of services in Scotland from those in England and Wales.

The National Health Insurance Scheme rescued the medical profession in Britain from the humiliations of 'contract practice.' In the NHI Scheme, the undertaking between doctor and patient was by mutual agreement, in essence, a private contract. The scheme offered reasonable security of employment and an income that varied from almost £250 for the average practitioner in a rural area to over £700[100] in a few large city practices. For almost all general practitioners in Scotland this was a very desirable package; some 2,000 had joined at once, long before the leaders of the BMA in London had concluded their battles over remuneration. Panels in Scotland were made up twice as fast as in England. At a stroke, on 1 January 1913, the great majority of Scottish doctors had become dependent on the state for their employment.[101]

The remit of the Scottish Commission was 'little more than a declaration of intent.'[102] The Commission could make whatever decisions it thought appropriate for Scotland, however. Since there were few established Friendly Societies in Scotland, the Commission promoted new County Approved Societies. It also adjusted the services and benefit levels given by the Approved Societies to local conditions in Scotland – 'sparseness of

---

100 Figures calculated from the First Report of the Insurance Commissioners, *BMJ*, i, 1913, p. 69.
101 They remained the lowest paid profession with the exception of teaching, and still, according to Bernard Shaw, 'hideously poor' (*Doctor's Dilemma*, 1927).
102 Gilbert, *op cit.*, p. 421.

population, difficulties of communication, or other special circumstances.' The Scottish Commission found its own solution to such problems as the position of share fishermen who were not clearly employees or self-employed; of farm workers who, by custom, already received some support when sick;[103] of Highland crofters who were both self-employed and employees. The NHI Scheme was important in the separate organisation of medical services for Scotland. In July 1936, Arthur Greenwood said, in a question to the Minister of Health:

> The social services that had been built up over the three or four generations were one of our greatest national achievements but they had not been conceived as a perfectly co-ordinated system. They had been built up clumsily to meet instant social evils.[104]

His comment came within a very few weeks of the publication of the Cathcart Report. It was an epitome of judgements made in the Report but expressed with a bluntness that would have been considered impolitic by the Cathcart Committee.

103 A difficulty that led to the incident described by A. Fenton in *The Turra Coo* (Aberdeen, 1989).
104 *BMJ*, ii, 1936, p. 204.

7

The Hospitals

I t was widely recognised during the inter-war years that there were inadequacies in Scotland's hospital services, due principally to a shortage of beds.[1] This had been the conclusion of a number of reviews carried out since the creation of the Scottish Health Board.[2] From its first years, the Board had encouraged the voluntary hospitals, the local authorities and the several medical organisations in Scotland to co-operate in making the best use of all available resources. It had become widely accepted that there must be a single deliberate and active policy in Scotland for the creation of a more effective hospital service. The Cathcart Committee was able to build on this consensus in producing its plan for the future.

In England and Wales there was no such consensus. There the development of hospital services had a history that made disharmony inevitable. Evolution over centuries had produced different hospital systems with very different priorities, causing rivalries and gross inequalities in hospital provision across the counties and boroughs. Although Scotland remained on the sidelines as interests clashed south of the border, the compromises eventually reached in the resolution of England's problems in the creation of the National Health Service were to be influenced by the proposals made by the Cathcart Committee for Scotland.[3] It was also inconceivable that Cathcart's scheme could have been put in place in Scotland without reference to decisions being made for England and Wales. It was highly improbable that Westminster would legislate for fundamentally different hospital services for two parts of the United Kingdom. The full significance of the recommendations made by the Cathcart Committee for Scotland is therefore best understood against the background of events in England.

Hospitals in England and Wales

The leaders in hospital services in England and Wales, in standards if not in

1 'Beds' in this context includes the staffing and equipment to service them to a satisfactory standard.
2 *A Scheme for Medical Services for Scotland* (MacAlister Report) 1920, Cmd. 1039; *Report of the Hospital Services Committee* (Mackenzie Report), HMSO 1926; *Report on Hospital Services* (Walker Report), HMSO 1933; *Annual Report of the Department of Health for Scotland* 1934, Cmd. 4837, pp. 91–97.
3 Discussed in Chapter 8.

numbers, were the large city voluntary hospitals. After the First World War their numbers had increased and England had become 'littered'[4] with small voluntary hospitals. These small hospitals had proliferated particularly in rural areas to serve small communities. Almost half of all the voluntary hospitals in the English provinces were of 40 beds or less.[5] It appeared to the Voluntary Hospitals Commission in 1937 that many of these small hospitals had been founded 'upon the mere whim or caprice of some person with money to leave.'[6] In many cases the donor's generosity had been encouraged by local general practitioners striving to prevent the loss of their patients to some larger centre to which they had no access to treat patients. After the initial endowment, it was often difficult to find funding for long-term maintenance. Local communities became saddled with institutions they could ill afford to support. Some hospitals flourished while others found it impossible to fulfil the obligations they had taken on themselves. The distribution of voluntary hospitals across England and Wales became haphazard. While there was overcrowding in some hospitals, there were empty beds in others. Standards tended to be poor as each minor hospital attempted to do the work of a major city general hospital in miniature. Hospitals often wasted money in equipping themselves for procedures they could not or should not attempt. In some areas hospitals had to compete to survive. It was not unusual for difficult cases to be accepted for treatment by 'specialist' general practitioners without the relevant training or experience.[7] On other occasions an appropriate specialist was not available since consultants in the English provinces based themselves in the large and prosperous centres of population.[8] The major voluntary hospitals in England's cities and large towns maintained the highest standards of care but in many hospitals across the country standards were at best uncertain.

While the voluntary hospitals in England were supported by endowments and donations, four out of five were also dependent on income from paying patients.[9] In the years immediately after the First World War there was a dramatic drop in income from all sources. It was the threatened financial embarrassment of the London teaching hospitals that, in 1921, prompted the Ministry of Health to set up a committee under the chairmanship of Lord Cave to investigate the financial position of all the voluntary hospitals in England and Wales.[10] Over half the

4 B. Abel-Smith, *The Hospitals* (London, 1964), p. 406.
5 The *Medical Directory* for 1935 lists 605 voluntary hospitals in the English provinces of which 280 were of 40 beds or less and only 42 of 200 or more.
6 *Report of the Voluntary Hospitals Commission* (Sankey Commission), 1937, para. 51.
7 *Ibid.*
8 The *Medical Directory* for 1935 lists twelve teaching hospitals with a total of 5,566 beds.
9 Hospitals receiving paying patients in 1935 are indicated in the *Medical Directory.*
10 *Report of the Ministry of Health Voluntary Hospitals Committee* (Cave Report), HMSO, 1921.

voluntary hospitals were found to have deficits on their normal income. Income from gifts and investments had suffered most in the downturn; their contribution to income had fallen from 88% in 1891 to 55% by 1921.[11] More than ever the voluntary hospitals were forced to rely on income from paying patients. As an immediate rescue package, the Cave Committee recommended a support grant from Treasury funds of £1 million for 1921, possibly to be repeated in 1922. A further £250,000 was recommended for upgrading and extensions. The recommendations of the Cave Committee were rejected. The Government agreed only to a once-and-for-all sum of £500,000 and appointed a commission[12] under the chairmanship of Lord Onslow to manage the allotted fund. The Onslow Commission set up area committees to advise on the local distribution of Government moneys and to encourage and organise appeals for additional funds in each local area. However, the local committees soon found that the £500,000 allocated by Government as a rescue package was more than adequate.[13] By 1924 it was clear that the Cave Committee had overestimated the problem; the revenue of the voluntary hospitals had not continued to fall as Cave had predicted. However, the managers of the voluntary hospitals persuaded the Onslow Commission that, to meet the increasing demand for hospital services, some 10,000 new beds would be required in England and Wales. Government was asked for a special grant to allow this projected deficiency to be made up by the voluntary hospitals. However, the Minister of Health, Neville Chamberlain, ruled that any further allocation of Treasury funds was impractical in the existing financial situation.

Since improvement of hospital services could not be achieved by expansion, Onslow hoped that the local area committees already set up by his Commission would be willing to remain in being to co-ordinate a more efficient use of the existing hospital resources in their areas. But few local committees complied. Although attempts at co-ordination among voluntary hospitals were made in a very few major centres,[14] in general the voluntary hospitals continued to work in competition with each other. The British Hospitals Association, formed in 1884 to promote the interests of the voluntary hospitals, was well aware of the dangers of indiscriminate and over-ambitious competition. But the Association was not well supported and hospitals were slow to join. As its Secretary commented, 'the hospitals consistently closed their eyes to danger patent to all except themselves.'[15] But slowly the provincial voluntary hospitals

11 C. Webster, *The Health Services Since The War*, i (London, 1988), p. 4.
12 *Report on the Voluntary Hospitals Accommodation in England and Wales*, 1925, Cmd. 2486.
13 J. Pater, *The Making of the National Health Service* (London, 1981), p. 13.
14 Liverpool, Manchester, Sheffield and Oxford (G. Finlayson, *Citizen, State, and Social Welfare* (Oxford, 1994), p. 240.).
15 Abel-Smith, *op. cit.*, p. 411.

came to understand that their future was under threat, and in 1935 the British Hospitals Association decided that there would be support for a commission

> ... to take into consideration the present position of the voluntary hospitals of the country; to enquire whether in view of the recent legislative and social developments it is desirable that any steps should be taken to promote their interests, develop their policy and safeguard their future, and to frame such recommendations as may be thought expedient and acceptable.[16]

While the voluntary hospitals were threatened by competition among themselves, there was also an increasing threat from a new hospital system. The Local Government Act of 1929 had launched, in England and Wales, a process of reform of local authority hospitals. The reforms had been long in coming. In 1909 the Minority Report of the Royal Commission on the Poor Laws and Relief of Distress had condemned the hospital services provided under the Poor Law as a grave public scandal. It had recommended the creation of a unified service to be provided by counties and county boroughs through their health committees. That recommendation was not followed. In the 1920s, in the *Lancet's* judgement, the Poor Law hospitals were still little better than the rubbish heaps of practice. In 1929 the Local Government Act, in line with the recommendations made 20 years before, concentrated the responsibility for public health and Poor Law medical services in the hands of a single local authority in each county and burgh. The Act also allowed each local authority greater freedom in conducting its own affairs. The system of percentage grants, previously given at the discretion of the Minister of Health for each individual local service, was discontinued and replaced by a system of block grants to be used at the discretion of the local authority. Local authorities were urged to use their new powers to improve their services. As a vital component of this improvement, local authorities were invited to submit schemes for the appropriation of Poor Law medical institutions administered by their Public Assistance Committees to allow for their upgrading as general hospitals administered by their Public Health Committees.[17]

Although there was a general awareness that hospitals now coming under the control of the new local authorities were less than satisfactory, in 1929 the Ministry of Health had little information on the true extent of the

---

16 *Report of the Voluntary Hospitals Commission* (Sankey Commission), *op. cit.*, p. 5.
17 Technically the Local Government Act allowed for the separation from the Poor Law of those services which could be discharged under other enactments such as the Public Health Act 1875, the Maternity and Child Welfare Act 1918, the Public Health (Tuberculosis) Act, 1921 and the Blind Persons Act, 1920.

problem. From the autumn of 1930 members of the medical staff of the Ministry conducted a survey of all local government hospital services in England and Wales. Their report was completed in 1935.[18]

In retrospect the report was unsatisfactory. Over the five years the Ministry failed to set clear standards by which services should be assessed. In 1932 the Ministry decided that it would be inappropriate to determine the number of hospital beds required in each local authority area on the basis of the size of the population to be served but it failed to decide on an alternative.[19] There was also continuing uncertainty about the standards of patient accommodation to be required of public hospitals. Only in 1933 was a committee appointed under the chairmanship of Sir Amherst Bigge to determine what should be set down for 'the treatment of disease . . . tak[ing] account of modern methods of construction.'[20] This committee had not completed its deliberations in 1935.

For their part the Local Authorities were slow to make use of their new powers. Improvements were expensive and borrowing required the sanction of the Ministry of Health. In September 1931, Ministry of Health Circular 1222 made it clear that, due to 'the difficulties in the present financial situation', consideration should only be given to schemes for the improvement that was so urgently required 'on grounds of public health.'[21] The financial situation eased later but in 1933–34 borrowing by Local Authorities for hospital improvements allowed by the Ministry was limited to £302,359, reduced for 1934–35 to £275, 701. Income from patients also seemed threatened by the changes in administration. The Poor Law local authorities could be sure that they would receive the appropriate payments from the patients, or from their relatives, for treatment received in hospitals under their administration. But the mechanism for recovering any part of the cost of treatment in hospitals appropriated and administered under the Public Health Acts was far from certain.

Apart from these financial considerations, many County Councils had other reasons for their reluctance to submit schemes for appropriation. As the Chief Medical Officer, Sir George Newman, explained:

> The problem consists essentially in converting a number of isolated units intended to serve portions of the county into a system to serve the county as a whole. In some counties the situation is complicated by the reluctance of patients to be moved out of their own area. The institutional care of the sick in the counties also differs somewhat from

18 *Annual Report of the Ministry of Health*, 1934–35, Cmd. 4978, p. 97.
19 *Annual Report of the Chief Medical Officer*, 1932, p. 168.
20 *Annual Report of the Chief Medical Officer*, 1933, p. 204.
21 *Annual Report of the Ministry of Health*, 1931–32, Cmd. 4113, p. 46.

the county boroughs, as in the rural institutions the number of patients with acute illness is generally small since they are usually sent into Voluntary Hospitals.[22]

By 1932, only 27 of the 97 boroughs in England and Wales had submitted schemes for the appropriation of Poor Law hospitals and none of the 48 counties. Over the next two years further schemes were approved for a further small number of borough and a very few county schemes.[23] In 1935 the Ministry reported on the total number of hospitals and hospital beds in England and Wales now provided under the Public Health Act and those still administered by Public Assistance. In Table 17.1 these numbers are shown along with the corresponding figures for the hospitals maintained by voluntary organisations.

Table 7.1 **Hospitals in England and Wales, 1934–1935**

	Local Authority Hospitals			Voluntary Hospitals	
	No.	Beds		No.	Beds
Public Health	326	57,129	General	663	49,673
Public Assistance	532	86,365	Specialist	325	22,283
Total	858	143,494		988	71,956

Sources: *Annual Report of the Ministry of Health*, 1934/35; *Annual Report of the Chief Medical Officer*, 1933

These bed numbers give no indication of the standard of medical care delivered by each of the hospital services. The drive for modernisation that was causing necessary expense for the managers of the voluntary hospitals was discouraged by most local authorities; many local authorities had not completely abandoned the attitudes of Poor Law administrators. As the *Lancet* pointed out, the municipal hospitals were also at a financial disadvantage in being unable to control admissions of, or to discharge, the chronic sick; they were therefore committed to the continuing expense of their long-term care.[24] Teaching hospitals also took every opportunity to shed their uninteresting and unprofitable cases to the nearest municipal hospitals. Although the appropriated public hospitals were now directed by medical superintendents rather than by masters, they continued to be under-funded and under-staffed; professional standards remained poor. Patients in the Public Health hospitals and their associated clinics were cared for by fewer than 500 full-time doctors with part-time assistance from a further 2,000. This was an impossibly high patient/doctor ratio. The

22 *Annual Report of the Chief Medical Officer*, 1932, *op. cit.*, p. 162.
23 *Annual Report of the Ministry of Health* 1934–35, *op. cit.*, p. 99.
24 *Lancet*, i, 1935, p. 888.

quality of medical staff employed was not good. Salaries were low, working conditions were poor and few doctors were unwilling to be 'first and foremost local government officers and doctors only secondarily.'[25] Nursing staff was usually inadequate; in many hospitals the ratio was one nurse to 13 patients.[26] Poorly motivated by their administrators, understaffed and inadequately equipped, the municipal hospitals did not deliver a good standard of care.

The overall figures published by the Ministry of Health in 1935 did not reveal the great disparities in the distribution of hospital services, voluntary and local authority, which existed across England and Wales. In the west the population of Devon was chiefly served by 34 small voluntary hospitals (average 44 beds) with only one public health hospital of 570 beds.[27] On the other hand, in Lancashire in the north there were 14 public health hospitals with a total of 10,975 beds and two Poor Law hospitals providing a further 3285 beds; the voluntary sector provided little more than half (7681) of the general hospital beds in the county dispersed in 37 small hospitals. In the east, Lincolnshire was served entirely by 14 small voluntary hospitals; Norfolk had no Public Health hospitals but a quarter of the county's general hospital beds were provided by a single Poor Law hospital.

In 1935 the reform of the old Poor Law medical services in England and Wales was very far from complete. Nevertheless the voluntary hospitals were now beginning to rally to the British Hospitals Association to protect their interests against what was now perceived as the growing competition and threat from the new local authority general hospitals. Ominously the Chief Medical Officer felt it necessary to urge that there was 'no reasonable cause of war between them.'[28]

In London the development of hospital services had a history separate from that of the services in counties and county boroughs. London was a special case.[29] Under the provisions of the Act of 1929 the functions of the 25 Metropolitan Boards of Guardians and the Metropolitan Asylums Board[30] were transferred to London County Council (LCC). The LCC, which had no previous responsibility for institutions providing in-patient medical care, now became responsible for a total (including infectious disease and mental hospitals) of 76 hospitals and over 42,000 beds. Antici-

25 E. Grey-Turner and F. Sutherland, *History of the British Medical Association* (London, 1982), p. 158.
26 *Annual Report of the Chief Medical Officer*, 1932, p. 164.
27 *Medical Directory*, 1935.
28 *Annual Report of the Chief Medical Officer*, 1932, p. 196.
29 Ministry of Health reports and all other relevant publications such as the *Medical Register* and the *Medical Directory* deal separately with London and the English and Welsh provinces.
30 The Metropolitan Asylums Board was responsible for fever hospitals.

pating the provisions of the Act, the LCC had earlier set up a new sub-committee of the Public Health Committee (later the Hospitals and Medical Services Committee) to undertake the 'gradual reconstitution'[31] of a number of their institutions to create hospitals of sufficient 'status' to offer a general medical and surgical service to the public in London. In 1929 the Ministry of Health accepted that the transformation of the Boards of Guardians' institutional services into a unified municipal hospital service for London would prove difficult due to the extent and complexity of the services involved. However, the new Public Health Committee for London was able to appropriate immediately 29 Poor Law hospitals (28,000 beds) and 12 Public Assistance Institutions (9,500 beds) for upgrading. A small number of other institutions (including a former military hospital) were also acquired by the Committee under a separate provision of the 1929 Act. Almost all these appropriated institutions were large, varying in size from 260 to 1,500 beds, and not of the standard that would be expected of a modern voluntary hospital. Many were 'antiquated both in design and equipment. Uniformity of staff was of course necessarily absent.'[32] As in the provincial local authority hospitals, there were deficiencies in the standards of the nursing staff, and doctors were few in number and generally without specialist training.[33] The process of upgrading these hospitals would be costly. Nevertheless, and in spite of the national financial stringency between 1931 and 1933, the LCC was able to begin a long-term programme of major works together with an annual programme of minor upgrading. The bed capacity of the local authority general hospitals was increased and further institutions were appropriated. New wards were created and 11 operating theatres and six X-ray departments were installed. Five hospitals were provided with some form of laboratory service of their own and five group biochemical laboratories and one histological laboratory were set up to serve all LCC hospitals. From 1932, whole-time staff became somewhat better motivated; although still under the direction of a medical super-intendent, they were allowed clinical responsibility for patients under their care. From 1933 part-time consultants and specialists were appointed on a sessional basis.[34] In July 1933 the foundation stone was laid at the LCC's Hammersmith Hospital for a new Post-Graduate Medical School which it was hoped would open in 1935.[35] In a further effort to lessen the distance

31 *Annual Report of the Ministry of Health*, 1934–35, Cmd. 4978, p. 54.
32 *Ibid.*, p. 56.
33 The Lambeth Hospital, for example, had 1310 beds all under the direction of a single medical superintendent who, although licensed, was not a graduate and had no higher training or qualification.
34 Consultants received a payment for each session of two to three hours work at the hospital.
35 *Annual Report of the Ministry of Health*, 1933–34, Cmd. 4664, p. 8.

between municipal hospitals and mainstream medical practice, it was arranged that Public Health hospitals would be opened to London's teaching hospitals to provide clinical experience for medical students. (Unfortunately the offer was not received with enthusiasm; by 1935 only six students had taken advantage of the arrangement.[36])

By 1935, although the process of upgrading was far from complete ('completion of the process could not be expected to take place in the short time which has elapsed since the transfer'[37]), much had been achieved. The care of the chronic sick was concentrated in 21 hospitals (6882 beds) administered under the Poor Law and the LCC could now claim to provide a service for the 'acute sick' of London in their 40 Public Health hospitals (21,000 beds). The service was not yet of high quality. Teaching hospitals still took every opportunity to shed their unwanted cases to the nearest local authority hospitals. (The London Hospital, for example, discharged cases to the old Poor Law hospitals now re-incarnated and renamed St. Peter's, St. Andrew's and St. Leonard's Hospitals.)[38] Employment by the local authority still did not attract the best medical staff. Understandably Public Health hospitals were not popular with the public. Not only was the standard of care seen to be poor but also patients were liable to pay for treatment on the basis of a means test, a process most working-class people found highly objectionable. Nevertheless the service was improving and growing; LCC general hospitals now provided more beds per head of population than the combined resources of the voluntary and Public Health hospitals provided across England and Wales.[39]

In London, hospitals were not only part of a public service, they could also be entrepreneurial businesses and a form of charity. Excluding the great teaching hospitals in 1935, there were 82 small general and special hospitals; 17 were supported entirely as charities; 65 provided services for paying patients.[40] Although the voluntary hospitals attracted many of their patients from outside London, they were nevertheless threatened by the growth of the LCC's municipal hospitals which were increasing in sophistication and already had almost twice as many beds.[41] Although under the Local Government Act of 1929 the voluntary hospitals were allowed representation on the local authority committees responsible for development of

36 *Ibid.*
37 *Annual Report of the Ministry of Health*, 1934–35, Cmd. 4978, p. 66.
38 A. E. Clark-Kennedy, *The London* (London, 1963), p. 236.
39 LCC public hospitals provided 5 beds per thousand of the population of the County of London; the number provided by voluntary and public health hospitals in England and Wales was 3.8.
40 *Medical Directory*, 1935.
41 The total number of general, maternity and special beds in England and Wales was 13,000.

London's Public Health hospitals in their districts, this was thought to be a sufficient safeguard against encroachment. In 1935 the voluntary hospitals looked to the London Regional Committee of the British Hospitals Association to protect their interests.

The London teaching hospitals were a separate case. They were not part of the LCC hospital service. Nor did they belong comfortably to the company of the small voluntary hospitals in London or in the provinces of England and Wales.[42] These twelve independent institutions had long histories and distinguished reputations but for a time at the end of the First World War even they were financially unsound. Income had increased since 1913 but operating costs had risen by at least twice as much.[43] The London Hospital and King's College Hospital were forced to close beds; the Middlesex and St George's could only finance two-thirds of their expenditure from income. It was their temporary financial embarrassment that had prompted the Ministry of Health to set up the Cave Committee, and they shared in the financial help secured by the Committee. But in the crisis they also sought their own salvation. Patients were required to contribute to their care in accordance with their means, and private wards were added. In one year between 1920 and 1921 the contribution of patients' payments to income rose from 10% to 25%. Paying patients were recruited from outside London and by 1931 their charges made up 37% of total income. Each hospital had its own fundraising campaign, usually chaired by a member of the aristocracy (e.g. Viscount Connaught at Guy's, Lord Knutsford at the London). Some received large private donations such as Lord Nuffield's gift of a new block at Guy's. By the early 1930s the London teaching hospitals were again prospering. In 1933 the Westminster Hospital abandoned its pre-war plans to move to Wandsworth or Clapham and in 1935 opened a new hospital on its old site close to Harley Street. The Middlesex Hospital rebuilt on its central site at a cost of a million and a half pounds in 1935 and St George's planned to do the same. By the mid-1930s the London teaching hospitals were in good heart and had confirmed their presence 'near the fashionable centres of consulting practice.'[44] Uniquely supported by the City, The King's Fund, the Royal Colleges, the House of Lords and with ready access to Ministers, the London teaching hospitals saw no reason to throw in their lot with the voluntary hospitals as a whole. When a

---

42 Teaching hospitals in nine provincial centres did maintain a marsupial connection with the London teaching hospitals, sharing, to some extent, their aspirations and attitudes.

43 The Prince of Wales commented that: 'these hospitals will still have to keep up their income at a figure nearly two and a half times what it was before the end of the war.' H. C. Cameron, *Mr Guy's Hospital* (London, 1954), p. 389.

44 Abel-Smith, *op. cit*, p. 408.

committee (London Voluntary Hospitals Committee) was set up at the prompting of the King Edward's Hospital Fund for London to represent the interests of all the voluntary hospitals, the teaching hospitals insisted on their own special representation through the Conference of Teaching Hospitals.

By 1935 the teaching hospitals, the other voluntary hospitals and the LCC were all prospering to a degree not shared in the provinces. All recognised that change was inevitable, but there was no coming together of minds. As Pater, at the time an official at the Ministry of Health and an 'insider' witness to events, has recorded, between the voluntary hospitals and the local authorities 'the climate was not so much that of co-operation as of cold war.'[45]

This uncertain progress towards an efficient hospital service for England and Wales was soon to be disrupted by preparations for war. But by then the Ministry of Health had come to its own view of the way forward. Before his death in 1920, Sir Robert Morant, the Ministry's first Permanent Secretary had prepared a memorandum[46] setting out a plan for the future. In Morant's plan, conceived when the voluntary hospitals were in financial difficulty, it was assumed that voluntary hospitals were doomed and that all future hospital provision would inevitably be in the hands of the county and county borough councils, acting through health committees composed in part co-opted experts. By 1935 circumstances had changed and this plan had been abandoned. The Ministry of Health now accepted that 'co-operation between the local authorities and the governing bodies and medical staff of voluntary hospitals[47] is not merely a desideratum but an imperative need, and this is likely to continue in increasing degree in the future.'[48] It was proposed that local authorities should accept responsibility for the hospital treatment of all infectious diseases (including tuberculosis), for maternity, for children, for 'lunacy' and for the treatment of the necessitous. However, it was proposed that local authorities should be permitted to discharge these responsibilities, in whole or in part, by contracting them out to voluntary hospitals. This was to be the normal practice where treatment involved 'expensive materials, particular apparatus or highly specialised skills.'[49] For the Ministry, Sir George Newman advised that local authorities should not attempt to duplicate all the facilities available in voluntary hospitals. Since it

---

45 Pater, *op. cit.*, p. 16.
46 PRO MH 80/24.
47 In Morant's scheme influential medical input to management was to be through 'experts' on local health committees. The Chief Medical Officer suggested that doctors should have a major part in the administration of their own hospitals.
48 *Annual Report of the Chief Medical Officer*, 1933, p. 193.
49 *Ibid.*, p. 198.

was accepted that voluntary hospitals would not be in a position to provide for all acute cases, it was advised that local authorities should make provision for similar cases to those treated in voluntary hospitals but only where this was not to 'engage in wasteful competition.'[50]

In 1935 there were five distinct groupings – the London teaching hospitals, all other voluntary hospitals in England and Wales, the London County Council hospitals, the provincial local authority hospitals and the Ministry of Health – each with its own interests and its own view of the way forward. There was no consensus in sight.

Hospitals in Scotland

In Scotland the situation was quite different. By the 1930s the various bodies supporting and serving the hospital services had already established a habit of co-operation. The Cathcart Committee could confidently plan to build on much that had already been agreed.

Historically, in Scotland the state had made little provision for the institutional care of the sick poor. In 1919 the few poor houses that had been built since the middle of the nineteenth century came under the administration of the Scottish Board of Health.[51] The Board soon 'had under consideration the whole question of the accommodation in poor law institutions.'[52] Some older buildings were found 'unsuited to modern requirements' and were sold. Plans were made to transfer inmates out of some larger poorhouses to allow the buildings to be adapted for use as hospitals for infectious disease, for mental defectives or for convalescent patients. In Glasgow, the Govan Poorhouse was adapted to become the Southern General Hospitals, a Poor Law hospital operating as a general hospital alongside the city's three existing purpose-built Poor Law hospitals.[53] Consultants – physician, surgeon, obstetrician, paediatrician, psychiatrist, ophthalmologist, ENT surgeon, and dermatologist – were appointed to bring the Poor Law hospitals in Glasgow to 'a standard equal

50 *Ibid.*, p. 196.
51 In 1850 there were 21 poor houses (6058 beds) in Scotland. By 1900 the number had increased to 65. *Report of the Royal Commission on the Poor Laws and the Relief of Distress in Scotland*, 1909, Cd. 4922, p. 855.
52 *Annual Report of the Scottish Board of Health*, 1920, Cmd. 1319, p. 236. The efforts of the Scottish Board of Health to make better provision for the poor were aided by the Poor Law Emergency Provision (Scotland) Act of 1921 which as a temporary measure allowed parish councils to grant relief to the able-bodied poor. This power was continued annually by the Expiring Laws Continuation Act until confirmed by the Poor Law (Scotland) Act of 1934. Between 1914 and 1934 the number entitled to aid under the Poor Laws quadrupled.
53 Stobhill Hospital, Eastern District Hospital (Duke Street) and Western District Hospital (Oakbank).

to the best general hospital.'[54] A working association was established in Edinburgh between the voluntary and the Poor Law hospitals in the academic year 1919–20 when clinical teaching of medical students was introduced in the Poor Law institutions. In 1920 the Medical Research Committee (forerunner of the Medical Research Council) set up a unit in Edinburgh, at Craiglockhart Poorhouse Hospital, to work on infant nutrition. In 1928 the Town Council of Aberdeen had already assigned the town's Poor Law hospital as a municipal general hospital in the Northeast Regional Hospital scheme. This co-operative scheme had been founded in 1925 by Aberdeen County Council, Aberdeen County Education Authority, Aberdeen Royal Infirmary and the medical faculty of Aberdeen University to ensure that the most effective use was made of the medical services in the north-east.[55]

To an extent the Scottish Board of Health had anticipated the Local Government (Scotland) Act of 1929. Its successor, the Department of Health for Scotland, continued the reform of hospital service along the lines already set by the Board. The Department continued to insist that wherever hospital developments or reorganisations were being planned by a local authority, the local voluntary hospitals must be consulted. 'As a result of this policy, the relations with the managing bodies of the voluntary hospitals have become increasingly intimate and friendly.'[56] It was found that much of the reorganisation and extension could continue without recourse to the provisions of the 1929 Act. Glasgow Corporation continued to administer and upgrade its hospitals. Responsibility for medical care in Glasgow's Poor Law hospitals was delegated to the Public Health Committee but continued as a charge against the Poor Law. The success of the programne to 'seed' these hospitals with consultants from the teaching hospitals was later recognised by the establishment of the Chair of Materia Medica at Stobhill Hospital in 1937. Reform was already in progress across Scotland under existing legislation, and only the local authorities of Edinburgh, Dundee, Aberdeen and Bute chose to use the provisions of the Act of 1929 to appropriate Poor Law accommodation for general hospital use. In Edinburgh three Poor Law institutions were appropriated to become the Western General Hospital, the Northern General Hospital and the Eastern General Hospital; in 1932 the clinical professors of Edinburgh University were appointed as clinical directors and university staff were appointed for clinical and teaching duties in these hospitals. Maryfield Hospital was appropriated and upgraded in Dundee. In Aberdeen, Woodend Hospital

---

54 *Annual Report of the Scottish Board of Health*, 1923, Cmd. 2156, p. 172. The first appointments were made to Stobhill Hospital in 1923.
55 *Annual Reports of the Scottish Board of Health.*
56 *Annual Reports of the Scottish Board of Health*, 1923, Cmd. 2156, p. 172.

was formally appropriated as a Public Health hospital but still as part of the Northeast Regional Hospital scheme. In Bute, part of the Lady Margaret Hospital for infectious disease was appropriated for use as general medical and surgical wards.[57]

In 1934 the Department of Health completed a survey of hospital accommodation in Scotland. In all there were 449 hospitals and a total of 31,250 beds.[58] Of these, 179 (11,520 beds) were special hospitals for those patients – infectious disease, maternity, paediatric, orthopaedic – for whom the local authorities had a statutory duty of care under the Public Health (Scotland) Act of 1897, the Maternity and Child Welfare Act of 1918 and the Local Government (Scotland) Act of 1929. Still under the Poor Law, 55 mixed poor houses provided 3270 beds. In all, the local authorities administered nine general hospitals (3,880 beds) – four in Glasgow still technically administered under the Poor Law and a total of five in Edinburgh, Dundee and Aberdeen under the Public Health Acts. By 1934 all of these general hospitals had well-established associations with their local medical schools and were being assisted by members of their clinical staffs.[59]

The Scottish Board of Health and the Department of Health for Scotland had increased the number of general hospitals administered by the local authorities and had presided over an improvement in their standards of care. However, in 1935 most general hospital services[60] in Scotland were still provided by 206 (12,575 beds) voluntary hospitals.[61] In the main centres the larger voluntary hospitals were also the teaching hospitals of the university medical schools. Scotland's voluntary hospitals had grown up over more than two centuries, established and maintained by their local communities. As a result the distribution of hospitals and hospital beds in Scotland corresponded closely with the distribution of the people. Some 65% of voluntary hospital beds were in large hospitals, each with an average of 707 beds, in the four major cities. Some 22% of voluntary hospital beds were in the county towns and other large burghs in hospitals with bed capacities between 100 and 250. Six smaller burghs had their own hospitals with between 40 and 80 beds. The remaining 8% of Scotland's beds were scattered in

57 *Annual Reports of the Department of Health for Scotland.*
58 This did not include institutions for certified lunatics and mental defectives but did include Poor Law institutions with beds for the sick poor.
59 *Annual Reports of the Department of Health for Scotland.*
60 General medicine and surgery but excluding the new specialities, e.g. neurosurgery and plastic surgery.
61 Most beds were used by surgical services. Some 500 beds were allocated to maternity cases. The allocation of medical beds fluctuated according to circumstances.

small cottage hospitals of 6 to 30 beds in the most rural parts of the country.[62]

Scotland had no teaching hospitals as separate and independent institutions on the model of the London teaching hospitals. From their beginning, the medical faculties of Scotland's universities had relied for their clinical teaching on the great voluntary hospitals of the cities in which they were based. Scotland's hospitals came to fall naturally into a regional pattern. Four regions centred on the four great cities and their medical schools; the fifth was the more remote and diffuse region centred on Inverness, with the Royal Northern Infirmary as its central hospital but dependent for the most specialised services on the university centres. In 1923 the Scottish Board of Health had recommended that these regional formations should be formally recognised with committees appointed to co-ordinate the activities and development of all hospitals, voluntary and local authority, within each region.[63] This recommendation was not accepted and no statutory structure was put in place. But functional alignments continued to develop. Although unofficial, these alignments were well founded not only as pragmatic arrangements within recognised geographic areas but also on the personal relationships that were to be expected where the great majority of the medical profession in each area were graduates of the local medical school. It became the practice of the Scottish Board of Health and its successor, the Department of Health for Scotland, to recognise these groupings as functioning entities; in its Annual Reports the Department of Health adopted the practice of listing all hospitals by Region (Northern, North-Eastern, Eastern, South-Eastern and Western).[64] The value of these regional groupings between voluntary and local authority hospitals was recognised by Government in 1924. The Ministry of Health proposed that an inquiry to be conducted by the Voluntary Hospitals Commission in England and Wales should be extended to include the voluntary hospitals in Scotland. The Scottish Board of Health rejected this proposal since, in its view, limiting the inquiry to voluntary hospitals would prejudice its usefulness in Scotland and would be contrary to Scottish practice.[65] This was accepted by Government, and in May 1924 the Hospital Services (Scotland) Committee was set up under the chairmanship of Lord Mackenzie to review all hospital services in Scotland both local authority and voluntary.

The Mackenzie Committee remarked on the phenomenal increase in the

62 *Medical Directory*, 1935.
63 NAS HH 65/549.
64 E.g. *Annual Report of the Department of Health for Scotland*, 1934, Cmd. 4837.
65 NAS HH 65/50.

demand for hospital treatment, especially for surgery, since the beginning of the century.[66] The Committee found that in 1926 Scotland's hospitals were over-stretched: it was estimated that an additional 3,600 beds were required. The Committee recommended that the voluntary hospitals should increase their capacity by 3000 beds, financed half by the hospitals themselves and half by Treasury funds. It also recommended that local authorities should increase the number of beds for maternity and paediatrics (for which they had some statutory responsibility) by 600, again with support from central Government. Mackenzie regretted that the Poor Laws hospitals contributed so little and, anticipating the Local Government (Scotland) Act of 1929, suggested that they should be transferred to the administration of the local authorities, not only to provide patient care but to take a full part in medical teaching and research.

Scotland's hospitals were reviewed again in 1933 by the Consultative Council on Medical and Allied Services under the Chairmanship of Sir Norman Walker.[67] Walker brought together the recommendations of the Scottish Board of Health in 1923 and the MacKenzie Committee in 1926 and took their proposals to a further stage. Walker again recommended that the regional arrangements in Scotland should be formally recognised and that there should be a single hospital system in each region co-ordinated by a body representing each region's voluntary hospitals, local authority hospitals and medical schools. Walker stressed that such an arrangement could only succeed if there was equality in the equipping and staffing of Scotland's hospitals and uniformity in payment of staff and charges made to patients. While the Walker Report did not lead immediately to any administrative or legislative action, its principles were accepted by the Department of Health and adopted as the basis for its future policy.[68]

In 1935 Scotland's voluntary hospitals continued to be over-stretched. The problem is illustrated by the experience of Edinburgh Royal Infirmary, Scotland's largest voluntary hospital.[69] Like other voluntary hospitals, the Infirmary was operating at a deficit which had to be made good from investment income. Over ten years, ordinary income had increased from £107,200 to £128,649 (20%).[70] The cost of each in-patient had increased only from £7 10s to £7 18s (5%). However, the annual number of in-patients had increased from 17,024 to 20,695 (22%) and the number of out-patients had increased even more. Waiting lists had increased from 2,261 to almost 3,500. The financial difficulties of the Edinburgh Royal Infirmary,

66 *Report of the Hospital Services Committee* (Mackenzie Report), 1926.
67 *Report on Hospital Services* (Walker Report), 1933.
68 *Annual Report of the Department of Health for Scotland*, 1934, Cmd. 4837, p. 93.
69 LHB/4/122–138.
70 Income had fallen temporarily in 1929 and again in 1932–34. Ibid.

and the voluntary hospitals generally in Scotland, was not due to the rise in cost of modern medical treatment as has often been claimed. An increase in cost of treatment of only 5% could easily have been accommodated by a rise in income of 20%. The essential problem was the increasing demand for hospital services, not only for in-patient care but even more for consultant advice at out-patient clinics and still more for emergency treatment or minor surgery in the casualty department.

The increase in demand for hospital treatment had been first created in the second half of the nineteenth century by the new effectiveness of surgery improved by anaesthesia and antiseptic and aseptic techniques. Into the twentieth century the demand for beds in hospitals continued to be vastly greater for surgery than for medical treatment. As surgical procedures became more sophisticated, fewer could be performed in the patient's home (traditionally on the kitchen table). Patients and doctors alike looked more and more to the voluntary hospitals for all but the most minor surgical treatment. The operation of the National Health Insurance Scheme increased the load on hospital surgical services still further. Cases that might benefit from surgical treatment were discovered in increasing numbers as the insured population gained greater access to general practitioners. Even minor operations, which could have been competently performed in the patient's home by his or her own doctor, were not chargeable against the Insurance scheme. Cases were therefore increasingly referred to the nearest voluntary hospital where treatment was free. The increased demand for surgery did not only come from the insured population. The NHI Scheme brought general practitioners more into contact with the families of the insured, leading to the discovery of more problems to be referred for free hospital treatment; in the 1930s up to 44% of patients on the waiting list of Edinburgh Royal Infirmary were children awaiting removal of tonsils and adenoids.[71]

Voluntary hospitals in Scotland were prohibited by their charters or instrument of creation from recovering even part of the cost of treatment directly from their patients.[72] In 1935 Edinburgh Royal Infirmary and voluntary hospitals generally in Scotland were recovering from the lean years of the Depression although more slowly than voluntary hospitals in England and Wales. While income from legacies, donations and subscriptions increased well in line with increases in England and Wales, the increasing volume of free treatment was a drain on financial resources. In

71 LHB/4/124.
72 'In general the voluntary hospitals [in Scotland] have no power of recovering the costs of maintenance and treatment. Some are debarred by their charters or other instruments of creation from claiming any payment or are restricted to treating only the necessitous poor.' DH 8/1101.

England and Wales, where the great majority derived income directly from paying patients, voluntary hospitals benefited financially rather than suffered from the increasing demand for hospital care. Nevertheless, in spite of this disadvantage the Scottish Committee of the British Hospitals Association was able to join in the satisfaction of the main body of the Association when it reported that although the annual expenditure of the voluntary hospitals in Britain had increased to £15,000,000, income had increased to £16,000,000 and that over the previous five years £2,500,000 had been invested in new buildings. Sir John Fraser[73] was able to report that over the previous ten years the bed complement of Edinburgh Royal Infirmary had been increased by 16.9%. However, the waiting list had increased by 71.4% over the same period.[74] Sir John asserted that the 'opening up of the municipal hospitals' after 1929 had not helped to relieve the burden of an ever-increasing demand for hospital services. (Over a number of years Sir John had drawn particular attention to the new and increasing burden of casualties from traffic accidents; the cost of their treatment was only rarely recovered from the insurance companies.) The Board of Managers of the Infirmary agreed with the British Hospitals Association that 'the Approved Societies had not recognised in a practical way or to any considerable extent the services which the hospitals rendered to their members.'[75] The Chairman of the Board of Managers admitted that the increasing activities of the Infirmary were 'straining the financial resources to the utmost.'[76] Edinburgh Royal Infirmary's situation in the 1930s was not unique. It was shared by the other voluntary hospitals in Scotland.[77] In 1936 the British Hospitals Association welcomed the proposal in the Cathcart Report that the voluntary hospitals in Scotland should increase their bed capacity by 3,000 supported by a Treasury grant of £900,000.[78]

In spite of increasing financial pressure the voluntary hospitals in Scotland were in no immediate danger of becoming insolvent and looked to increased support from new public appeals.[79] In 1935 local authority hospitals were not in a position to provide the necessary supplement to the overstretched services in the voluntary hospitals. Patients in the former Poor Law hospitals were being required to pay for treatment as determined by a means test. This together with the social stigma still attached to

---

73 Professor of Surgery and a manager of Edinburgh Royal Infirmary.
74 *BMJ*, ii, 1936.
75 LHB 1/60/1.
76 LHB/1/70/29.
77 Histories of other voluntary hospitals in other parts of Scotland record the same situation, e.g. D. Dow, *Paisley Hospitals* (Glasgow, 1986) and T.C. Mackenzie, *The Story of a Scottish Voluntary Hospital* (Inverness, 1946).
78 *BMJ*, i, 1936, p. 42.
79 *The Scotsman*, 5 May 1938 and 31 December 1938.

hospitals that had not yet thrown off the image of the Poor Law made admission to local authority general hospitals very unattractive to patients. General practitioners were also well aware that, although local authority hospitals had improved in the few years since appropriation, they could not yet pretend to the standards of care, particularly surgical care, available in the large voluntary hospitals. Nevertheless, the Department of Health was confident that the hospitals that had been removed from the Poor Law would continue to improve 'as opportunity arises and would in time become an equal partner with the voluntary hospitals in a co-operative hospital services for Scotland.'[80]

The Department therefore regretted that, overall, the reorganisation of local authority hospital services since the Act of 1929 had been 'slow and, on the whole, disappointing.'[81] 'Years of financial stringency have left authorities generally with some arrears of hospital provision.' Reorganisation had been 'a slow business, often involving protracted negotiations between several authorities with conflicting interests and, it may be, long standing antipathies.'[82] There were still 3270 hospital beds in mixed poorhouses 'long out of date, and in most of them the lighting, the heating and ventilation arrangements are not adapted to hospital requirements. Few of them have proper operating facilities and the number of resident medical staff is less – often very much less – than in other institutions for the sick.'[83]

The Department of Health was very clear and forceful in its comments on future progress:

A rational reorganisation demands, first, a survey by each local authority of its hospital needs and of the resources it possesses or can utilise; second, collaboration with neighbouring authorities and with managers of local voluntary hospitals in drawing up a long term plan of development; and, third, consideration of each hospital need, as it arises, with reference to the determined plan. If a hospital service at once efficient and economical is ever to be built up in Scotland, local authorities will have to bring themselves, sooner or later, to planning ahead; to considering with their neighbours how wasteful duplication and overlapping can be avoided; and generally, to securing that every step they take, however small, will contribute to an effective service not merely for themselves but for the hospital region of which they are a part.[84]

80 *Annual Report of the Department of Health for Scotland*, 1934, *op. cit.*, p. 94.
81 *Ibid.*, p. 97.
82 *Ibid.*, p. 95.
83 *Ibid.*, p. 94.
84 *Ibid.*, p. 97.

In spite of the slow progress being made by the local authorities the Department of Health for Scotland remained confident that the policies set by the Scottish Board of Health, and developed in the Mackenzie Report and the Walker Report, would eventually prove successful. The Cathcart Committee did not propose any break from these policies nor did it consider it necessary to conduct yet another review of hospital services; the Committee accepted that the 'central problem is the inadequacy of hospital facilities.' As a measure of the inadequacy Cathcart referred, not to the number of beds in relation to the numbers of the population, but to the unanimous reports from general practitioners of their difficulties in arranging admission for their patients. Delay for acute cases was negligible but there were unacceptable delays in medical admissions for diagnosis and treatment and even greater delays for surgery. On average the delay for ENT surgery was 70.1 days, for hydrocele and variocele 62 days, for hernias 37 days, for gynaecology 35.5 days, for non-malignant tumours 29.3 days, for haemorrhoids 23.3 days, for gastric and duodenal ulcers 20 days.[85] Cathcart endorsed the policy advocated by the Department of Health and supported by the representatives of the voluntary hospitals, that it should fall to the local authorities to fill the gaps in the existing hospital services. In Cathcart's judgement the delay in achieving the co-operative hospital service planned for Scotland was mainly due to the 'financial difficulties' of the local authorities.

Cathcart recognised that the voluntary hospitals performed a great public service, had a fine tradition and enjoyed the confidence of the people. It was therefore in the interests of the state to avoid any action that would weaken their position. To ask them to meet the existing shortfall by increasing their bed capacity, even with the support of a capital grant from Treasury funds, would, in the long term, impose on them a serious burden of maintenance that they might not be able to carry indefinitely. In view of their particular dependence on legacies and donations, Cathcart proposed that the position of the voluntary hospitals should be eased by granting them immunity from legacy and succession duties and remission from local rates. It was also thought that they should receive a grant in support of their teaching facilities; this would be appropriate and would cost the state very little.

Cathcart also recommended that the Department of Health should be given powers to require, rather than to encourage, local authorities to bring their hospitals up to a standard that would allow them to take their full part in co-operative hospital service for Scotland in which one group of hospitals

---

85 Cathcart's comment has resonance today: 'The shortage has continued for a long time and it may be that in some quarters there is a tendency to get used to it.'

would not 'be regarded as inferior to the other and all the hospitals should be administered in the same spirit and should aim at the same standards':

> In short, the hospitals of all kinds, whether they are general or are limited to a specialism, whether they are managed by a statutory body or by a voluntary board of management, must be viewed as a whole and over wide regions; that must be regarded as one service. This conclusion is now commonplace; it is stated in much of the evidence submitted to us. To execute a policy based upon it, however, some adjustments of law and of administration are necessary.

The Committee agreed that an effective system of central supervision must be established. Something more was required than the existing statutory obligation on local authorities to 'take account of' the voluntary hospitals in any reorganisation or extension of their services. The Committee therefore adopted the proposal, made by the representatives of the teaching hospitals in Glasgow, that the voluntary hospitals in Scotland should be officially recognised by the state as an essential component of the country's health services and that as a corollary they should accept the supervision and guidance of the Department of Health for Scotland. The Committee proposed that regional hospital service committees, representing voluntary and statutory hospitals, should be set up by statute for each of the five regions in Scotland. These were to be advisory bodies to facilitate co-operation within the regions; all developments recommended by these regional committees were to be submitted to the Department for approval. The Department, in its turn, must maintain a close relationship with the regional committees. For co-operation between statutory and voluntary hospitals it was necessary to place both groups of hospitals on an equal footing. All hospital services were to be regarded as a public health function and completely dissociated from the Poor Law. No hospitals were to remain in the control of the Poor Law authorities.

The Cathcart Report drew attention to the differences imposed by history on the development of hospital services in Scotland and in England and Wales. The historic reluctance of the state in Scotland to provide for the institutional care of the sick poor had imposed on the voluntary hospitals the civic duty to care for the poor and to give greater emphasis to their charitable functions. It had never been intended, or even made possible, that the voluntary hospitals in Scotland should exploit any opportunity for entrepreneurial success. This was one of the major distinctive characteristic of medical provision in Scotland which, in 1919, were accepted as justification for separate administration of medical services. When the Ministry of Health was set up to administer services in England and Wales, a Scottish Board of Health of six members, none a civil servant, was appointed to be responsible for the 'co-ordination of measures conducive to the health of the people.'[86] The Board had adopted a pragmatic approach to securing an effective service for the community, accepting that the desired results could best be achieved by consensus and by nurturing every possible resource. The Ministry of Health on the other hand, under the domination of its first Secretary, Sir Robert Morant, was more ideological.[87] Morant proposed that the Government should do nothing to halt what seemed, in the years immediately after the First World War, to be the inevitable demise of the voluntary sector, while with the support of central Government, hospital services became entirely the province of local government. By the 1930s the Ministry, advised by its Chief Medical Officer, Sir George Newman, had reversed its policy. The voluntary hospitals had not continued to decline as forecast. There had been no need for the assistance proposed by Lord Cave in 1921. For the Ministry of Health, Newman now envisaged a two-tier system; voluntary hospitals were to be encouraged to continue to establish their position as the leaders in providing the best of modern equipment and the highest levels of expertise. However, 'the voluntary hospitals are not in a position to provide for all acute cases and the local authority is therefore compelled to make provision for similar cases to those treated by the voluntary hospitals.'[88] The views of the Ministry in the 1920s and again in the 1930s were widely known and were contentious. The British Voluntary Hospitals Association was suspicious of any encroachment of local authority hospitals on the services of its members in acute medicine and surgery. London County Council, now well on the way to creating a large, modern and sophisticated hospital service, resented the suggestion that the highest levels of service should be the prerogative of the voluntary hospitals. Most provincial county councils, on the other hand, were in no position to provide even the second-grade hospitals in the numbers proposed by the Ministry. The London teaching hospitals were unwilling to abandon any of their independence, their privileges or their unique financial resources. In England powerful forces were gathering and conflict was inevitable. As the discord continued and became more bitter in the 1940s, it did not spread to Scotland. In Scotland history had not created the divisions or the powerful factions that existed in England. Over the years a consensus had developed in Scotland and that consensus found its expression in the Cathcart Report. As will be discussed in Chapter 8, the Cathcart Report was not only important for Scotland but also pointed the way to a solution of the conflicts in England.

86 NAS HH/1/467.
87 Morant was a friend of the Webbs and Fabian in his outlook, but the Fabian Society has no record that he was ever a member.
88 *Annual Report of the Chief Medical Officer*, 1933, p. 198.

8

General Practitioner Services

The general practitioner was to be at the heart of the Cathcart Committee's scheme for the promotion of health in Scotland. The state was to be responsible primarily for the creation of social conditions and an environment that would promote rather than destroy health and to provide medical care through an efficient hospital service and specialist public clinics for all those whose health had failed. In Cathcart's scheme the role of the general practitioner (GP) would be as advisor to patients persuaded by a state programme of education to take full charge of the promotion and maintenance of their own health. The general practitioner was also to act as guide to his patients when ill, assisting them in taking advantage of the full range of available medical services. No longer was the general practitioner to confine his role to the management of the day-to-day failures in health of those in a position to consult him. For Cathcart's health policy to succeed it was essential that the new general practitioner services should be freely accessible to every member of the public.

In the 1930s the services of a general practitioner were beyond the financial reach of a great many people. This was not only a major problem in itself but also contributed to the failure of the local authority medical services. 'The statutory services presupposed that the persons concerned have the services of a general practitioner.'[1] However, the families most in need of assistance were generally the same families that could not afford the services of a general practitioner. The Cathcart Committee found that the advice given by the staff of the local authority services was often futile, sometimes because it was ignored, but usually because of the unaffordable cost of finding a doctor to administer the appropriate medical treatment.

When the Cathcart Committee was convened, the National Insurance Scheme made the services of a general practitioner available to only 40% of the population. In the industrial districts some employers, particularly in the mining industry and public works, arranged for deductions to be made from the wages of their employees to provide medical treatment for their dependants. In most areas GPs also organised their own schemes of 'Public Medical Service' in which regular weekly payments secured treatment for

1 Cathcart Report, p. 158.

those who were not otherwise insured.[2] Those who had lost or had never had medical benefit could, in theory, resort to the Poor Law for medical attention. In practice most of those who were poor and without medical benefit either received treatment from a general practitioner without payment or did not call a doctor except in extreme circumstances.

It had long been recognised that this fragmented and unsatisfactory arrangement should not be allowed to continue. In 1924 a Royal Commission was set up 'to inquire into the scheme of national health insurance established by the National Insurance Acts, 1911–1922 and to report what changes, if any, should be made in regard to the scope of that scheme and the administrative, financial, and medical arrangements set up under it.'[3] The Royal Commission agreed that whatever changes were to be made in the insurance system in the future, the general trend should be towards the development of a unified health service. The Royal Commission did not feel that it was within its remit to set out a policy for the medical services of the future but made it clear that, in its view, the principle of unification must be accepted. In February 1926 it proposed only some very modest changes, 'confining itself to the nuts and bolts of insurance practice.'[4] The deficiencies of the general practitioner service continued. A large proportion of the 60% not covered by the NHI scheme were unable to pay for medical treatment from their own resources. This resulted, not only in the failure to relieve distress and to prevent unnecessary death, it also left many disorders quiescent rather than cured. Since many of the untreated were children, the failures of the medical service created an accumulating store of ill health and disability in the adult population.

The absence of general practitioner support had its effect on the efficiency of the statutory medical services. Although Child Welfare Centres were not, and were never intended to be, clinics for sick children, patients were often brought to them inappropriately. Defects discovered at medical inspections by the School Medical Service were notified to the parents, in the expectation that they would arrange for treatment by a general practitioner; in the absence of affordable GP services many children did not receive the treatment prescribed.[5] The infectious disease hospitals also suffered; patients were often admitted at a late, even terminal, stage of illness as a result of a reluctance to call a doctor; other cases that might have been managed at home were admitted only because of the patients' inability

2 A general practitioner scheme set up in Airdrie in 1933 was typical. Medical attendance, treatment and drugs were provided for a weekly fee of 6d. *Glasgow Medical Journal*, cxix, 1933, p. 61.
3 *Report of the Royal Commission on National Health Insurance*, 1926, Cmd. 2596.
4 *BMJ*, i, 1926, p. 491 and p. 103.
5 *Annual Report of the Scottish Board of Health*, 1924, Cmd. 2416.

to pay for a general practitioner. The effectiveness of the Tuberculosis Service was reduced; a large number of patients went untreated because they were unable to retain the services of a general practitioner for the whole period of what was almost inevitably a long illness.

In response to these inadequacies of the general practitioner service, some local authorities began to expand their own services. Maternity and Child Welfare schemes, originally intended for mothers with children under one year, were extending to include children up to the age of five or more, and advice was accompanied by elementary treatment. The School Medical Service, which was required to provide treatment only for the 'necessitous,' began to bring a wider interpretation to 'necessitous' and there was increasing pressure for the School Medical Service to join hands with the Maternity and Child Welfare Services. Services provided under the Poor Law were also increased as the interpretation of 'destitute' was allowed to become more generous.

In 1932 the situation was exacerbated by the new National Insurance Act. In Scotland the Act deprived some 35,000 people who had been unemployed for long spells of their entitlement to medical benefit. Together with their families these long-term unemployed now increased the pool of people unable to pay for medical treatment. In Glasgow alone the number of able-bodied unemployed and their dependants entitled to Poor Law medical services rose from 20,000 to 96,000.[6] Many, almost certainly the great majority, were unwilling to accept the stigma of pauperism and to resort to free treatment under the Poor Law. Some found that their 'panel' doctors were willing to continue to provide treatment even after payment for their services from the NHI scheme had been withdrawn. But large numbers turned to the outpatient departments of the voluntary hospitals, putting intolerable pressure on their services. Local authority clinics came under pressure to provide treatments well beyond their proper responsibilities.[7] More patients with infectious disease could not afford treatment at home, creating a bed crisis in the hospital service.

In 1933 Sir Alexander Macgregor, the Medical Officer of Health in Glasgow, and Glasgow Corporation felt compelled to make special arrangements to meet what had become a crisis. A full-time service of doctors and nurses was set up to operate from clinics in the 'industrial' districts of the city, to provide free care for those poor who were unable to pay for

6 A. Macgregor, *Public Health in Glasgow 1905–1946* (Edinburgh, 1967), p. 144.
7 At a conference on the Public Health Services, Alfred Cox, later the Secretary of the BMA, gave a paper on 'The Encroachment on Private Practice.' He claimed that the local authority clinics and the hospitals were being abused and that the work could be done by general practitioners at less cost to the public purse. *Lancet*, ii, 1935, p. 1479.

treatment but were not officially on the Poor Roll. The medical staff was composed almost entirely of Glasgow general practitioners who already had some form of part-time appointment with the local authority but were willing to become full-time medical officers for the duration of the crisis.[8] At its peak this service achieved 72,000 domiciliary visits and 302,000 clinic consultations in a year.[9] This service was unique and beyond the means of other local authorities. In Scotland generally the distress of the 1930s had greatly increased the number of those for whom, for financial reasons, the services of a general practitioner were simply not available.

A New Role for the General Practitioner

The MacAlister Report[10] had already concluded in 1920 that the change from a 'system that dealt with aggregates and their hygienic environment' to a 'system that includes the medical care and treatment of individuals' that had begun in the early years of the century had not proceeded to any single or well-ordered plan. MacAlister advised that Scotland should, indeed must, have a general practitioner service available to all the family rather than only to the breadwinner.

After more than a decade no action had taken place on MacAlister's recommendations. In 1931 the Department of Health again drew attention to the lack of co-ordination in the health services and particularly to the 'difficult problem of co-operation of the private general practitioners in the statutory health services.'[11] The Department of Health convened a meeting with representatives of the local authorities and the Scottish Committee of the BMA inviting them to set up a small committee to 'pursue the matter in detail.' This was agreed and the committee began work in 1931. To the Department it had also been 'apparent for some time that there are fields of medical investigation in which the private practitioner could make a valuable contribution, and that something has been lost to medical research in the past by the failure to fully appreciate the practitioner's point of view and to utilise his experience.' A standing committee of the Department and representatives of the Scottish Committee of the BMA was set up in 1931 to investigate and keep under review the true extent of morbidity in Scotland. At that time the only statistics available were those extracted from the operation of the NHI scheme; it was now planned to improve the usefulness of these statistics by including the wider experience of general practice. By

---

8 In 1938 the munitions programme began to absorb the unemployed. The service reverted to its task of caring for those on the Poor Roll. It later provided the core of a geriatric service.

9 Macgregor, *op. cit.*

10 *A Scheme of Medical Services for Scotland* (MacAlister Report), 1920, Cmd. 1039.

11 *Annual Report of the Department of Health*, 1931, Cmd. 4338, p. 13.

1933, when Cathcart was exploring the possibilities for reform, the Department was confident that both its committees on general practice were proceeding successfully and their objectives were already in sight.

In 1931 the Department had reported that the vital and morbidity statistics were 'not so favourable' as they had been in previous years. Later, as the social distress caused by the Depression continued, health problems increased even further. The number of separate illnesses treated by general practitioners under the NHI scheme increased from 113,037 in 1930 to 400,052 in 1933, a rate of 227 for every 1000 patients insured.[12] The pattern of morbidity also began to show some new and disturbing trends. The continuing marked fall in the severity of and the number of deaths from infectious disease was no longer causing a fall in the death rate; the overall death rate was increasing.[13] The marriage rate and the birth rate had fallen to record lows but the number of attempted abortions was increasing, with a sharp rise in the number of maternal deaths from septic abortion.[14] A study in Port Glasgow, one of the communities most affected by unemployment, found that the health of the children was clearly deteriorating.[15] From Glasgow, the town with the highest proportion of its population on poor relief (17%) in the United Kingdom,[16] it was reported that an exceptionally large number of patients were being admitted to mental hospitals, 'most of whom were acutely ill.'[17] As the health crisis continued across Scotland, it seemed possible that, following the precedent in Glasgow, a general practitioner service might emerge on an *ad hoc* basis as, one by one, local authorities found themselves forced to set up schemes of their own. A second state general practitioner service would then have come into being, operating alongside, but independent of, the NHI scheme. Cathcart decided that a drift in that direction must be prevented since it would perpetuate the principal defect already found in the existing local authority medical services; operating under the constraints of local rates, developments would be haphazard, creating a service that would be uneven across Scotland as some areas went ahead faster than others. It was also foreseen as inevitable that there would be wasteful overlapping and friction between two state-supported general practice services acting under separate administrations. Cathcart found that:

12 *Annual Report of the Department of Health for Scotland*, 1930, Cmd. 3860, p. 193, and 1933, Cmd. 4599, p. 142.
13 Report from the Medical Officer of Health for Glasgow. *BMJ*, ii, 1933, p. 704.
14 *Glasgow Medical Journal*, cxxvii, 1937, p. 292.
15 *Glasgow Medical Journal*, xxiii, 1935, p. 8.
16 Liverpool came second at 11%. The rate for Scotland as a whole was 10.4% while in England it was 4.32%. *Reports to the General Assembly of the Church of Scotland*, xiv, 1935, p. 463.
17 *BMJ*, ii, 1934, p. 131.

The case presented to us for organised provision for the dependants of the insured is irresistible, both on grounds of national health policy and on the narrower grounds of immediate administrative expediency in order to maintain the efficiency of the existing medical services, and to obtain full value from them . . . We therefore regard it as imperative for the State to frame a policy to meet the medical need of the dependants of insured persons and others and to lay down the lines along which the medical service should develop.

Cathcart proposed that the general practitioner services should be extended on the basis of the National Health Insurance scheme which already served 1,900,000 people in Scotland and employed the vast majority of Scotland's 5,162 doctors.[18] Cathcart recommended that statutory provision for general medical attendance should be extended not only to the dependants of insured persons but should include all others in similar economic circumstances. Cathcart stressed that, as far as possible, the same general practitioner should care for the whole family and should act as its health advisor and liaise with the statutory health services. This idea had been well received when first put forward in the MacAlister Report in 1920. The Cathcart Committee therefore expected that it would again find support in 1936, especially since 'we were not prepared for the remarkable concentration on it, by local authorities as well as medical and other bodies, as the outstanding present need in any reform of the statutory medical services.' A call for an openly available and comprehensive general practitioner service was included in the evidence submitted to the Committee by the Scottish Association of Insurance Committees, the Insurance Committees of Edinburgh, Glasgow and Aberdeen, the National Conference of Friendly and Approved Societies, the Convention of Royal Burghs, the County Councils Association, and the Town Councils of Glasgow and Aberdeen.

The new role for general practice was also proposed by all the bodies representing the medical profession. The Royal College of Physicians of Edinburgh stated that 'the family doctor must, in the opinion of the College, remain the pivot of all schemes which concern the national health; his responsibilities should be expanded.'[19] This view was repeated in the submissions of the Royal College of Surgeons of Edinburgh, the Royal Faculty of Physicians and Surgeons of Glasgow, the Scottish Committee of the BMA, the Medical Practitioners Union, the Lanarkshire Medical

18 This figure, which includes 832 women, is drawn from the local lists published in the *Medical Directory* of 1935. Many doctors holding hospital appointments as specialists also acted as general practitioners; many who were essentially general practitioners held appointments at voluntary hospitals. It is therefore not possible to distinguish clearly between consultants and general practitioners.

19 Cathcart Report, p. 152.

Practitioners Union,[20] and the Society of Medical Officers of Health in Scotland. The Society of Medical Officers of Health stressed particularly the importance of the general practitioner in health education. 'To be efficacious health education should be as personal as possible. The family doctor would appear to be the most suitable person to undertake this work.'[21]

In Scotland, there was consensus among the representatives of all branches of the medical profession – general practitioners, hospital consultants and local authority doctors, not only on the place of the general practitioner but more generally on the need to 'make common cause' in the creation of a modern medical service.[22]

Employment by the State

Cathcart's scheme for an extended general practitioner service would only be possible if the practitioners agreed to accept employment by the state. Differing views on the preferred basis of employment were discussed in the Report. Some younger medical graduates were known to favour a full-time salaried service; in theory medical officers would be carefully selected and appointed within a career structure appropriate to civil servants. Full-time contracts would ensure pensionable employment with provision for periods of annual leave and leave for further medical training. There would also be opportunities for promotion. The advocates of such a service believed that it would reduce to a minimum any temptation to put personal interest before the interests of the patient or the service.

Cathcart accepted the contrary argument that a full-time service would militate against the full application of modern concepts of the practice of medicine. If a salaried service within the civil service was to offer an attractive career, medical officers would be in constant movement and promotions and transfers would involve frequent changes of personnel from one district to another. Medical officers, it was argued, would never remain long enough in one area to acquire the intimate knowledge of the patients and their home circumstances that would allow them to provide a service comparable to that provided by private practitioners. The suggested disadvantages of inadequate supervision and discipline were discounted

20 The largest of Scotland's many local general practitioner societies.
21 Cathcart Report, p. 155.
22 Ibid., p. 154. Historians have painted a different picture in England. 'Between the wars, when the foundations of the NHS were laid, the doctors were not united but split between three rival interests, each of whom hoped to dominate the emerging service: the voluntary hospitals, the insurance based panel doctor system and the local authority health services.' H. Perkin, *The Rise of Professional Society* (London, 1990), p. 445.

on the evidence of the Highlands and Islands Medical Service which had 'demonstrated the practicability of ensuring satisfactory supervision in a service based on contract with private practitioners.' It was further argued that in time, in a salaried service, contracts would be gradually adjusted and improved, reducing spells of duty, increasing periods of leave and creating more promoted posts. It was predicted that in the long run a salaried service would prove to be the more expensive option.

Cathcart concluded that the basis of employment should be, as in the National Health Insurance scheme, by contract for part-time services remunerated by capitation fees. The principle of free choice of doctor was to be preserved. This was considered to be essential in modern practice. 'Confidence between doctor and patient has become more important with the increasing frequency of psychoneurotic conditions and other ailments, the growing appreciation of early diagnosis and treatment and the function of the doctor as advisor on hygienic living as well as the treatment of disease.' It was also recommended that the training of the general practitioner should be widened 'to encourage the preventive outlook and equip him fully for the role of health advisor.' 'The need for change in medical training is widely recognised in the medical profession.'

Standards in General Practice

Cathcart's review of the general practitioner service was confined to its availability and scope; there was little reference to quality. No official or other assessment had been made by that time and the Committee attempted none. In general, the public seemed to accept whatever service could be found. But during the 1930s there were many protests in the correspondence columns of the *BMJ* and the *Lancet* from young doctors protesting about the impossibility of putting into practice what they had been taught in medical school.[23] Many of the more senior general practitioners echoed the despair of a correspondent to the *Lancet* in 1933: 'the more highly equipped a man is for the task and the more conscientious and thorough he is in his work the more steadily and surely will the conclusion be borne in on him that the labour he has been set to do is intolerable and beyond the wit of man to accomplish.'[24]

Much of the hankering for reform among the medical profession in Scotland came from this dissatisfaction with the standards then being achieved in general practice. Senior members of the profession had

23 A. J. Cronin, a Glasgow medical graduate, vividly described the limitations and frustrations of working-class practice in Wales in his novel *The Citadel* in 1937.
24 *Lancet*, ii, 1933, p. 265.

witnessed little evidence of progress in line with the advances in medical science. Recent graduates from the Scottish medical schools were frequently disappointed and disillusioned by experience as assistants in practice, particularly if that first experience was south of the border.[25] The only study to describe conditions in general practice in the United Kingdom in the 1930s was not published until 1950. The author, J. S. Collings, found that the little change that had occurred over the years between the wars had been for the worse.[26] He concluded that, during those years, general practice as an institution had been in retreat from the dominance of modern medical practice in the hospitals and the introduction and expansion of the statutory medical services since the beginning of the century.

On the situation in England, Collings concluded that the overall state of general practice was bad and deteriorating. In industrial areas where the demand for good medical care was greatest and most urgent, general practice had 'reached a point where it is at best a very unsatisfactory medical service and at worst a positive source of public danger.' While shortcomings were often attributed to the volume of work, this was judged to be a convenient rationalisation of an otherwise embarrassing situation. The working environment of the industrial practice provided no comfort or convenience for the patient, and the doctor was so limited by lack of space, equipment, and organisation that good practice was impossible. 'In the circumstances prevailing, the most essential qualification for the industrial general practitioner, from the standpoint of public safety, is ability as a snap diagnostician, an ability to reach an accurate diagnosis on a minimum of evidence, objective or subjective.' Treatment was more limited even than diagnosis. 'It is rare indeed to see a practitioner in an industrial area open an abscess, put in a suture or indeed undertake any procedure requiring sterilisation of instruments.' Medical treatment was usually the 'bottle-of-medicine' from a stock mixture. No records were kept. Relieved of responsibility for school and pre-school children, for antenatal care and midwifery, and more inclined to attend rather than care for the aged, the general practitioner was no longer a family doctor. Collings found that, broadly speaking, the doctors were of two types, the 'mercenaries' and the 'missionaries.' Among the missionaries were men of outstanding character

25 This comment summarises the views expressed in recorded interviews of doctors in practice at that time. Those interviewed on this subject are listed in the Bibliography.

26 The study was carried out by J. S. Collings, a research fellow in the Harvard School of Public Health who had graduated in medicine in Australia and had experience in general practice in New Zealand and Canada. His report was published in the *Lancet* in 1950 (*Lancet*, i, 1950, p. 555). Its findings were endorsed in a leading article that stated: 'The issue has been placed squarely before us.'

and ability who had gone into practice to 'do good.' Among the mercenaries were some who 'by our accepted standards, are judged undesirable.' However, mercenaries, with good skills of snap diagnosis, were, in the circumstances, more effective than the missionaries. Under the conditions of industrial practice even the 'good' doctor had little opportunity to exercise the humanistic, psychological and educational functions which were essential to good family practice:

> The important point is that this form of practice constitutes the pattern for most industrial areas, and the pattern is accepted by doctor and patient alike. It is far from the ideal of family doctoring on the one hand, and of modern scientific medical practice on the other; yet it is still wilfully identified with both these.

The pattern of general practice in rural areas of England was found to be somewhat better. At a distance from large hospitals and fully developed local authority services, the pattern of practice was determined largely by the personal choice and initiative of the doctor himself. Rural practitioners often undertook a high level of diagnostic responsibility. Some, especially those with access to reasonable cottage hospital facilities, could work to much the same level as a consultant physician. Others could at least equip themselves to a useful standard. But the majority adopted the same empirical methods as doctors in industrial practice. Similarly, doctors in rural areas could perform even major operations if they had access to a well-equipped cottage hospital, or minor operations in their own surgeries. Some rural practitioners continued to do some of the midwifery in their areas. However, in general, medical treatment tended to be on the same 'bottle-of-medicine' principle as in industrial practice. Indeed many rural practices were little different from a run-of-the-mill industrial practice. The greatest difference was that the rural general practitioner dealt with patients of all ages and not primarily with the working section of the community. The range of the work undertaken in different practices varied but the rural practitioner still approximated to the ideal of the family doctor. However, few rural doctors aspired to meet the demands of modern medical science and practice. Collings found that, in the final analysis, rural practice in England was an anachronism that had retained few of the virtues of the past.

In Scotland, Collings found that the quality of general practice was higher and he had special praise for the practices in the north and west which formed part of the Highlands and Islands Medical Service. 'This service enjoys a high reputation internationally as well as locally. It is held up as an example of a well organised medical service giving medical care of high quality.' However, not all rural practices in Scotland reached this standard:

There were some where the continued failure to establish and maintain standards of medical care, and the continued acceptance that general practice is good for its own sake, has deadened the critical faculty and sensitivity of the best general practitioners, and has resulted in the decline of standards of practice to a dangerously low level.

Collings found that the worst in industrial practice in Scotland was at least equal to the 'good' in England. Although the surgeries were as forbidding as in England, they were better equipped. Every practice had an examination couch; sterilisers were almost always available and instrument cupboards were well stocked. A conscious effort was nearly always made by the doctor to conduct some sort of useful physical examination. In absolute terms, these were by no means good examinations but they were purposeful and at least eliminated some dangerous possibilities. As a rule the minor laboratory tests, essential for reliable diagnosis, were done. Patients were not referred to out-patient departments with quite the same readiness and lack of inquiry or thought as in the industrial practices in England. There was also a conscious-ness of the need for records, and these were always kept in some form. In the practices where lists were full (4000) and the doctors were busy, there was nothing like the congestion or lack of organisation found in comparable practices in England. Collings found the influence exercised by the doctors on the family to be notably stronger and sometimes of educational value.

While the difference in practice in the two countries was principally one of degree, there were important differences in form. In Scotland dispensing practice had never reached the same proportions as in England, and the 'bottle-of-medicine' mentality had not been developed by the doctor or accepted by the patient. In Scotland the doctor had retained some respon-sibility for mothers and children and, in general, had remained much more the family doctor than in England.

But the greatest difference between the doctors of the two counties was one of attitude:

The attitude of most general practitioners to both local and central authority, as represented by city and county health departments and the Department of Health for Scotland, seems more reasonable and co-operative than that that of English doctors to the corresponding authorities there. Though it could be not be said that the relationships are by any means ideal, for the most part they were at least workable.

The explanation that has been offered me for this difference – that it is merely a matter of size – is not good enough. The relationships in country towns in England are often worse than comparable relation-ships in big cities in Scotland. There is a basic difference in attitude of mind.

This difference in attitude is reflected in other ways. In England discussion with general practitioners on the new health service usually centred on the size of capitation fees, the number of patients on the list, mileage rates, basic salaries, and so on, until it was steered into professional channels. In Scotland I found much more spontaneous interest in professional issues such as the quality of medical service, the relationship of general practice to hospital and specialist services, and the development of health centres.

I do not wish to give the impression that I am attributing all good to the Scottish doctor and all bad to the English. That is not the case at all. But there is an appreciable difference.

I was similarly impressed by the difference in attitude to general practice (in the two countries) among specialists who had thought deeply about general practice. In England there was little genuine respect for general practice or the average general practitioner. Much more respect was shown by the corresponding Scottish specialists, and their criticisms of general practice were almost always constructive and sympathetic. Similarly the attitudes of representatives of organised medicine towards the new service seemed to me more objective in Scotland than in England.

While general practitioners in Scotland in the 1930s had retained some of the traditional characteristics of the family doctor, even in Scotland the average general practitioner was not the doctor that Cathcart had in mind for the general practitioner of the future. To Cathcart, it seemed desirable that in a new service the working practices of general practitioners should be supervised.[27] And in preparation for their extended role as health educators, medical attendants and liaison with special services, appropriate changes in their training were clearly necessary.

The Prospects for Consent

Cathcart proposed that the general practitioner service should be developed on the basis of an extended National Health Insurance scheme. Since the scope of the medical services and the terms of employment of doctors in that scheme were uniform across the United Kingdom, it was inconceivable that Cathcart's scheme could be introduced only in Scotland. The necessary legislation, which could only be agreed in London, must be found accaptable south of the border. While there were sound reasons to suppose that the medical profession in Scotland would be very ready to accept the

27 Cathcart Report, p. 304.

proposed new role, there were equally good reasons to suppose that it would be less welcome in England.

In Scotland the idea of a new role had been taking root for some years. MacAlister's 'exposition of some general principles' that should govern general practice had been accepted by the Scottish Board of Health as a guide for future policy and these principles had been promoted in the Scottish medical schools between the wars.

Traditionally the medical profession in Scotland was predisposed by its training and its established ethos toward public service. In the 1930s there was a more immediate factor that made employment by the state increasingly attractive. Opportunities for employment in Scotland were becoming fewer. In the years from 1927 to 1933 the number of doctors employed in England had increased by over 11%, while in Scotland over 500 jobs had been lost.[28] At the same time the number of doctors being trained in Scotland continued to increase. In Glasgow, clinical teachers found that the number of their medical students was continuing to rise beyond the number that could be assured of the necessary clinical experience. (In 1939 it was eventually found necessary to restrict the number of students in Glasgow to a total of 240 from the United Kingdom and 60 from overseas.[29]) Throughout the 1930s the opportunities for Scottish graduates to find employment in their own country were diminishing. In the circumstances the prospect of employment in a state-maintained service was becoming increasingly attractive in Scotland.

In England the medical profession was neither disposed to become the servant of the state nor was it difficult for medical graduates in England to find employment where job opportunities were increasing. There was little incentive to make radical changes. In 1920, the Consultative Council on Medical and Allied Services of the Ministry of Health had produced an interim report on *The Future Provision of Medical and Allied Services* (the Dawson Report).[30] Dawson's scheme for England and Wales was similar to MacAlister's scheme for Scotland (though significantly more hostile to a salaried service). But as Pater records, 'the conclusions of the interim report carried little weight because they were opposed by a substantial body of opinion on the council, and the production of the report was rushed so that the dissidents were prevented from expressing their opposition.'[31] The Minister of Health was hesitant in his acceptance of this interim report, issuing only a brief statement referring to the possibility of reform of the Poor Law. A final report was never produced. The Dawson Report was

28 *Medical Directory*, 1927–1933.
29 *Minutes of the Royal Faculty of Physicians and Surgeon of Glasgow*, 23 July 1939.
30 *The Future Provision of Medical and Allied Services* (Dawson Report), 1920, Cmd. 693.
31 J. Pater, *The Making of the National Health Service* (London, 1981), p. 10.

recalled during the final planning of the National Health Service in the 1940s but there is nothing in the Annual Reports of the Ministry of Health or the Annual Reports of the Chief Medical Officer to suggest that the Dawson Report, with its new role for the general practitioner, received active support in England during the 1930s. Nor is there evidence that the Ministry of Health made any attempt to emulate the Department of Health for Scotland in working to achieve the co-operation among the various sections of the health services in England which might lead to the creation of a new unified (or even co-operative) medical service sponsored by the state.

In the schemes proposed for Scotland, initially by MacAlister and now in the 1930s by Cathcart, it was essential that the general practitioner should become more absorbed into public service and employment by the state. There were good reasons to believe that this shift would be more readily acceptable to doctors educated in Scotland than by those who had been schooled in a different tradition in England.[32] Over the years teaching was modified in keeping with changes in medical science and practice. But in its principles it continued unchanged, and instruction in each new branch of medicine, as it established its place in the widest concept of medical practice, was included in the curriculum. A Scottish degree became recognised as an excellent qualification for a career in various forms of medical practice. Many Scottish graduates made their careers in public health,[33] in the armed services, and in the colonial medical services.[34] (In 1935, 15 of the 29 Medical Officers of Health in the administrative County of London were Scottish graduates; Scottish graduates made up 25% of the total medical personnel of the Naval, Military, Indian and RAF Services.[35] When the Indian Medical Service was at its highest strength, 30% of its medical officers were Scottish graduates.[36]) A few achieved success in entrepreneurial private practice in London and Harley Street. But the great majority, not only those who remained to practise in Scotland, continued in the Scottish tradition in which service to the state or to medical science could confer a status that could only be achieved in England in entrepreneurial private practice. The medical schools in Scotland had been first promoted by the state in the shape of the local authorities, and for the benefit of the state. They generated a discourse and rhetoric in which public service was highly regarded. It may be argued that the students entering the medical schools were already more predisposed to employment

32 Chapter 2.
33 *Medical Directory*, 1935.
34 The remaining 75% were made up of medical officers from Ireland, England, India, New Zealand, Canada and Australia.
35 *Medical Directory*, 1935.
36 D. G. Crawford, *Roll of the Indian Medical Service* (London, 1930).

by the state than students south of the border. While the breadth of the curriculum and the quality of the instruction were the outstanding attractions, the Scottish medical schools also offered the added advantages of ease of entry, religious tolerance and economy of fees and living expenses.[37] Scottish students were drawn from a wider spectrum of society than those of the English, particularly the London, medical schools. In 1901 the *Edinburgh Medical Journal* reported:

> Through the munificence of Mr. Andrew Carnegie cost of academic training had been lessened by the payment of the education fees in the case of students of Scottish Nationality and also those who have attended any scholastic institution under the inspection of the Scotch Education Department of whatever nationality during at least two years after the age of fourteen.[38]

The interest on Carnegie's endowment of £2,000,000 was to provide bursaries to students 'in the hope that only those who require help will apply although no question as to the circumstances are asked from the claimant.'[39] The bursaries so openly available from the Carnnegie Trust had an immediate effect on recruitment to Scottish universities. By 1910, at Glasgow, the percentage of working-class students had risen to 24%, a proportion that continued thereafter throughout the 1930s.[40] The usual ambition of a child of working-class parents was to become a teacher. The longer training for medicine required, in addition to the support of the Carnegie Trust, considerable financial sacrifice by the parents. The proportion of working-class students in the medical school was therefore less than the general level in the university. Nevertheless medical students at Glasgow and the other Scottish medical schools were not regarded, and did not regard themselves, as an elite. They received their medical training in a culture that did not regard entrepreneurial success as the most laudable of ambitions.

In Scotland, general practitioners, who made up the great majority of the medical profession, operated in a society culturally and economically distinct from that in England. The profession in Scotland had its own place in society, its own system of values and its own characteristics – notably a higher proportion of women[41] and a much higher proportion of

---

37 In 1901 annual fees at Glasgow were £126 and at Aberdeen £113. Fees at Oxford were £220 and at Cambridge £200. *Edinburgh Medical Journal*, x, 1901, p. ii.
38 *Ibid.*
39 *Ibid.*
40 K. Collins, *Go and Learn: The International Story of Jews and Medicine in Scotland* (Aberdeen, 1988), p. 28.
41 The proportion of women in Scotland was 16.2% and in England 9.4%. Figures derived from the local lists of the *Medical Directory* for 1935.

university graduates.[42] But in spite of the shared characteristics of its members, the profession in Scotland did not function as a corporate entity. The great majority of doctors practised independently, either alone, possibly with an assistant, or in a very small partnership. Their loyalties were to the local community rather than to any central organisation. For professional guidance and direction general practitioners looked to the local university centre at which, in most cases, they had been trained. There was no one national centre in Scotland on the model of Harley Street to which patients from all over England and Wales were referred for an ultimate authoritative opinion. That part of Scottish society that might have supported such a centre of fashionable practice had, for many years, taken 'the social high road to London.'[43] Politically the medical profession in Scotland had no established or influential leadership. Only a small minority of Scottish general practitioners had any continuing association with the Royal College of Physicians of Edinburgh, the Royal College of Surgeon of Edinburgh or the Royal Faculty of Physicians and Surgeons of Glasgow.[44] Although these corporations together made up one of Britain's most important licensing bodies, they were principally concerned with the maintenance of standards in specialist and consultant practice. Although called from time to time to respond to questions of national importance, they were not inclined to be politically pro-active. Politically the medical press in Scotland, the *Edinburgh Medical Journal* and the *Glasgow Medical Journal*, echoed the activities of the Royal Colleges and the Royal Faculty which sponsored them, but gave first place to their roles as scientific journals.

General practitioners in Scotland related more to local associations than to any national body. Since the middle of the eighteenth century 135 local medical associations had been formed in Scotland;[45] in the mid-1930s some 37 were still in being. The objectives of these associations varied from those few with a very specific professional purpose (e.g. the Edinburgh Missionary Society was formed to train medical students for mission work overseas or at home) to those which were no more than closed dining clubs (e.g. the Harveian Society, initially limited to 30 Fellows of the Royal Colleges in Edinburgh meeting for an annual dinner and oration). The great majority were founded 'to provide friendly and social intercourse between members

42 In England the proportion of non-graduates was 32.5% and in Scotland 6.4%. *Ibid.*
43 N. T. Phillipson, 'Nationalism and Ideology', in J. N. Wolfe (ed.), *Government and Nationalism in Scotland* (Edinburgh, 1969), p. 170.
44 Founded in 1599, the Royal Faculty of Physicians and Surgeons of Glasgow changed its title to the Royal College of Physicians of Glasgow in 1962.
45 The societies are listed by J. Jenkinson, *Scottish Medical Societies, 1731–1939* (Edinburgh, 1993).

of the medical profession'[46] and 'for the purpose of writing and discussing medical subjects.'[47] The medical subjects might include the presentation of difficult or interesting cases or the presentation of a scientific paper. These societies also met, as occasion arose, to agree such local matters as staffing arrangements for the local voluntary hospital, local schedules of fees, or salary levels to be paid to assistants. In the 1930s they also met to co-ordinate resistance to the increasing encroachments on their practices by the rising auxiliary professions of pharmacy and midwifery.

The interests of these societies remained essentially local. There was little inclination among them to come together to form a national body. An Association of Scottish Medical Practitioners was formed in 1859 to help in the enforcement of the Medical Act of 1858 but within a year it was in 'a state of suspended animation.'[48] In 1865 a number of medical societies in the north came together as the North of Scotland Medical Association; the Association gradually faded away to become extinct after some 25 years, leaving its constituent local societies still in existence. The arrival of the British Medical Association in Scotland in 1872[49] was not greeted with enthusiasm. Many societies regarded it as a threat to their independent existence; some, on the other hand, mooted the formation of a Scottish Medical Association to recognise and maintain the distinct nature of the profession in Scotland.[50] The BMA gained ground only slowly even after the Scottish Committee of the BMA was set up in 1903. As the number of BMA branches increased in Scotland, the local associations continued to retain some interest in political matters, often in opposition to the policies of the BMA.[51] Within a few years the Scottish Committee was itself dis-satisfied with its relationship with the central body of the BMA in London; the Scottish Committee felt that the Association was not taking as active a role in watching Scotland's interests as it might.[52] The Scottish Committee therefore tended to pursue its own line when necessary in the interest of medical services in Scotland. In sharp contrast with the confrontation between the BMA and the Ministry of Health in London, the Scottish Committee established and continued in a constructive relationship with the Scottish Board of Health from 1919 and with its successor the Depart-ment of Health for Scotland from 1929.

46 Quoted from the objects of the Western Medical Club. *Ibid.*, p. 203.
47 Quoted from the objects of the Glasgow Medico-Chirurgical Society. *Ibid.*, p. 161.
48 *Edinburgh Medical Journal*, vi, 1860, p. 775.
49 Founded originally as the Provincial Medical and Surgical Association, the BMA had been functioning in England since 1832.
50 Jenkinson, *op. cit.*, p. 81.
51 *Ibid.*, p. 82.
52 E.g. Memo from the Scottish Committee to the Council of the British Medical Association. LHB 1/60/15.

Membership of the BMA was not high in Scotland. In 1935 only 50.9% of doctors in Scotland were members.[53] For most doctors the chief attraction of membership was the *British Medical Journal* which, apart from publishing scientific papers, acted as the profession's employment agency[54] and gave notice of matters of essential importance to medical practice. It also reported on the activities of the central body of the BMA. For most general practitioners, even for members of the BMA, the journal was the only contact with the political apparatus of the BMA. Few members were active within the Association or attended meetings. A review of the minute books of the branches and divisions of the BMA in Scotland in 1935 shows that attendance at meetings averaged some 4% of the membership (2% of the medical profession) in Scotland. The largest numbers attended meetings in the cities; in Ross and Cromarty, where the membership was 43, no meetings could be convened in that year. Poor attendance at meetings did not necessarily indicate a lack of interest; general practitioners, especially those in single-handed practices, found it difficult to travel to meetings, leaving their practices unattended. There was therefore a severe, even crippling, lack of communication within the BMA. Although the membership could hear of the activities of the leaders as reported in the *British Medical Journal*, the leadership could only gather the opinions and hear of the problems of the very few members with the leisure to attend meetings.[55]

The views of the individual general practitioners were of crucial importance. The health policy advocated by the Cathcart Committee could only go forward with their support. Without their active participation the whole scheme would be impossible. The representatives of all the medical bodies in Scotland had indicated to the Cathcart Committee that the policy would find willing co-operation. However, there was no organisation through which the views of general practitioners, dispersed independently across Scotland, could be accurately assessed although there was good reason to expect that Cathcart's proposals would be welcomed. In the Highlands and Islands Medical Service general practitioners in Scotland had already shown that, given the opportunity to join a state scheme, they were more than ready to take it. From at least 1931 the Department of Health had gone forward on that assumption.

However, the re-structured general practitioner service advocated by Cathcart could not be put in place in Scotland alone. Planned as an extension of the NHI scheme, it could not go forward except as a national

---

53 *Annual Handbook of the BMA.*
54 It was known to the children of one former colleague as 'daddy's job book.'
55 There was no arrangement for postal voting.

plan agreed at Westminster. In England there could be no certainty that the medical profession would be willing to give the necessary backing to such a scheme and there was good reason to suspect that it would not. The precedent of the resistance to the NHI seemed ominous. But in England in 1911, as in Scotland, the rank-and-file of the profession had not had a clear opportunity to make their views known or to confirm their individual support for those who had taken it upon themselves to speak on their behalf. There was no reason to suppose that, in creating an extension of the NHI scheme, those speaking for the profession in London would be more accurate in voicing the views of the rank-and-file. In the United Kingdom the attitude of general practitioners to a new and extended role in a scheme which involved employment by the state could only become known with certainty when its individual members were given the opportunity to join. But there was reason to suppose that the new form of general practice would be welcomed in Scotland.

9

Publication and Response

The *Report of the Committee on Scottish Health Services* was published as a Blue Book on 2 July 1936. There was little reaction from the general public. For months the attention of the public had been taken up by the failure of the League of Nations to prevent Mussolini's invasion of Abyssinnia and its implication for world peace. On 2 July 1936, newspapers were given over to reports of the Foreign Secretary's mission to Geneva in an attempt to restructure an organisation in imminent danger of falling apart. Leader writers deplored the 'mad folly of the arms race in Europe.'[1]

In this gathering crisis the *Times* and the other London broadsheets carried only summaries of the Cathcart Report and without comment. However, the medical press recognised the importance of the Cathcart Report as the most comprehensive inquiry ever carried out into the provision of community health care in Britain. The *Lancet* urged that it should be carefully studied since 'health problems transcend national frontiers and have in them much that is common in all countries.'[2] The *BMJ* was even more positive: 'This publication should mark the setting up – perhaps at no distant date – of a comprehensive national health or medical service.'[3] The *BMJ* saw similarities to the scheme proposed by the BMA in its pamphlet, *A General Medical Service for the Nation*, in 1930.[4] Now that such a scheme had been again 'recommended by an influential composite Committee for application in Scotland', the *BMJ* hoped that there would be some parliamentary action. At the very least the extended general practitioner service could be introduced in Scotland as an experiment.[5]

In Scotland, it was not only the medical press that recognised the significance of the Cathcart Report. The *Scotsman* was clear that what was being proposed was 'a State medical service.'[6] The *Glasgow Herald* welcomed the plan but pointed out that such a radical extension of state services would require 'much public discussion for a long time.'[7] The

1 *Scotsman*, 2 July 1936.
2 *Lancet*, ii, 1936, p. 27.
3 *BMJ*, ii, 1936, p. 27.
4 The BMJ overstated the similarities. The BMA proposed an extension of state services but without such a shift in philosophy. However, both plans pointed in the same direction.
5 This had been suggested as a possibility by the Cathcart Committee (Report, p. 283).
6 *Scotsman*, 2 July 1936.
7 *Glasgow Herald*, 2 July 1936.

medical profession was more confident that the plan would be carried out in due course. At a large special meeting in Edinburgh it formally recorded

> . . . its sense of the great value of the service rendered by the Committee on Scottish Health Services in their detailed and comprehensive study and analysis of the health problems in Scotland and the preparation of this most valuable report. The meeting is in agreement with the principles of the recommendations in the Report for improvement in the health services and venture to hope that legislative action may be taken at the earliest possible moment to give effect to the proposals of the Committee.[8]

However, the medical profession and the national press in Scotland agreed that, although much to be desired, the creation of a new state medical service was not the immediate priority. In 1936, there were more pressing matters. The maternal mortality rate was higher than it had been ten years before. Taken together, the number of maternal deaths, still births and neonatal deaths was greater than the number of deaths from cancer and heart disease and even greater than the total number of deaths from infectious disease. In 1935, the *Report on Maternity Morbidity and Mortality in Scotland* had exposed the full extent of this loss of life and had identified the crucial deficiencies in the existing maternity services. As promised in its election manifesto in the summer of 1935, the Government had introduced a Midwifery (Scotland) Bill that would, it was hoped, put an end to what had become a national scandal. In 1936, it seemed right to give precedence to saving the lives of young mothers of families over plans for the introduction of a state health service at some indefinite time in the future.

In 1936 and 1937 the BMA in Scotland held no special meetings to discuss the Cathcart Report, and its recommendations were not included on the agendas of the regular business meetings of its local Divisions. In the first months following the publication of the Report, these meetings were entirely taken up by discussions of the proposed new maternity services. Then, within a few months, there was a new focus of attention, the preparations for war. By the end of 1936 BMA members were being called to attend special meetings to discuss preparations for poison gas attacks. From October 1937 even larger numbers of general practitioners, in some cases over 500, gathered for more formal instruction in Air Raid Precautions. Special meetings were called to make the necessary arrangements for the maintenance of adequate local general practice services in preparation for the expected loss of large numbers of doctors to military service. For the

8 *Transactions of the Medico-Chirugical Society of Edinburgh*, cxvi, 1936–37, p. 1.

medical profession and the general public in Scotland, a plan for a health service in a very uncertain future had become an irrelevance.

However, even at this troubled time, Scotland's representatives in Parliament did not allow the matter to drop. Only 12 days after its publication, they created an early opportunity to voice their support for the recommendations of the Cathcart Report during a meeting of a Committee on Supply. The business of the day was to agree the allocation of funds to the Department of Health for Scotland for the coming year. It was made clear to members that, during a debate on Supply, while Scotland's health and health services were open for discussion, advocacy of new projects that would involve new legislation would be out of order. In spite of that ruling, it soon became evident that on that day it was the Cathcart Report, rather than the salaries and expenses of the Department of Health, that was uppermost in the minds of Scottish members of Parliament and the Secretary of State for Scotland.

In opening the debate, Sir Godfrey Collins briefly reviewed the development of medical services in Scotland over the previous fifty years and outlined his policy for the future. His statement was in effect a summary of the Cathcart Report and, in many passages, expressed in the same words. He accepted the verdict of the Cathcart Committee that the existing machinery of government, although it had done splendid work in the past, was 'not fully adapted to conditions today.'[9] The Committee had submitted proposals for reform. At a debate on Supply it would be out of order for him to announce the Government's intentions for legislation, but he assured members that his administration would act, and 'in doing so we think we are interpreting aright the mind of Scotland.'[10]

Even without a precise statement on legislation, the Scottish members understood the Secretary of State to have given the Cathcart's scheme his 'blessing.'[11] His statement was welcomed by J. C. M. Guy for the Conservatives, by Sir Archibald Sinclair for the Liberals and W. McL. Watson for the Labour Party; in the debate that followed the Report did not become an issue between political parties. Tom Johnston, the chief spokesman for the Labour Party, suggested that, in view of the importance of the matters raised in the Cathcart Report, members should limit their speeches to 15 minutes to allow as many as possible to take part in the discussion. In all, the unusually large number of 28 members of all parties were given an opportunity to speak[12] and every aspect of the Report was picked up

9 *Ibid.*, col. 1903.
10 *Ibid.*, col. 1904.
11 *Ibid.*, col. 1988
12 Labour, 12; Unionist 5; Conservative, 3; Liberal 2; Liberal National, 2; Labour Co-op, 1; National Liberal, 1; Conservative Unionist, 1; National Unionist, 1.

for discussion by at least one member. It soon became clear that, within days of its publication, the Cathcart Report had not only been accepted by Scottish members of Parliament of all parties as the ultimate analysis of Scotland's poor health but that it would also be the touchstone in the process of organising for improvement.[13]

Sir Godfrey Collins died only three months after its publication. He was succeeded as Secretary of State by Walter Elliot who was no less eager to promote the Report's recommendations. At the opening of the new parliamentary session in November 1936, the King's Speech included a promise that a comprehensive effort was to be made to improve the health of the nation and that proposals would be submitted to Parliament in due course.[14] Replying on behalf of the Conservative Party, Florence Horsburgh welcomed this as an assurance of the Government's intention to bring forward legislation in 'response to the Cathcart Report.'[15] Within a few months Walter Elliot assured Scottish members of Parliament of his intention to carry out some of the recommendations in the Cathcart Report immediately and that action on 'many more' would follow as soon as possible.[16] After Walter Elliot became Minister of Health in 1938, this pledge was kept by his successors as Secretaries of State.

The Cathcart Report was not published at a propitious time for ambitious, expensive and potentially controversial reforms. The country's health services had to be prepared for war. On 17 February 1937 the Prime Minister was authorised by Parliament to borrow £400,000,000 for defence expenditure. Even if sufficient funds had still been available, immediate implementation of those recommendations in the Report that required new United Kingdom legislation was not possible. In England and Wales they were not ready. There was not even the beginning of agreement on how hospital services should be organised for the long term; the antagonisms that would inevitably be aroused by fundamental reorganisation would be damaging to the process of organising the hospital services for war. The extension of the general practitioner service proposed by Cathcart was bound to be highly controversial in England where medical practice was conducted in a more entrepreneurial spirit than in Scotland. Discord had to be avoided at a time when the willing co-operation of general practitioners was required in preparing for emergency care of the massive number of

13 'As a result of the discussion today, the Secretary of State will arise like a giant refreshed, and as far as the future is concerned, he will be a modern Wallace, cleaving his particular opinion into the minds of the Anglified Government Front Bench with which this House is faced at the present time.' J. Cassells (Lab.), *ibid.*, col. 1915.

14 *Hansard*, cccxvii, HC 3 November 1936, col. 9.

15 *Ibid.*, col. 15.

16 *Hansard*, cccxxv, HC 24 June 1937, col. 1403.

civilian casualties expected in the coming war. United Kingdom legislation for a fundamental reform of the health services was out of the question.

Progress in Scotland

In June 1937, the Secretary of State announced that in Scotland the Department of Health would press ahead with those of the Cathcart reforms that could be carried out under existing legislation or extensions to existing legislation.[17] Further reorganisation of the services was still possible under the Local Government Act of 1929 and could be achieved with the support of the new Commissioner for Special Areas in Scotland.[18]

Some reforms, particularly the recommended improvements in the environmental services, could be mediated through the local authorities. From 1937 some priority was given to the massive and long-standing problem of housing. Surveys begun under the Housing (Scotland) Act of 1935 established that 250,000 new houses were required to replace unfit houses and to relieve overcrowding. Scotland's local authorities had anticipated that only 55,500 houses would be completed by 1941. In 1936, the Secretary of State put pressure on local authorities to step up their building programmes.[19] He also announced that local authorities would no longer be allowed to build small houses of one or two rooms.

In 1937, a revival in the Scottish economy and the demands of a growing armaments industry diverted building workers to other and more highly paid employment. At the same time there was a sharp increase in the cost of building materials. In 1937 the number of houses completed was less than in 1936. However, in 1938 three new Acts – the Housing (Financial Provisions) (Scotland) Act, the Housing (Rural Workers) Act, and the Housing (Agricultural Population) (Scotland) Act – and the support of the Commissioner for Special Areas gave new encouragement and financial support for house building. Before the outbreak of war 150,000 new houses were completed,[20] many fewer than the number required but almost three times the number envisaged before the publication of the Cathcart Report.

Progress was also made in correcting the deficiencies in drainage and water supply. The Department of Health put pressure on local authorities to co-operate in making the best use of natural water resources which were

17 *Hansard*, June 1937, *op. cit.*, col. 1403.
18 The Special Areas Act of 1934 set up a Commission to co-ordinate and promote public works in the most distressed areas in the U.K. It was one of Sir Godfrey Collins' achievements that a separate Commissioner was appointed for Scotland.
19 *Hansard*, July 1936, *op. cit.*, col. 1902.
20 Approximately 70% by local authorities, 0.6% by the Scottish Special Housing Association Ltd and public utility societies, the remainder by private enterprise. *Ibid.*, p. 21.

clearly adequate for all foreseeable needs and for the necessary engineering work to make full use of the existing Treasury grants, especially those offered through the Special Areas Fund. Already in 1938, the Secretary of State was able to report that two large regional schemes were in place and that 71 other new water schemes had been agreed.

There was also scope for immediate extension of medical services. Improvement in the nutrition of children, better co-ordination of local authority clinics could all be achieved under existing Scottish legislation. Some extension of the general practitioner services was written into the Maternity Services (Scotland) Act. This Scottish Bill, which eventually became law in May 1937, had been more ambitious and wider in scope than that being prepared for England and Wales and had been ready since early in 1936. However, fearing that publication of the Scottish Bill might create a demand for a similar extension of services in England and Wales, the Minister of Health had asked for the Scottish Bill to be delayed until his own Bill had passed the House of Commons.[21] When the Scottish Act finally came into force, it was soon strengthened by the Registration of Stillbirths (Scotland) Act in 1938. Further extension of the general practitioner service to cover thousands of young people was made possible by the National Health Insurance (Juvenile Contributors and Young Persons) Act of 1937.

On the reorganisation of the hospital services the Secretary of State was able to report in 1937 that important progress had been made.[22] The five regions to be served by Scotland's 474 hospitals (219 voluntary, 255 local authority) had been defined.[23] Within this new regional organisation, only four of Scotland's 55 local authorities had not yet agreed to submit schemes for rationalising their hospital services. Progress had only been slow where 'unfortunately large burghs did not see eye to eye and would not combine in a joint scheme with a county council.'[24]

By 1938, seven new local authority hospitals were nearing completion. In Greenock the local authority had rejected plans for a new municipal hospital in spite of an offer of financial support from the Commissioner for Special Areas, on the grounds that local hospital accommodation was

21 PRO, CAB 23/82 36(36) 7th; NAS HH61/787.
22 *Hansard*, June 1937, *op. cit.*, col. 1430.
23 (1) Northern Region – Counties of Inverness, Ross and Cromarty, Sutherland, Caithness and Orkney. (2) North-Eastern Region – Counties of Aberdeen, Kincardine, Banff, Moray and Nairn, and Shetland. (3) Eastern Region – Counties of Angus, Fife (north and east), and Perth and Kinross. (4) Counties of Midlothian, Peebles, Roxburgh, Selkirk, West Linton, Berwick, Clackmannan, East Lothian and Fife (south and west). (5) Counties of Lanark, Renfrew, Dunbarton, Stirling, Ayr, Dumfries, Kirkcudbright, Wigtown, Bute and Argyll.
24 *Hansard*, June 1937, *op. cit.*, col. 1403.

already satisfactory. (A judgement with which the Department of Health profoundly disagreed.[25]) In addition to local authority hospitals, new voluntary hospitals were being planned in Ayrshire and in Fife. When hospital accommodation came to be surveyed in the early years of the war it was judged to be adequate, even to cope with the expected additional load of civilian casualties.

By the measure set by the Cathcart Report, hospital services had not reached their target; there were still waiting lists. Nevertheless, significant progress had been made. The regional arrangement of hospitals had found general acceptance and, to a varying degree, within these regions co-operation had been established among local authority and voluntary hospitals.

In 1937 the creation of the extended general practitioner service was also under way.[26] The National Health Insurance (Juvenile Contributors and Young Persons) Act of 1937 had added 133,500 people between the ages of 14 and 16 years of age as new panel patients on general practitioners' lists. The National Health Insurance (Amendment) Act of 1937 added those people employed by relatives who had previously been excluded from the NHI scheme. The increased level of employment in Scotland added a further 200,000.[27] By 1939 general practitioner services had been extended to include some 2,500,000 people – well over half the population – and the new maternity service was available to every woman in Scotland.

The Maternity Services (Scotland) Act provided that any woman who wished to be confined at home could have the services of a general practitioner and a certified midwife throughout her pregnancy, labour and lying-in period. A consultant obstetrician was also to be available at any time at the request of the general practitioner. Where it had been introduced, the service was running smoothly and had proved to be popular. However, under the Act, the new service was to be administered by the local authorities and by 1939 only 14 schemes were fully operational in Scotland's 55 local authority areas with a further nine approved but not implemented. Some local authorities had been slow to interest themselves in the scheme but in most areas the delay was caused by difficulty in negotiating contracts with local general practitioners. These difficulties were eventually resolved and by 1941 the maternity service was successfully established across Scotland.

The Cathcart Report had expressed concern about the poor nutritional state of Scotland's children and had recommended that the scheme, in which

25 *Annual Report of the Department of Health for Scotland*, 1938, Cmd. 5969, p. 115.
26 *Hansard*, June 1937, *op. cit.*, col. 1403.
27 *Hansard*, July 1939, *op. cit.*, col. 1150.

the Milk Marketing Boards in Scotland offered to supply milk to school-children, should be encouraged and developed.[28] In 1938 some 294,000 school children in Scotland were receiving a daily ration of one third of a pint of milk. Since the Secretary of State was advised that milk supplements during childhood would in time improve the general nutrition, not only of children but eventually of the whole population, he proposed to increase the daily milk supplement to the seven-eighths of a pint.[29]

The formulation of a general policy on nutrition was delayed until further investigation had been completed. The Cathcart Committee had thought it probable that, although there was no widespread or gross malnutrition[30] in Scotland, improved feeding would nevertheless raise the standard of health. The Department of Health awaited the results of an investigation to be carried out with the support of the Carnegie Trust. Sir John Boyd Orr was to make a dietary and clinical survey of 1000 families to study the effects of food on physical and psychological development and especially on the mental development of children. The Ministry of Labour was investigating the cost of the diets of families across the United Kingdom. It was expected that these various investigations would take two years.

The Department of Health accepted the Cathcart Report's proposals for health education. However, its very detailed programme of health education in schools could not be put in place immediately. Changes to teacher training and revision of the school curriculum would take some years to accomplish and would require the agreement and support of the Education Department and the teaching profession. The programme also called for very considerable capital investment in the improvement and extension of school buildings and the construction of new schools. Financing the programme presented great difficulties for the local authorities. Nevertheless no opportunity for an initiative in health education was neglected. During the Empire Exhibition in Glasgow in 1938 the Under Secretary of State, Henry Wedderburn, presided at two full-day public sessions devoted to health education.

In the few years before the outbreak of the Second World War important progress was made towards the establishment of a more effective and comprehensive health service in Scotland. However, the implementation of Cathcart's recommendations was inhibited by the financial, administrative and political constraints of the time. Then, in 1939, the pace of change increased. At the height of the Second World War Scotland's Chief Medical Officer assured an audience in Edinburgh that it had been 'indeed fortunate'

28 Cathcart Report, p. 191.
29 Annual Report of the Department of Health for Scotland, 1937, *op. cit*, p. 53.
30 In the 1930s 'malnutrition' was only diagnosed when the effects of nutritional deprivation were apparent on a single superficial inspection.

that, at the outbreak of war, the Department of Health had the advantage of a full and recent review of the medical services in Scotland.[31] The Cathcart Report 'was one of the best products of its kind and its scope extended over every aspect of the health services of the country.'[32] The Cathcart Report, with other factors 'such as the ease with which the country divides itself into regions suitable for hospital administration, the convenient size of Scotland as a national unit and the whole hearted support given to the Department of Health by local authorities, by voluntary hospitals and by all branches of the medical and nursing professions had combined to minimise the difficulties of providing a national hospital service for wartime purposes.' The Chief Medical Officer for Scotland saw this all-round spirit of co-operation as a happy augury for the post-war reorganisation of the country's health services, 'which most people are agreed is necessary.' Already in 1942 he was confident that Scotland had at hand something more than the scaffolding of a first-class national hospital service.

The Emergency Hospital Service had been conceived at a Cabinet meeting in September 1938.[33] The plans were drawn up by Walter Elliot, then the Minister of Health, and John Colville, the new Secretary of State for Scotland. They had been warned to expect that, in Great Britain as a whole, civilian casualties from air raids might total 17,500 killed and 35,000 wounded every day[34] during the first two or three weeks of the war.[35] Since the existing hospitals could not hope to cope with such numbers, it was proposed that huts should be constructed to accommodate additional hospital beds, 20,000 in England and the proportionately much greater number of 6,000 in Scotland. In April 1939 these numbers were doubled. Under the Civil Defence Act, 1939 the Emergency Hospital Service in Scotland became the responsibility of the Secretary of State. In Scotland the service soon created an opportunity to expand the facilities for general surgery, orthopaedic surgery, general medicine and obstetrics.[36] New hospitals were built 'from the ground upwards,' existing hospitals were upgraded, some small hospitals were extended by constructing hutted annexes, two hotels and a teacher training college were converted into surgical hospitals, 62 large private houses were converted into auxiliary hospitals and four convalescent homes were taken over.[37] In all, the number

31 Honeyman Gillespie Lecture given at Edinburgh Royal Infirmary, 30th July 1942.
32 A. Davidson, 'The Contribution of the Emergency Medical Service to Medicine and Surgery in Scotland', *Edinburgh Medical Journal*, xlix, 1942, p. 555.
33 I. Levitt, *The Scottish Office* (Edinburgh, 1992), p. 355.
34 This forecast was based on the experience of the Spanish Civil War and the assumption that in modern warfare the bomber would always get through.
35 PRO, CAB 24/284 CP (39) 77.
36 Davidson, *op. cit.*, p. 556.
37 *Ibid.*

of beds in the Emergency Hospital Service in Scotland reached a total of 20,527. Of these, 16,574 were general hospital beds and 3953 were for convalescents. By 1942 the Emergency Hospital Service (EHS) had more than doubled the number of general hospital beds in Scotland.[38] In addition to the many specialists who gave their services gratuitously, at its height the EHS employed 1149 doctors, 1,277 nurse, 823 assistant nurses and 3,121 nursing auxiliaries.[39]

In terms of general hospital services the Department of Health for Scotland was now the largest hospital authority in Scotland, administering nine base hospitals and 66 auxiliary and convalescent hospitals. The EHS conformed to the regional structure already in place. A Regional Hospital Office in each of the five Regions administered the EHS hospitals and co-ordinated the activities of the voluntary hospitals and local authority hospitals in the Region.[40] It had soon become apparent that the number of civilian casualties forecast for the first months of the war had been a wild over-estimate. The doubling of the number of general surgical and medical beds in Scotland to accommodate vast numbers of casualties had quite unexpectedly created space for new services.[41] The Department of Health took the opportunity to establish special units for neurosurgery, peripheral nerve surgery, orthopaedics, maxilliofacial surgery, effort syndrome, ophthalmic surgery and thoracic surgery. These units were distributed, again on a regional basis, in 17 separate hospitals. These were all new developing services that could never have found a space in the pre-war voluntary hospitals and would never have been contemplated in local authority hospitals.

In 1936, the Cathcart Report had found that pulmonary tuberculosis, although falling in incidence, was 'still formidable, especially among adolescents and young adults.' Inevitably, after a marked decline over several years, the incidence of tuberculosis in Scotland increased sharply in the first years of the war.[42] Tuberculosis wards that had become redundant in the 1930s had been commandeered at the outbreak of war as accommodation for the expected vast number of casualties. When it became evident that they would not be needed for that purpose, they were returned to the tuberculosis service to accommodate its increasing patient numbers.[43] The accommodation for the in-patient treatment of tuberculosis

---

38 Calculated from the figures given by Dr Davidson, the Chief Medical Officer for Scotland. *Ibid.*, p. 555.
39 *Ibid.*
40 Davidson, *op. cit.*, p. 556.
41 *Ibid.*
42 *Health Bulletin*, ii, 4, 1943, p. 33.
43 'Tuberculosis in Wartime', *Annual Report of the Department of Health for Scotland*, 1942, Cmd. 6308, p. 14.

in Scotland was reviewed; 350 beds were added to the existing units and a new central unit was set up in an EHS hospital. Although the circumstances had not been foreseen, these developments were in line with the recommendations in the Cathcart Report that new centres should be set up for 'modern treatment' of tuberculosis.

Cathcart had also proposed that centres should be created for the investigation of 'disabilities of industrial origin' and for treatment and rehabilitation of 'any disabilities that may be found.' This suggestion was taken up in the Clyde Basin Scheme.[44] The areas chosen for this comprised the counties of Dunbarton, Renfrew, Lanark and the City of Glasgow; 44% of the total insured population of Scotland lived in this area and their pre-war sickness rate had been particularly high. Accommodation was made available in the EHS hospitals at Killearn (640 beds) and Law (1,280 beds) and in their associated convalescent homes. The necessary specialist skills were provided by the clinical staff of Glasgow University. General practitioners were asked to refer any of their patients, particularly young adult workers, who showed signs of a possible breakdown in health but did not yet suffer from overt organic disease. By 1944 almost 13,000 patients (52% female) had been referred. Most complained of tiredness, vague aches and pains or loss of appetite. A large number were suffering from anxiety states. Overall 44% of those referred to the Clyde Basin Scheme were found to be suffering from treatable disorders; 22% were admitted to hospital; 22% were admitted for convalescence.[45]

Not all the capacity created for the Emergency Hospital Scheme was taken up by war casualties or by the new specialist services. Under an arrangement between the Department of Health and the British Hospitals Association (Scottish Section), first made in the summer of 1941 and extended from 16 January 1942, arrangements were made which allowed patients on the long waiting lists of voluntary hospitals – medical and surgical (but excepting chronic cases) – to be treated in EHS hospitals. No charge was made to the patient but, on his behalf, the voluntary hospital concerned made a payment that was uniform irrespective of length of stay.[46] In the first years of the scheme, 5695 patients were admitted from voluntary hospital waiting lists.

Under the Civil Defence Act of 1939, the Department of Health was given powers to co-ordinate 97 voluntary and 29 local authority hospitals in addition to the EHS hospitals under its direct control.[47] The operation of this total Emergency Hospital Scheme, organised in the five Scottish regions, became the responsibility of a Hospital Officer answerable directly to the Department

44 *Annual Report of the Department of Health for Scotland*, 1942, Cmd. 6372, p. 30.
45 *Ibid.*, p. 6.
46 *Health Bulletin*, i, 2, 1942, p. 13.
47 *Annual Report of the Department of Health for Scotland*, 1942, *op. cit.*

of Health. In 1942 it was already clear that 'a striking feature of the Emergency Hospital arrangements was the co-operation between all interested hospital authorities and their staffs.'[48] An important aspect of that co-operation was the sharing of resources, with ready transfer of patients within the system according to patient needs and the availability of specialist skill and equipment. All hospitals in each Region were served by an Emergency Bacteriology Service set up under the Civil Defence Act establishing four central laboratories and nine subsidiary laboratories. An emergency Blood Transfusion Service, organised by the Department of Health at the outbreak of the war, served every hospital in Scotland. In March 1940 the Scottish National Blood Transfusion Association was constituted and assumed control of the service as a voluntary body subsidised by government grant. In a very short time, with the creation of the EHS, the Department of Health for Scotland had become the hospital authority directly controlling the greatest number of general surgical and medical beds and almost all the new specialist services in Scotland. The Department of Health had also achieved an effective degree of functional integration of all three hospital systems in Scotland – the voluntary, local authority and Department of Health hospitals. Each of the five hospital regions was centred on a university medical school, and clinical departments of the cities' universities had been set up in local authority hospitals in Aberdeen, Edinburgh, Glasgow and Dundee and the University of Aberdeen provided services for the Highlands and Islands Medical Services Board. By 1942, an effective working partnership had been created in which each hospital system had its own valued place.

Progress toward the creation of the comprehensive general practitioner service envisaged by Cathcart faltered in the early years of the war but did not come to a complete stop. The extensions to the National Insurance scheme after 1937 had created new opportunities for co-operation between the school health service and the industrial health service.[49] The general practitioner's entrée to the families of his insured patients was opened further by the new maternity service after 1937. In practice, however, it quickly became impossible for these opportunities to be fully taken up and promoted. Preparations for war had already begun as early as 1935 with the establishment in Whitehall of a Department for Air Raid Precautions. The Scottish Central Emergency Committee (SCEC) of the BMA was revived[50] in 1936 to organise

48 Davidson, *op. cit.*, p. 559.
49 The Secretary of State included these new relationship in the intended benefits of the National Health Insurance (Juvenile Contributors and Young Persons) Act. *Hansard*, cccxxxviii, HC 20 July 1938, col. 2234.
50 First formed in Edinburgh in May 1915 and disbanded at the end of the First World War. J. R. Curry, *The Mustering of Medical Service in Scotland, 1914–1919* (Edinburgh, 1922), p. 26.

general practitioners' part in ARP classes and anti-gas instruction. These duties added to general practitioners' already growing commitments and many doctors soon began to feel that their workload was becoming excessive.[51] In July 1939 the difficulties for general practice increased as the SCEC began to allocate doctors to the services or to civilian practice. Soon 33% of all doctors on the Medical Register in Scotland were serving in the armed forces.[52] Since the SCEC had a duty to ensure that civilian general practitioner services were maintained, the proportion of general practitioners allocated to the armed services was less than that from the profession as a whole. Nevertheless the number of general practitioners in civilian practice was reduced by 18%.[53] Although the general recruitment to the armed services reduced the number of men on doctors' lists in Scotland by 13.9%, this was compensated by an increased number of women. During the war years the total number of persons entitled to the services of a general practitioner under the NHI scheme remained virtually unchanged. But for a change in the income limit for participation in the scheme from £252 to £420 in January 1942, the number would have increased sharply. Incomes had increased significantly in the early years of the war and a proportion of the population was now able and obliged to pay for medical care. There were more private patients, and together with those already being treated under the NHI Scheme, the overall number of patients to be served by a severely reduced number of general practitioners increased. At the same time the scope of the demands on their service to be provided increased; the new maternity service gradually came into full operation; the war-time public health services demanded doctors' participation; the longer hours of work of industrial workers obliged general practitioners to extend surgery hours late into the evening; doctors were also required to be available for casualty duties in emergencies. From 1941 there was a shortage of medical and surgical supplies. In 1942 a memorandum was issued by the Department of Health stressing the urgent need to limit prescribing to essentials and for a wider use of alternative drugs.[54] Throughout the war general practitioners remained overstretched and under-resourced.

War inevitably brought a decline in the health of the population.[55] The volume of sickness among the insured population increased; on average each of these patients reported more illnesses.[56] Most complaints were of

51 P. Bartrip, *Themselves Writ Large* (London, 1996), p. 220.
52 *Annual Report of the Department of Health for Scotland*, 1945, Cmd. 6661, p. 16.
53 *Ibid.*, p. 13.
54 *Ibid.*, p. 10.
55 Paradoxically the suicide rate fell from 102 per million at the height of the Depression to 76 during the war. *Health Bulletin*, ii, 1948, p. 29.
56 *Annual Report of the Department of Health for Scotland*, 1942, Cmd. 6372, p. 11.

minor illness[57] but life-threatening illness also increased. Infectious disease became more prevalent in the population as a whole. The incidence of cerebrospinal fever (meningitis) rose sharply in the first winter of the war from a pre-war level of approximately 300 cases each year to a peak of 2,580 in 1941 and remained high throughout the war.[58] Wartime living conditions increased the incidence of pulmonary tuberculosis from 4,657 in 1939 to 7,518 by the end of the war.[59] The incidence of syphilis increased from a pre-war level of a little over 2,500 each year to a wartime peak of 5,340; the number of cases of gonorrhoea, almost 5,000 cases annually before the war, rose to a peak of 6,500. Much of the increased burden of illness was in the non-insured population, particularly among children. Deaths from diphtheria almost doubled in 1940;[60] in the West of Scotland there were persistent outbreaks of dysentery during 1941 and 1942; in the east there was an epidemic of paratyphoid in 1941; an epidemic of milkborne scarlet fever late in 1941 affected many parts of Scotland.[61] Deaths from these illnesses became somewhat fewer after 1943 but cases of dysentery and meningitis in children increased again in 1945.[62] Outbreaks of smallpox affected both children and adults in Fife in 1942.[63] In the nurseries that had become a new feature of the Public Health service during the war there were frequent outbreaks of diarrhoea caused by giardia lamblia. Nutritional problems were not entirely prevented in children; there were cases of scurvy in 1942.[64] In a health survey of mothers and children in Scotland's four major cities, 16% did not reach the standard of 'good.'[65] In all cities many children were found to be verminous and suffering from contagious skin diseases.[66]

The official statistical indices recorded the sharp decline in Scotland's health from the first months of the war. In the first quarter of 1940 the death rate had already increased by 30% over pre-war levels. In the first 21 months of the war the estimated excess of deaths in Scotland was over 10,000 of which only 2,000 could be attributed to enemy action. The chief causes were acute infectious disease, tuberculosis, accidents and bronchitis

57 The Department of Health discontinued its central recording of incapacitating illness among the insured population in 1939.
58 *Annual Report of the Department of Health for Scotland*, 1942, *op. cit.*, p. 32.
59 *Annual Report of the Department of Health for Scotland*, 1945, Cmd. 6661, p. 6. The number of deaths in Scotland from tuberculosis during the war years was 26,528 (i.e. more than the 21,942 British and Empire soldiers who died in the Boer War).
60 *Health Bulletin*, i, 1942, p. 30.
61 *Health Bulletins*, 1942–52.
62 *Annual Report of the Department of Health for Scotland*, 1946, Cmd. 7188, p. 31.
63 There were 103 cases with 25 deaths.
64 *Health Bulletin*, i, 1942, p. 31.
65 *Health Bulletin*, ii, 1943, p. 45.
66 Glasgow introduced five mobile 'cleansing units' in 1942.

and pneumonia. Only the new maternity services could claim improved results during the war: the maternal mortality rate fell from 4.9 in 1938 to 2.7 in 1945 and the infant mortality rate from 70 in 1938 to 53.8 in 1945.

The deterioration in health was attributed to the 'many and varied stresses' of war, and reached a peak in the winter 1940–41.[67] Thereafter there was a gradual recovery, beginning in 1942 and continuing until 1945. The improvement had been difficult to achieve and much of the load had fallen on a reduced number of general practitioners. In meeting their increased commitments, general practitioners had to endure an increase in working hours, disturbed sleep and difficulties in travel in the blackout. There had been no opportunity for retraining in the skills required for Cathcart's comprehensive general practitioner.

Nevertheless, wartime circumstances had carried general practice some way towards the model described in the Cathcart Report. The organisation of the country's medical services for war had brought the general practitioner into closer contact with local authority and hospital services and at the same time the GP had become, in some degree, the doctor to the whole family. Cathcart had found that general practitioners 'at present do not share what is called the preventive outlook'[68] and were not trained to advise on positive health. An Inter-Departmental Committee on Medical Schools appointed in 1942 recommended that, in future, medical students should be trained in the management of health as well as the diagnosis and treatment of disease.[69] Its report was a further step towards creating the new general practitioner service of the Cathcart Report. Cathcart's concept was given further support in the *Report of the Medical Planning Commission* in 1942 (below).[70] Progress toward the general practice envisaged by Cathcart was temporarily hampered by the extraordinary demands of the time but his ideas not only survived but also attracted increasing support.

Sir George Newman famously observed in 1907 that 'the centre of gravity'[71] of the state's responsibility for the health was shifting from the protection of the population as a corporate whole to the promotion of the health of the individual. In the circumstances of war that shift was necessarily reversed. In the Second World War, rather than negating the progress made toward the implementation of the recommendations of the Cathcart Report, this reverse created an opportunity for further reform. Cathcart had recommended that, while there was perhaps a case for certain

67 *Annual Report of the Department of Health for Scotland*, 1945, Cmd. 6661, p. 4.
68 Cathcart Report, p. 167.
69 *Report of the Inter-Departmental Committee on Medical Schools*, HMSO, 1944 (the Goodenough Report).
70 *BMJ*, i, 1942, p. 743.
71 G. Newman, *The Health of the State* (London, 1907), p. 7.

local arrangements, there should be a comprehensive sanitary code administered centrally to 'secure uniformity.'[72] From 1939 the Department of Health assumed powers to become that central administration. The Department exerted its authority by the powers already vested in the Secretary of State for Scotland, by his additional powers under the Defence (General) Regulations and (in the words of the Chief Medical Officer for Scotland[73]) by exhortation.[74] The Department organised and strengthened measures to protect the health of the community from the hazards that might be expected in wartime. Local authorities were directed in measures to control infection. The existing regulations for vaccination against smallpox were enforced; new schemes of immunisation against diphtheria and whooping cough were introduced.[75] Depots were established for the distribution of antitoxin against botulism. Schemes were arranged for the containment of outbreaks of scarlet fever and preparations were made in expectation of cases of typhus and rabies. Water supplies for all communities of over 3,000 were chlorinated. Measures were put in place to make milk safe, either by pasteurisation or by other means. Measures were introduced to reduce the contamination of air. In October 1943 guidelines were issued to ensure the best use of the limited supply of penicillin.[76] Efforts were made to maintain good standards of nutrition. Milk was made more readily available in schools and during holidays. School meals were no longer restricted to children of poor families or those who had to travel long distances to school, and meals were provided at boys' and girls' clubs, and at community centres. From December 1942 cod liver oil and fruit juices were distributed to children.[77] These achievements were administered centrally and attained a large degree of uniformity.

In addition to these traditional approaches to public health, in November 1941 the Department of Health launched a campaign on 'Making the People Health Minded.'[78] As in the Cathcart Report, the usefulness of pamphlets, posters, public lectures, and even of the cinema, in health propaganda was treated by the Department of Health with considerable scepticism. 'As a first step towards bringing the ordinary man and woman to a more health-

72 Cathcart Report, p. 5.
73 Written in a typescript circular that preceded the issue of the first Health Bulletin (RECPE Archive).
74 This exhortation was by official memoranda and, after June 1941, by the regular issues of the *Health Bulletin*, a publication launched by the Chief Medical Officer for Scotland and distributed at first only to Medical Officers of Health, but later to a much wider readership.
75 *Health Bulletin*, i, 2, 1941, p. 5.
76 *Health Bulletin*, ii, 6, 1943, p. 78.
77 Department of Health for Scotland, Circular 201/1942.
78 *Health Bulletin*, i, 2, 1941, p. 23.

minded attitude,' Medical Officers of Health across Scotland were urged to follow the example of a scheme first launched in Edinburgh.[79] in which members of the casualty services were trained to conduct discussion groups in their areas, acting 'as missionaries in the new campaign and to encourage a common sense application of the basic principles of sound and healthy living.'[80] In 1942, in co-operation with the Scottish Education Department, plans were made to introduce hygiene as a subject in teacher training. Schemes of health education were gradually introduced in nursery schools, primary schools and post-primary schools on the model described in the Cathcart Report. More immediately, from 1943, classes on 'Mothercraft' and 'Housewifery' were included in the curriculum for girls in Scotland's secondary schools.

From 1936 and into the early years of the war the Department of Health had pressed ahead as far as possible with the creation of a new comprehensive state health service based on the Cathcart Report. In the 1930s the Ministry of Health had denied the need for reforms of the health services in England and Wales and, after 1939, was slow to adjust to wartime conditions. In August 1940, the British Medical Association[81] took it upon itself to set up a Medical Planning Commission to 'study wartime developments and their effects on the country's medical services both present and future'[82] in the United Kingdom. The Commission defined the desired objectives for the post-war medical service as:

a) To provide a system of medical services towards the achievement of positive health, the prevention of disease, and the relief of sickness.

b) To render available to every individual all necessary medical services, both general and specialist, and both clinical and institutional.

In an interim report the Commission reiterated many of the criticisms of the existing medical services made in the Cathcart Report, particularly Cathcart's censure of the lack of co-ordination of local authority services.[83] Quoting the Scottish Board of Health's MacAlister Report, the BMA Commission endorsed the principle that 'the organisation of the national health services should be based upon the family as the normal unit and on the family doctor as the normal medical attendant and guardian.'[84] Refer-

79 *Ibid.*
80 *Ibid.*
81 The work of the Commission was carried out by six committees that included representatives of the Royal Colleges and the Royal Scottish Corporations.
82 'Interim Report of the Medical Planning Commission', *BMJ*, i, 1942, p. 743.
83 *Ibid.*, p. 744.
84 *Ibid.*, p. 745.

ring again to the Cathcart Report, the BMA Commission repeated its recommendation that the general practitioner should 'be concerned not only with diagnosis and treatment but also with the promotion of health and the prevention of disease.'[85] The Commission at last conceded that the National Health Insurance, which the BMA had roundly condemned in 1911,[86] had 'proved a greater success than was anticipated' and that it should now be extended and developed as recommended by the Cathcart Report. On hospital reform, the Commission commended the actions of the Department of Health for Scotland which, for several years, had 'advocated joint action for hospital purposes by local authorities and voluntary bodies over wide regions with teaching centres as their base.'[87] The Commission now put forward possible models for the introduction of the 'Group Medicine and Health Centres'[88] that had been advocated in Scotland in the MacAlister Report in 1920 and again in the Cathcart Report in 1936.

The Medical Planning Commission produced an interim report in June 1942. No further report was issued. The Commission had been forestalled by the Government. On 9 October 1941, responding to a question in the House of Commons, the Minister of Health gave the first indication that reform of the health services in England was being considered. However, reform was to be confined to the hospital services:

> It is the objective of Government . . . to insure that by means of a comprehensive hospital service appropriate treatment shall be readily available to every person in need of it. It is accordingly proposed to lay on the major local authorities the duty of securing, in close co-operation with the voluntary hospitals engaged in the same field, the provision of a service by placing on a more regular footing the partnership between the local authority and voluntary hospitals on which the present hospital services depend.[89]

While the voluntary hospitals and 'the more specialised services at teaching centres'[90] were to continue, the local authority system was to absorb the EHS hospitals and be recognised as the dominant partner. This was a rational proposal for England and Wales where, in terms of size, the local authority system was already the major player, providing most of the hospital accommodation, including that for general medicine and surgery.

---

85 *Ibid.*
86 In 1911 the National Health Insurance Scheme had been 'roundly condemned, by the BMA'. Bartrip, *op. cit.*, p. 153.
87 *Ibid.*, p. 745.
88 *Ibid.*, p. 748.
89 *Hansard*, ccclxxiv, HC 9 October 1941, col. 1116.
90 *Ibid.*

In England and Wales the Emergency Hospital Service was, relatively, only a third of the size of that in Scotland[91] and had not been used so extensively to supplement the pre-war services or to foster the new specialist services; it could therefore be readily taken over by local authorities.

Such a plan was clearly impractical for Scotland where the voluntary hospitals had always been the main suppliers of the core hospital services of general surgery and medicine and where the number of beds for these core services provided by the local authorities was now only a fifth of the number of beds available in EHS hospitals. Local authorities in Scotland, unlike those in England and Wales, had never been given powers to develop the ancillary services, even such basic services as out-patient clinics and ambulance services, so necessary for any fully functioning general hospital.[92] Outside the major cities, local health authorities in Scotland had no experience in managing a modern general hospital.

Nevertheless the Minister of Health had made it clear that the Government's policy was to apply to Scotland as well as to England and Wales, although 'certain differences in the Emergency Hospital Service and in the method of financing voluntary hospitals in Scotland are being given consideration.'[93]

This new Government policy was a direct contradiction of the proposals in the Cathcart Report, which represented the consensus view in Scotland. Tom Johnston, the Secretary of State for Scotland, had now to examine the problems posed for Scotland by the Minister of Health's statement. He appointed Sir Hector Hetherington, Principal of the University of Glasgow, to chair a Committee on Post-War Hospital Problems in Scotland. Sir Hector hoped to avoid any unnecessary discord. In a letter to Tom Johnston on 23 December 1941, he wrote: 'In selecting members I have tried to avoid people who might be regarded as being too closely committed to the view of the Voluntary Hospitals or the Local Authorities.'[94] But even before his committee had begun its work he was warned by W.R. Fraser, Secretary of the Department of Health, that the soundings 'of the principal interests'[95] indicated that the longstanding consensus in Scotland was in some danger of becoming unsettled. Both the voluntary hospitals and the local authorities had been disturbed by the Minister of Health's statement and both were suspicious of the committee now being set up to interpret that policy for

91 PRO, CAB 24/284 CP(39) 77; PRO, CAB 27/659 EHO 1(39)2.
92 Sections 181(2) (a) and 197 (1) of the Public Health Act, 1936 that provided these powers in England and Wales, did not apply in Scotland.
93 *Hansard*, 1942, *op. cit.*
94 DC 8/1101, Letter from Sir Hector Hetherington to the Secretary of State, 23 December 1941.
95 DC 8/1101, Letter from W. R. Fraser to Sir Hector Hetherington, 27 December 1941.

Scotland. Sir Hector, in a letter to the Secretary of State in December 1942, accepted that his task would be 'difficult and thorny.' It was not open to his Committee to design a hospital service from scratch. 'The ground is already very well occupied with institutions of all kinds, many of them with years of distinguished service.' There was also 'the special and most interesting question of the future of the Government [EHS] hospitals of which, so far as I know, the Department of Health has made a great success.'[96] In Sir Hector's view the options open to his Committee had been severely restricted by the Government's decision announced by the Minister of Health on 9 October, and 'I take it that by that decision we are bound.'[97] Later he found that his difficulties had been increased even further by the publication of the Beveridge Report which had 'added a certain definiteness to several points in the original statement by the Minister of Health.'[98]

The Hetherington Committee struggled to find an acceptable solution. After a year, in December 1942, Tom Johnston wrote to Sir Hector: 'I need hardly point out that the early publication of your Committee's report has now become a matter of importance, and I am sure the committee will be anxious to assist us by letting us have it as soon as possible.'[99] On 14 April 1943 Johnston wrote again. He accepted that the Beveridge Report and various official statements about the post-war National Health Service were creating difficulties for the committee. 'But I am alarmed to think that we shall not have a report from you before August. Until I get your report I cannot go very far in discussions with the Voluntary Hospitals and I am afraid that consultations in England may get so far ahead that nothing which the Committee might say will make any difference . . . I am satisfied that a provisional or summary report could not fail to exert a greater influence on the discussions than would a full-length report in four months time.'[100]

In June the Committee had still not reached a conclusion but had indicated that it had it in mind to recommend that the EHS hospitals should be handed over to the local authorities. In a letter on 7 June Tom Johnston asked the Committee to reconsider. 'Since I have become Secretary of State, I have been impressed with the great value which the possession of State hospitals has been to us in facilitating experiments and pioneering work in various directions . . . These experiments have wide public and medical practitioner support, and their cancellation would be

96 DC 8/1101. Draft of letter from Sir Hector Hetherington to the Secretary of State, December 1941.
97 Ibid.
98 Ibid.
99 DC 8/1101. Draft of Letter from the Secretary of State to Sir Hector Hetherington, December 1942.
100 Ibid.

regarded as disastrous. I suggest that the difficulties of direct ownership by the Department of Health side by side with voluntary and local authority owned hospitals could easily be obviated by a sort of Public Corporation management of these state hospitals.'[101] On 21 June Tom Johnston gave more details of the Public Corporation he had in mind. He suggested

> an organisation on lines similar to the Scottish Housing Association which consists of persons invited by the Secretary of State to form an association for a particular purpose, the association being registered under the Companies Act. It might consist of from six to ten members, probably with a paid chairman and it would of course have the necessary administrative, technical and clerical staff.
>
> The business of the corporation would be to take over and administer such of the State's own hospitals as were not required for other purposes. It would be subject to general directions from the Secretary of State, the most important of the directions no doubt being one which defined its scope in terms of pioneer and experimental work in certain fields.
>
> The Corporation would be expected to co-operate, in the exercise of its functions, with other interests, particularly in such matters as the transfer of suitable patients, the joint use of certain consultants and specialists, etc. We should hope that suitable arrangements could be made with the Universities and other recognised Teaching Bodies for the use of material for both undergraduate and postgraduate study.[102]

Although the primary purpose of the Corporation's work would be to carry out pioneering work, it would also assist the other hospital services in introducing newly developed forms of treatment and provide assistance in reducing waiting lists. The exact financial arrangements would ultimately depend on the financial arrangements for the country's hospital services as a whole, but the Corporation would be substantially supported by the National Exchequer and would not have to depend on charitable funds or become a charge on local rates.[103]

The Corporation proposed by the Secretary of State could have been incorporated in Cathcart's recommendation that the hospital system should be based on the co-operation of voluntary and statutory hospitals and the public authorities. But the Hetherington Committee felt bound absolutely by the Government's stated policy for the United Kingdom. When its report

101 DC 8/1101. Letter from the Secretary of State to Sir Hector Hetherington, 7 June 1943.
102 DC 8/1101, Letter from the Secretary of State to Sir Hector Hetherington, 21 June 1943.
103 Ibid.

was eventually published on 13 October 1943,[104] the Secretary of State's proposal of a Public Corporation was ignored. In flat contradiction of Tom Johnston's proposal, the report recommended that the experiment of state-run hospitals should be discontinued and that the Secretary of State, acting through the Department of Health, should refrain from active participation in general hospital administration. The Secretary of State must maintain his position of impartiality, essential to his function as arbiter between all other parties within the health care system. The EHS hospitals were to go either to the voluntary or to the local authority sectors on easy financial terms. This was thought to be in line with Government policy that was predicated on the assumption that, in time, voluntary hospitals would inevitably run into financial difficulties and, one by one, they would then be taken over by the local authorities. In the meantime, in Scotland, harmonious and effective partnership between the voluntary and local authorities was to be secured by setting up advisory councils in each of the five regions. These councils were to have equal representation from the two hospital systems with an independent chairman and a group of medical assessors to represent local medical opinion. The advisory councils would have some administrative authority including control of admission to hospitals. Unpaid medical service in the voluntary hospitals would cease and there would be uniform salary scales in both hospital systems. A compulsory contribution scheme that would entitle patients to treatment and maintenance in hospital was to be set up as part of the social security scheme. Exchequer grants, administered by a Central Hospitals Fund, would be distributed to both voluntary and local authority hospitals to cover 60% of their expenditure.

The Report of the Committee on Post-War Hospital Problems in Scotland was a failure. It was late. Its financial arrangements were hopelessly complex; it was far from unanimous; it was disowned by its Chairman in a long and carefully argued Reservation of 12 paragraphs. More significantly, it was not well received by the Secretary of State. He presented its recommendations in a memorandum to Cabinet on 1 September 1943 without comment.[105] He had already let it be known in Cabinet and elsewhere that he hoped to retain Department of Health hospitals within the hospital system in Scotland. He was well aware that, in the short term at least, committing them to the administration of the local authorities was an entirely impractical proposition. For almost every local authority in Scotland the administration of general hospitals was a closed book. Johnston was also in no doubt that any suggestion of consigning the country's hospitals to the care of the local

104 *Report of the Committee on Post-War Hospital Problems in Scotland*, 1943, Cmd. 6472 (the Hetherington Report).
105 PRO, CAB 87/13 PR (43) 52; NAS HH101/2.

authorities, even in the long term, would be bitterly opposed by the medical profession in Scotland.

The Hetherington Report was a setback for Scotland. The long delay before it was submitted weakened the position of the Secretary of State during Cabinet discussions on the future of the health services.[106] It had failed even to consider an imaginative proposal by the Secretary of State for a new force in hospital services that would have been easily accommodated as a logical development within the general scheme proposed by Cathcart. The Cathcart Report still represented the preferred plan for Scotland, but for the moment it had lost some of its impact. The Hetherington Report seemed to suggest that the consensus in Scotland had weakened.

Suddenly in 1942 all discussions of the future of Britain's medical services had been given a new impetus and a new context with the publication of the Beveridge Report on Social Insurance and Allied Services. The welfare system devised by Beveridge was predicated on the assumption that it would be supported by a comprehensive National Health Service. In February 1943 the Government announced that it accepted that assumption. The Health Ministers (Ernest Brown, the Minister of Health, and Tom Johnston, the Secretary of State for Scotland) now embarked on a staged process of planning for the National Health Service. In the first stage the Ministers held informal and confidential discussions to test the feeling of interested parties, the local authority associations, the bodies representing the voluntary hospitals, the Royal Colleges and Royal Corporations. Groups, chosen from the relevant bodies, were set up to discuss in detail those aspects of a comprehensive service that would most affect them. These confidential discussions informed the Ministers of current views but the Ministers also made it clear that what they had in mind was not a revolution but 'part of a general evolution of improved health services which has been going on in this country for generations.'[107] The introduction of a single comprehensive service for all was to be regarded as the natural next development.[108] In presenting a White Paper in 1944, the Ministers (now Henry Willink as Minister of Health and Tom Johnston as Secretary of State for Scotland) drew attention to the various reports on the health services that had made significant contributions to the progress achieved in previous decades. The Dawson Report and the MacAlister Report were given credit for the proposal that the NHI scheme should be extended to cover all persons at the same economic level as insured persons and dependants of insured persons. The Cave Report and the Sankey

106 DC 8/1101.
107 Ibid.
108 *A National Health Service*, 1944, Cmd. 6502, p. 5.

Report had proposed the establishment of central and local bodies to co-ordinate hospital services and had recommended that voluntary hospitals should be supported by Exchequer grants. The contributions made by the BMA and the bodies representing the voluntary hospitals[109] and the factual report published by Political and Economic Planning were all briefly noticed. However, particular prominence was given to the Cathcart Report:

> The report is too comprehensive in scope to lend itself to brief quotation, but it is one of the most complete official surveys of the country's health services and health problems yet attempted. The recommendations of the Committee have already been the basis of legislation in particular fields.[110]

The White paper acknowledged the importance of the Cathcart Report in setting out a national policy that included the promotion of the fitness of the people, the integration of the existing separate medical services to form a single integrated medical service and based, as far as possible, on the family doctor.[111]

The White Paper reviewed the health services in the United Kingdom as they existed in 1944 in order to illustrate what had already been achieved towards the establishment of a comprehensive health service. The Highlands and Islands Medical Service was particularly commended as 'a unique effort in co-operation between the State and doctors in private practice which has revolutionised medical provision in the area.' The White Paper set out in some detail how this co-operation had been achieved and maintained. It also drew attention to the vital contribution to the success of the HIMS made by the 'similar improvement that has been effected by the nursing services.' Since its foundation the service had developed 'beyond the primary essentials, medical and nursing' to provide general medical and surgical hospital services, tuberculosis and other specialist services. In 1944 there was in place a 'comprehensive service which obviates the transfer of many patients to the mainland' but also included an air ambulance service when transfers were necessary. The success of the HIMS had been achieved at an annual cost of 'just under £100,000.'[112]

In the White Paper the Ministers declared their intention to create a service that would be comprehensive in two senses – first it was to be available to all and second it was to cover all necessary forms of health care from the care of minor ailments to the care of major diseases and disabilities.

109 British Hospitals Association, King Edward's Hospital Fund for London, the Contributory Schemes Association.
110 *A National Health Service, op. cit.,* p. 75.
111 *Ibid.*
112 *Ibid.*

It was to include the ancillary services of nursing and midwifery 'and of the other things which ought to go with medical care.'[113] Advice and attention – from family doctor to specialists and consultants of all kinds – must cover the whole field of medicine, at home, in the consulting room, in the hospital or the sanatorium or wherever else was appropriate. The service was to be free for all, apart from possible charges for certain appliances. The inclusion of mental health services would not be possible until the law on lunacy and mental deficiency was re-drawn but the Ministers aimed to reduce as far as possible the distinction between mental ill health and physical ill health.

In the White Paper the Ministers set out what they believed to be the best means of bringing the service into effective operation. The scope and objectives of the service were to be the same in Scotland as in England and Wales but there would necessarily be certain differences in method and organisation. The structure of the service in Scotland would take into account the uneven distribution of Scotland's population – 80% concentrated in the 17% of the area of the country across its central 'waist' while 32 of the 55 local authority areas had populations of less than 50,000. Principal responsibility for the operation of the new service would therefore not be devolved to Scotland's very disparate local authorities, but would rest with the Secretary of State. While the employing agency for general practitioners would be the Central Medical Board (as in England and Wales), the proposed health centres would be administered centrally by the Secretary of State and not by local authorities as in England. In Scotland, all other services would be arranged in five administrative regions; the units of organisation in England and Wales would continue to be the counties and county boroughs

In 1944, the White Paper was issued for discussion and for the formulation of separate Bills to create the National Health Service in England and Wales and in Scotland. It left many differences unresolved in England and Wales, making it inevitable that, in finalising a Bill, there would be acrimony and delay. The formulation of the Bill for Scotland promised to be relatively free of controversy. In Scotland there was a long-standing consensus that had found its expression in the Cathcart Report and in the White Paper itself and, in the Highlands and Islands Medical Service, Scotland already had thirty years' experience in administering a comprehensive health service.

113 *Ibid.,* p. 9.

10

Two Acts and Two Services

The first post-war General Election, in July 1945, brought in a Government determined to introduce the legislation for the National Health Service within its first session.[1] The new Cabinet saw the White Paper issued by the previous Government as an unsatisfactory 'muddle,' especially in relation to its proposals for the service for England and Wales. The conflicting interests of the local authorities, the voluntary hospitals and the different sections of the medical profession in England and Wales had been left unresolved. Within the Ministry of Health there was still a lingering loyalty to the idea that the administration of new service should be devolved, as far as possible, to the local authorities. 'No government would want such a service to be administered by the Minister direct or by a corporate body supervised by the Minister.'[2] This Ministry view was strongly resisted by the British Hospitals Association, the governing bodies of the voluntary hospitals and the medical profession. However, the medical profession in England and Wales was agreed about little else; various, and often conflicting, strands of opinion were represented by the BMA, the Royal Colleges and the Socialist Medical Association while the views of the great majority of the profession had never been canvassed and remained unknown. In this confused situation the Cabinet was itself divided. Herbert Morrison supported the stand of the officers of the Ministry of Health, arguing on behalf of the local authorities in general and the London County Council in particular.[3] His views were actively opposed by Christopher Addison and at least four other members of the Cabinet[4] and were not acceptable to Aneurin Bevan, the new Minister of Health. It is the struggle to resolve these entrenched differences in England and Wales together with the belligerence of the BMA in negotiating the terms of employment for doctors that has been the focus of attention for historians and lives on in folk memory as the story of the creation of the National Health Service in Britain.

The White Paper, as it applied to Scotland, was free from these conflicts. The scheme for Scotland was firmly based on the recommendations of the

1 J. Pater, *The Making of the National Health Service* (London, 1981), p. 107.
2 *Ibid.*, p. 26.
3 The London County Council was the largest hospital authority in Britain and could provide services that could no be matched by other local authorities.
4 *Ibid.*, p. 111.

Cathcart Report that represented a consensus that had evolved in Scotland over many years. Only one gap in the plan for Scotland remained. The failure of the Hetherington Report had left the plan without any clear indication of how the integrated hospital service in Scotland was to be administered.

On 5 October 1945, the new Minister of Health, Aneurin Bevan, presented a paper to Cabinet[5] outlining his plan for the solution to what had emerged as the major problem in the structuring the National Health Service for England and Wales and the only remaining gap in the plan for Scotland. He proposed to nationalise the nation's hospitals.[6] Only the teaching hospitals were not to be taken over. A week later he modified his proposal; teaching hospitals were not to be excluded completely but 'special provision should be made for them within the scheme.' Following the publication of the White Paper, the governing bodies of the teaching hospitals and their consultant staff had made it clear that they would remain opposed to nationalisation unless given a much greater share in the planning and control of the new service.[7] Bevan's undertaking to make 'special provision' for the teaching hospitals silenced the opposition of a powerful pressure group and secured support for the main body of his proposals in the House of Lords from Lord Moran and Lord Dawson.[8]

Each teaching hospital was to be administered by a Board of Governors responsible directly to the Ministry of Health and not to the Regional Board in its area. One-fifth of the membership of the Board of Governors could be nominated by the Regional Board but the teaching hospitals were otherwise to lie outside the administrative and financial structure of the hospital service which served the Regions in which they were situated. Local hospitals were therefore limited in their access to the best specialist expertise and equipment in their areas. Teaching and research were virtually confined to designated teaching hospitals and medical students in England and Wales were deprived of proper experience in infectious disease and in the care of the disabled and the chronic sick.

In the provinces of England and Wales the teaching hospitals of ten university towns and cities[9] were set apart from the Regional hospital system. In London this separate designation was even more divisive and had an effect on the functioning of the NHS in every part of England and Wales.

5 PRO CAB 21/2032 (CP (45) 205).
6 This possibility was already being considered by Scottish officials.
7 Pater, *op. cit.*, p. 107.
8 *Ibid.*, p. 124.
9 Birmingham, Bristol, Cambridge, Cardiff, Liverpool, Leeds, Manchester, Newcastle (Durham), Oxford, Sheffield.

Eleven undergraduate teaching hospitals[10] and sixteen postgraduate teaching hospitals[11] in London remained outside the general hospital scheme. This not only continued the dissociation of London teaching hospitals from other local hospitals but, by allowing the great majority of the undergraduate and postgraduate teaching and research to remain concentrated in London, it confirmed London as the single commanding centre of specialist practice and research in the whole of England and Wales. The London teaching hospitals were also allowed to retain endowments that were, in general, vastly greater than those of provincial hospitals. With greater financial resources, a reputation as leaders in maintaining high standards of practice and a considerable measure of administrative independence, London teaching hospitals perpetuated a culture in London from which Regional hospitals were excluded and with which even the teaching hospitals in the provinces could have only an ambivalent relationship.

Among the privileges allowed to the London teaching hospitals was the direct access of their Boards of Governors to the Minister of Health. Paradoxically, it was not the full-time academic staff, but the Harley Street consultants holding part-time appointments at the 27 teaching hospitals in London, that dominated their Boards of Governors and through them could bring influence to bear on Government. The influence of this same group was further strengthened in the composition of the Central Health Services Council, the influential body that not only advised Government directly but also determined the composition of all other advisory bodies within the NHS in England and Wales. The National Health Act, 1946 provided that of the 41 members of the Council 'six shall be the persons for the time holding the offices of President of the Royal College of Physicians of London, the President of the Royal College of Surgeons of England, the President of the Royal College of Obstetricians, the Chairman of the Council of the British Medical Association, the President of the General Medical Council and the Chairman of the Council of the Society of Medical Officers of Health.'[12] These *exofficio* members, each the formal spokesman of an outside body, made up a large and most powerful group within this very

10 Charing Cross, Guy's, King's, London, Middlesex, Royal Free, St Bartholomew's, St George's, St Mary's, St Thomas's, University College.
11 Hammersmith Hospital; City of London Maternity Hospital; Hospital for Sick Children; London Chest Hospital; Metropolitan Ear, Nose and Throat Hospital; Moorfields Eye Hospital; National Hospital for Diseases of the Heart; National Hospital for the Paralysed; Queen Charlotte's Hospital; Royal Eye Hospital, Royal National Orthopaedic Hospital, Royal National Throat, Nose and Ear Hospital; St John's Hospital for Diseases of the Skin; St Paul's Hospital for Urological and Skin Diseases; St Peter's Hospital for Skin and Urological Diseases; West End Hospital for Nervous Diseases.
12 National Health Services Act, First Schedule.

influential body.[13] General practice, consultant practice outside the teaching hospitals, local authority medicine, industrial medicine and the universities together were represented by only thirteen members. This was a continuation of the practice followed in England in appointing the Consultative Council on Medical and Allied Services from 1929 which allowed the management of state health services in England and Wales to be strongly influenced by medical pressure groups from outside the service structure.[14] In 1948, great, and arguably undue, influence over the activities and policies of the NHS again became vested in bodies outside the structure of the service and not exclusively devoted to its interests. Paradoxically, these influential groups, whose relationship with the National Health Service remained ambivalent, were often assumed to represent the attitudes and ambitions of a profession almost totally committed to the NHS.

Scotland was not drawn into these controversies and divisions. At the Cabinet meeting on 5 October 1945, George Buchanan, the Under-Secretary of State for Scotland, successfully argued against giving teaching hospitals special status and administration in Scotland. He was armed with a short memorandum to this effect, prepared at the Department of Health for Scotland by Sir Norman Graham and Sir Douglas Haddow, which was accepted without opposition.[15] It followed that the Scottish Heath Services Council set up by the Scottish Act was quite different from the Central Council, the equivalent advisory body for England and Wales. Its membership of 35 was made up of 18 medical practitioners (unspecified), three dental practitioners, two nurses, a midwife, two pharmacists, four non-medical members, two with experience of hospital management and two with experience of local government. No professional or other body outside the structure of the National Health Service was formally represented. The chief advisory body created for Scotland did not have members constrained in their commitment to the NHS by conflicting responsibilities to outside bodies.

In the NHS in Scotland the family doctor became 'the indispensable instrument of national health policy.'[16] Care was taken to ensure that local authorities were not in a position to influence the distribution or scope of general practitioner services. Experience had shown that a general practitioner service provided by local authorities would be 'unreliable and would

---

13 A further two members represented the mental health services.
14 The resulting conflicts have been described by Eckstein in *Pressure Group Politics, op. cit.*
15 'It was very short and it went through, much to our surprise. When he got back, George said that Attlee had congratulated him on this very short and encouraging paper. There was never any argument about it and we went ahead on that basis.' Sir Norman Graham, recorded interview.
16 Cathcart Report, p. 156.

operate unevenly.'[17] The Scottish Act was therefore designed to keep the responsibilities of the local authorities within the limits of their capabilities.

In Scotland services were organised in areas determined by functional considerations and designed to promote co-operation. The contract of employment of general practitioners was to be with central Government for part-time services and remunerated by capitation fees. In Scotland, the general practitioner service was to be administered by Executive Councils for areas of convenient size and population and not designed to be coterminous with local authority districts. As indicated in the White Paper, more extensive use was to be made of Health Centres than in England and Wales. They were to be provided by the Secretary of State as premises for general practice and to act as the points of contact in an integration of services – specialist consultant services, dentistry, pharmacy, and 'any of the health services which local or education authorities are required or empowered to provide.'[18] They were to be managed by local committees representing these services.

While the terms of employment of general practitioners in England and Wales matched almost exactly those in Scotland,[19] the organisation of Health Centres was to be critically different. In England and Wales, Health Centres were to be established, equipped, maintained and managed by the local authorities, an arrangement that promised to perpetuate the inequalities and unevenness that Cathcart had found to characterise all local authority services. Since local authorities were no more popular with doctors in England than in Scotland, it was also a potential source of conflict.

Hospital Regions in Scotland were designed to be large enough to provide the full range of hospital practice – including medical training, research and development – and with the support of all necessary services including ambulances, blood transfusion, bacteriology and other laboratory services. General practice and its associated pharmacy services were more conveniently organised in smaller Executive Council districts. Local authority medical services continued to operate in districts coterminous with districts served by other local authority services such as education and public health.

In finally submitting the Health Service (Scotland) Bill for the approval Parliament in December 1946, the Secretary of State for Scotland stated that his Bill was essential to the scheme set out two years before in the White Paper of 1944,[20] modified only in response to the decision to nationalise the

---

17 Ibid., p. 162.
18 *A National Health Service*, 1944, Cmd. 6502, p. 45.
19 In recognition of the differences in dispensing in the two countries, the Apothecaries Act of 1815, which applied only in England and Wales, was not repealed.
20 *Hansard*, xixxxi, HC 10 December 1946, cols. 995–1002.

hospitals, a decision made in October 1945. His statement was the only public acknowledgement that the Scottish Bill had been ready since early in 1946 but had not been presented to Parliament until an acceptable formula for agreement could be been found for England and Wales.

When it was finally published, the National Health Service Act for England and Wales was identical with that already drawn up for Scotland except for two very important additional paragraphs specially written in to accommodate the concessions that had proved necessary to resolve the conflicts of interest in England and Wales. Paragraph 46 of the National Health Service Act, 1946 allowed for the concessions made to satisfy the interests of the local authorities. Paragraph 15 excluded from the general scheme the London teaching hospitals and by extension the provincial teaching hospitals. All the differences in the structure of the services north and south of the border in 1948 flowed from these two paragraphs.[20] The Act for England and Wales had been achieved with 'a notable lack of consensus'[21] and two paragraphs in the National Health Service Act of 1946 had introduced fissure lines in the unified service for England and Wales. The NHS was introduced in England and Wales with 'a conspicuous lack of harmony.'

The National Health (Scotland) Act was drawn up and passed without conflict. The scheme to introduce a comprehensive state health service had been in preparation for more than a decade and the introduction of the service was in the hands of an already committed administration at the Scottish Office. In 1935, Sir Godfrey Collins had obtained Treasury permission to recruit officers of 'suitable quality, education and other wise'[22] to replace the civil servants of executive grade who had previously made up the staff of the Scottish Office. The first to be appointed as an Assistant Principal was T. D. Haddow, followed later by Norman Graham, James Hogarth and Ronald Fraser. James Ford, returning to the Scottish Office after service in the army throughout the war, found that although 'there had been no sweeping changes, the leopard had changed its spots. Before the war, senior civil servants might advise ministers on the things that should be done but never attempted to achieve much on their own account. In the 1940s, a new breed of civil servants began to manage and take initiatives.'[23] By 1945 the Scottish Office had a new structure. A. L. Rennie[24] was a member of the new team:

21 C. Webster, *The National Health Service: A Political History* (Oxford, 1998), p. 3.
22 I. Levitt, *The Scottish Office: Depression and Reconstruction 1919–1959* (Edinburgh, 1992), p. 16.
23 J. Ford, CB, MC, later Registrar General for Scotland.
24 A. L. Rennie, CB, Department of Health for Scotland, 1947–62, Assistant Secretary, Scottish Home and Health Department, 1963–69.

The older men had great experience and ability. While they continued in charge of often complicated tasks of implementation and management, the policy drive was in the hands of new men. In a crude generalisation, one could say that the management divisions and branches were headed by the older men, while policy areas were the province of the young Turks – Douglas Haddow, Norman Graham, James Hogarth and Ronald Fraser. The Scottish Departments exemplified the civil service tradition of serving Ministers of all parties but they also saw themselves as advocates for Scotland. The Scottish Office had a strong ethic that our purpose was to deliver the best service in Scotland that we could.

The Scottish Office now had the people that Cathcart had required 'for efficient administration and sound governance.' They were unruffled by the late and troublesome disputes in London and, from a distance, respected Aneuran Bevan's efforts to overcome them. Sir Norman Graham,[25] responsible for the introduction of the new hospital service in Scotland recalls:

The Cathcart Report, in effect, laid the foundation for the whole National Health Service. It made a great impact in Scotland and beyond . . . Bevan was a radical who took the very serious problems of the hospital service at the end of the war by the scruff of the neck. He had to face much opposition, especially from the consultants in the south, but they were placated by the provisions in the legislation that gave the teaching hospitals their own Boards of Governors and separate financial arrangements. When he produced his proposals for what was in effect nationalisation, Scottish Ministers welcomed them and the prospect that statutory and financial control would lead to an integrated hospital service. In Scotland the Department of Health already had more experience in hospital administration than their opposite numbers in the London. And at that time the Scottish teaching hospitals accounted for such a large part of the general hospital provision that it was generally accepted that they should be an integral part of the Regional structure.

Most of the leading people in the medical profession in Scotland realised the need for change. Compared with the situation in the south the Scottish legislation was, relatively, a downhill run. Ronald Fraser[26] agreed:

25 Sir Norman Graham, Kt, CB, FRSE, Principal Private Secretary to the Secretary of State for Scotland, 1944–45; Assistant Secretary, Department of Health for Scotland, 1945–56.
26 Ronald P. Fraser, CB, Assistant Private Secretary to the Secretary of State for Scotland, 1944–47; Cabinet Office, 1947–54, Assistant Secretary, Department of Health for Scotland, 1954–61.

The Cathcart Report came out in 1936. It was the first study of its kind and had the greatest input into the planning of the National Health Service. It was the fount of all knowledge. Considered in a Scottish context, I have always felt that there was a certain artificiality in the later arguments that developed between the government, the BMA and the consultants and specialists and so on. The emergence of the National Health Service was quite inevitable and that really on two levels, first on the political level and second on a purely practical level. It was pretty well inescapable given the political situation at the time. It was also inescapable when you think of the state of the game in general practice. And the voluntary hospitals had been reduced in the pre-war depression and in the war they were on their beam end, baled out by money put in by the government. If Nye Bevan had not existed we in Scotland would have found ourselves carried into a National Health Service just as we were in 1948.

In 'an evolution that had been built up over the years by a variety of authorities, voluntary and public,'[27] the Department of Health for Scotland had already made substantial progress towards the creation of the National Health Service before 1948. Within two years of the publication of the Cathcart Report, Scotland's hospitals were surveyed in preparation for war. In 1939, the Emergency Hospital Service (EHS) Scheme was set up under the Civil Defence Act and in a very short time Scotland's total hospital accommodation had been greatly expanded and space had been created for the introduction of new specialist services.[28] All hospital services in Scotland were now directed and largely financed by the state. A. L. Rennie remembers that:

> Scotland had a flying start in the NHS revenue allocations because the running costs of the EHS hospitals – disproportionately located north of the border – were fully met in the initial provisions of the service. The allocations for capital works reflected bids made by the two Health Departments in London and Edinburgh with the influence of the Goshen formula in the background – Scotland 11: England and Wales 81. Here the Scottish Department, pressed by the Regional Hospital Boards – in turn under strong pressure largely, but not entirely, from their teaching hospitals – was able to carry out proportionately more capital work than the Ministry in London could manage, with its much larger and more diffuse regional and local administrations to energise.

27 *Annual Report of the Department of Health for Scotland*, 1948, Cmd. 7659, p. 11.
28 Sir John Brotherston, 'The Development of Public Medical Care 1900–1948', in G. MacLachlan (ed.), *Improving the Common Weal* (Edinburgh, 1987), p. 84.

As the revenue required to run new hospital units came on stream (known as the 'revenue consequences of capital schemes' and at that time funded by the Treasury as an absolute additional revenue commitment) the gap in revenue allocations continued to widen.[29]

The country's general practitioners had also come under the direction of the state in 1939 through the agency of the BMA's Scottish Emergency Committee that had been given authority to allocate doctors either to the armed services or to civilian work. By 1948, general practitioners in Scotland already had years of experience of employment or direction by the state. James Hogarth, who, as an Assistant Secretary at the Scottish Office, had responsibility for general practitioner services in the early of the NHS, remembers other advantages:

> We were relatively well off in Scotland in having more doctors. Lists in Scotland were something like 2000 patients per doctor and 2,500 in the south. And we did have financial advantages. If Scotland needed a little money for something or other, the Treasury would say – 'well it's not very much really'. We were able to build up a surplus. It built up very gradually.
>
> Relations with the Ministry were perfectly all right, but we knew that certain officials were rather hostile to advantages that Scotland was receiving. The Chief Medical Officer was certainly not favourable to Scotland. Something of the same was true of the BMA. There was a degree of antagonism between the Scottish BMA and the United Kingdom BMA. General practitioners in Scotland didn't always agree with their colleagues in the south.
>
> In the Department of Health, we got on very well with the BMA and the other general practitioners. We were on first name terms and held meetings in each others' houses. If we wanted to discuss something at any time we rang them up. The Ministry was at a distance from their regional organisations and their contacts were more formal. We got a lot of special arrangements in Scotland because we could discuss them quite frankly and openly with the BMA and the profession generally.

The hospitals in Scotland were to be administered by five Regional Boards, and for each one an entirely new management structure had to be created. In March 1948, Robert Moore[30] was appointed as Secretary of the Eastern Regional Board at Dundee. He was then 32 years old. His previous experience was as Town Clerk of Port Glasgow for five years:

29 A. L. Rennie, *op. cit.*
30 Robert Moore, CBE, Secretary, Eastern Regional Hospital Board, 1948–60.

I had an administration to set up and the Board to organise. It was a hellish time but I enjoyed it. The first Chairman was the very socialist Lord Provost of Dundee and we had a few other local authority members and representatives of trade unions but you would never have known which party anyone belonged to. There was no political bias. The other Board members were mostly nominated by the consultants but there was never any strife. And I don't remember any relationship with the BMA. There were difficulties but never any real opposition.

There were regular meetings of all the Chairmen and chief officers of the Regional Boards in Scotland. We talked about common problems and that was very useful. Although they had no official standing at these meetings, Douglas Haddow and Norman Graham always attended. There was always regular contact with the centre. Douglas Haddow would send me drafts of circulars the Department was about to issue and ask 'what do you think of this?' Norman Graham would get the minutes of our Board meetings and ring me up and say 'what's all this bloody nonsense about?'. In Scotland we knew each other well and relationships were very good. In England they didn't know each other. People in the Regions weren't friendly with people in Whitehall. They weren't close enough and they didn't see each other often enough. The Ministry tended to be more dictatorial. Because everything was done in writing in England it was all much more formal. Sheer size created that kind of relationship.

It is now almost impossible to find any evidence of significant or substantial resistance to the introduction of the NHS in Scotland. It is even more difficult to find any evidence that those who eagerly joined the NHS in Scotland were greatly motivated by ideological or political persuasion. For most, even medical politics were irrelevant. Dale Falconer, formerly Scottish Secretary of the BMA, confirmed the lack of conflict in Scotland over the introduction of the NHS:

When the health service came in 1948 the BMA in Scotland played no part at all. The consultants and hospital people were not members. On the other hand the GPs were all members. But they were all very poor and they saw that they were going to be looked after by the National Health Service. So there was no need for the BMA.

For the great majority of doctors in Scotland, the NHS offered a new degree of security of employment, an opportunity to practise a higher standard of medicine, and for many, a more acceptable way of life. Ekke von Kuenssberg became a general practitioner in Edinburgh in 1943:

It was the kind of practice where you did all the day and night work yourself. Seeing a hundred patients a day was chicken feed. We were lucky if we got three hours sleep a night. And there was the blackout. Every street lamp had a dash of white paint at the base and you had to learn how to get anywhere three white marks on the right then two on the left and so on. It was clear to me that this pattern of general practice was impossible. The Cathcart Report had been on the horizon since 1936. After the war something had to happen or there would be an earthquake. The few who resisted the health service seemed to get more press and more attention than the majority. The BMA was against it but there was a difference between the BMA and the rest of us in practice. The local BMA was a self-perpetuating group with a perpetual chairman, elected year after year.

Alex Macewan had been a general practitioner in a busy town practice since 1932. He also had an appointment as surgeon to his local voluntary hospital. His practice was well established and prosperous and his hospital had 'no financial difficulties as far as I am aware.' He remembers that, among his acquaintance, it was not only the general practitioners themselves but also their wives, the essential but unpaid partners in most practices, who were attracted by the less harassed life style offered by the NHS.

Dr. J. C. Mercer, a general practitioner in a largely middle-class country practice, was glad to be relieved of a recurring anxiety in treating his less well-off patients:

I remember a young family I was looking after. Father was working and was insured. But it was his child who was ill. The question was that if I give an antibiotic they will have to pay for it. So will I give it now or wait another day to see what happens? Come July 1948 I did not to have to worry about the expense of medicine for the children.

For most people in Scotland the greatest and most immediate benefit of the new NHS came from the general practitioner services. Advice, appliances and even the most expensive of the effective new medicines were all free and immediately available.

The changes in the specialist and hospital services seemed, at first, to benefit fewer people and were less immediately obvious. Robert Moore remembers that on the Appointed Day in July 1948, the patients in his hospitals seemed unaware that any change had taken place. 'I had to tell them about it. Everything just ran on as before. Everyone turned up as usual. There was no impact.'

Nevertheless it was the hospital service that was transformed by the coming of the NHS. New forms of medical treatment and new specialist surgical services – plastic surgery, neurosurgery, orthopaedics – had been developed during the war years. Space had been created for these new activities in the hospitals built for the Emergency Hospital Service. In time there were enormous benefits for patients as the expansion of the new specialisms made them available, not only in a few centres of excellence, but across the country.

There were also great benefits for the medical profession. The NHS made it possible for a new generation of young doctors to train as specialists. Until 1948 there had been no structure of training and support for doctors hoping to practise as specialist hospital physicians and surgeons. For most medical graduates there seemed to be no way into a career as a hospital consultant. 'After all, the pre-war pattern was that you hammered away for years, supported by a wealthy wife, hoping that you could hang on long enough to get an appointment on the consultant staff.'[31] The NHS introduced salaried posts for trainee specialists. 'Registrars could proceed to become Senior Registrars and eventually consultants. It was possible, by simple mathematics, but the system was not perfect. It was a revolving door with some coming in and others going out. Quite a lot of people who had been led to believe that they would become consultants found that when the time came there was no place for them to go after they had been Senior Registrars. I think a lot of them went to Australia and Canada.'[32]

Despite the difficulties, the new training structure provided opportunities for able doctors to make their mark at a time of rapid progress in medical science and practice.

For some young doctors, it became possible to change a career path that had already seemed set. James Williamson,[33] after two years as an assistant in general practice in England – 'a miserable time. Medieval medicine in the middle of the twentieth century' – was able to return to hospital medicine and go on to make a major contribution to the elimination of pulmonary tuberculosis from Scotland in the 1950s and become one of the founders of modern geriatrics. Lord Kilpatrick,[34] like many others in Scotland, was able to study medicine only with the support of a grant from his Local Education Authority. He was aware of the success of the Highlands and Islands Medical Service and the career opportunities that a national extension of such a services would offer. As a student he welcomed the creation of

31 Professor John Forfar, MC, MD, FRCP, FRCPE, FRCP(G), FRSE, Professor of Child Life and Health, University of Edinburgh. Recorded interview.
32 Sir Norman Graham, op. cit.
33 James Williamson, CBE, DSc, FRECPE, Professor of Geriatric Medicine, University of Edinburgh. Recorded interview.
34 Lord Kilpatrick, Kt, CBE, MD, FRCP, FRCPE, FRCP(G), Professor of Medicine, University of Leicester, President of the General Medical Council. Recorded interview.

salaried training posts in the NHS; he could look forward to an academic career in medicine that would have been financially impossible before 1948.

There were new opportunities for women in medicine. Joyce Granger,[35] who had held an appointment in the Emergency Hospital Service during the war, was relieved of 'a growing fear of unemployment among women in medicine. It seemed that, after the war, it would be difficult for women. But with the NHS it wasn't an obvious problem.'

Established physicians like Christopher Clayson,[36] a consultant in the tuberculosis service, found that the coming of the NHS enhanced the potential of the posts they already held:

> I was in favour of the whole scheme from the beginning. There was to be a sudden great change. We consultants could see that we were going to be able to exercise considerable influence and that was very appealing. At that time the problem of tuberculosis was getting out of hand. There weren't enough beds. The number of beds in my sanatorium had to be divided between four local authorities and had to be allocated in proportion to the amount of money the local authorities were willing to subscribe. Some authorities were more worried about their rates and more parsimonious than others. The allocation had to be kept to. All that came to an end in 1948. The entire number of beds came under my complete control and could be used as I thought best.

The National Health Service offered new opportunities but access to these opportunities was often difficult. For those returning from years of military service overseas, to become established in the new service required determination and a willingness to adjust, for a second time, to a new career. Many who had served with distinction and, while still very young, had acquired a degree of authority, found themselves as neophytes in a new order. A few individual histories, chosen and quoted almost at random, illustrate the difficulties experienced by many who later went on to make their mark in the NHS.

John O. Forfar, MC, BSC, MD, FRCP, FRCPE, FRCPG, FRSE, Professor of Child Life and Health, Edinburgh University:

> I graduated from St Andrews University in 1941. I had taken an integrated course, a BSc in physiology and biochemistry as well as the MB ChB; I thought that this would give me a broader academic base. In 1942, I joined the army and was first posted to a Field Ambulance.

35 Joyce Grainger, FRCPE, Consultant Physician, Edinburgh.
36 Christopher Clayson, CBE, MD, FRCP, FRCPE, FRCPath, President of the Royal College of Physicians of Edinburgh, 1966–70. Recorded interview.

This seemed likely to be based in Britain so I volunteered to go overseas and was posted to the Royal Marines. In 1943 it was decided to establish the Royal Marine Commandos and I joined later as a volunteer. That ensured an active time, especially after Normandy, till the end of the war.

While I was in an army hospital, after the European war was over, I decided that I would go into hospital medicine. After two brief ex-service Registrar appointments I held a time-limited post as a Senior Registrar. When that finished I was out of a job for a time and became a sort of lab boy – not quite that but a very junior biochemist – until I got a permanent clinical appointment in Dundee.

I was then appointed consultant to an ex-municipal hospital in Edinburgh, one that now has an international reputation. People were a bit snooty about municipal hospitals and the war-time EHS hospitals at that time – although not so much in Scotland. There was also a marked difference in the south to private practice. I remember telling someone in London that I was working with a Professor of Medicine, thinking this would boost my ego. But I was told that in London academic status didn't matter. It was private practice that counted.

Ronald Girdwood, CBE, MD, PHD, FRCP, FRCPE, FRCPI, FRCPATH, FRSE, Dean of the Faculty of Medicine, Edinburgh University, President of the Royal College of Physicians of Edinburgh:

If it hadn't been for the war I would have become a surgeon. I qualified in 1939 and, as was the custom, spent a full year as an unpaid house physician in Stanley Davidson's ward. Then while waiting to be called up I worked in the outpatient department. Eventually I was posted to India and Burma where I was sent to investigate the severe and sometimes fatal anaemia among the Indian troops. This I found to be tropical sprue that had been thought not to occur in Indians. But it responded to blood transfusion and to liver extract I had sent out from the UK.

I was very much in favour of the National Health Service. I had heard of Beveridge's proposals while I was in the army. After the war I came back to the Royal Infirmary and in 1948 I got a Rockefeller Scholarship to the United States, to the University of Michigan. I was married and had two children but in the army we had become accustomed to be parted in this way. When I got to the States I had problems. I wasn't allowed to take any money at all out of the country. I had to be met at the boat by someone from the Rockefeller Foundation who gave me a few dollars. The Foundation was still paying at pre-war rates so, for two years, I was very hard up.

When the NHS started I was in the States. At Ann Arbor the people were all very friendly and I got on well with the doctors. But when they heard that I was in favour of the NHS, I was not allowed to speak publicly about it. There were one or two discontented British doctors careering around talking against the NHS. They were allowed to speak but the Head of the Department, although he personally didn't mind, said that if I spoke publicly in favour of a National Health Service it might affect his funding.

When I returned to Edinburgh, I still intended to be both a clinician and a research worker. In the NHS it would be one or the other. But in a University post I was able to do both. And the NHS did help. They had to increase university salaries to match those in the NHS.

John Smith, OBE, TD, MA, MB, FRCPE, FRCPG, FFCM, Deputy Chief Medical Officer, Scottish Home and Health Department:

When the war came I was doing my second house job with the Professor of Surgery in Glasgow. I happened to be in the TA, not as a doctor but as a gunner. I was very soon commanding a troop doing regimental training. Then, after six months or so, the War Office began to draft medically qualified people out of combatant units into the RAMC.

After eighteen months with a Field Ambulance, I was posted to a staff job. I didn't know about staff duties but I knew enough about the army to pick them up quickly. I found myself in Second Army Headquarters a year before we went to Normandy. Soon after we got to Normandy, I was moved up to ADMS, as chief staff officer to the DDMS and later to 21 Army Group in the autumn of 1944. I finished as DDMS (Operational Plans) and a full Colonel just before I was 32.

During the war I was not in the least aware of Beveridge or the prospect of a National Health Service. But when the word got about I was already interested in medical administration. We had something over 30,000 beds in Northwest Europe – more than there were in Scotland. I came back to Glasgow Royal Infirmary and then, after about eighteen months, the Department of Health advertised for someone to strengthen their hospital services team in view of the coming Health Service. I wasn't involved with the [preparation of the National Health Service (Scotland)] Bill but I was involved in preparing the run up to the Appointed Day in July 1948.

Mark S. Fraser, MB, FRCPE, Consultant Paediatrician, WHO Professor of Paediatrics, Baroda Medical College, India:

My father was a doctor, my brother was a doctor, his wife was a doctor; it was always rather assumed that I would be a doctor. I went to Edinburgh in 1937. When the war started we were all advised to continue at Edinburgh until we qualified. I joined the RAF in 1942 and spent the next three and a half years mostly in India.

Beveridge came out in 1942 but we took no notice. We never heard of the welfare state until 1944. In 1945, when everyone expected Churchill to be re-elected, I wrote home that it seemed that everyone I knew in the forces in India was going to vote socialist and that I thought I would too. This distressed my father.

I didn't think much about the health service until 1948. I knew there was a great debate going on and I saw all the stuff in the *BMJ* but I was too busy studying for the College exams. On the other hand, I think the people of my generation were convinced it was a damn good thing. We had been to places like the slums of the Cowgate as students. We had seen the grim poverty in which people lived and the fact that they had no access to a doctor unless they could pay – and they couldn't pay. We thought on the whole the social re-organisation by the Attlee government was a good thing and the health service was part of it. Once I worked in it I was very happy about it. Especially the idea that people who had previously had very little access to medicine were now getting it free.

I have come to think of that as a golden time. We were happy to be back home with our families and that colours your outlook on life. It was a time of optimism.

It was that sense of optimism and the consensus view that the NHS was a 'damn good thing' that allowed the NHS in Scotland to overcome the difficulties of inadequate resources, an antiquated infrastructure, and the overwhelming demands of an enthusiastic public.

Ian D. Campbell, MB, FRCPE, Chief Administrative Medical Officer, Lothian Health Board, former Hon. Physician to Her Majesty the Queen:

I qualified at Edinburgh in 1939. I did my house jobs in Bradford and intended to have a year as a ship's doctor before taking a house job in obstetrics with a view to becoming a family doctor in the highlands of Scotland. But the war blew all that away. After a delay in my call-up, I joined the Rame in January 1941. I went first to a Field Ambulance unit in Londonderry and then to a similar unit in the 6th Armoured Division. In 1943 I was posted to a beach landing group and after commando-type training and beach-landing exercises throughout the UK. I eventually landed in normandy on the morning of D-day-6 June

1944, having advanced trough France, Belgium and Germany to the Elbe, when hostilities with Germany ceased, I was posted to a field ambulance in the 3rd Brit. Div. which was moving to Kentucky to be part of a Commonwealth, training for a landing on the Japanese mainland. Then the bombs fell on Hiroshima. I was then a Lieutenant Colonel commanding a Field Ambulance and although expecting to be demobilised, we were sent to the Middle East to act as a buffer force between the Jews and the Palestinian Arabs. Altogether I was in the army for five and a half years.

We had heard about the NHS toward the end of the German war. An emissary was sent out from the Ministry of Health – Dr Charles Wilson [later Lord Moran] – to talk to all the young doctors who would be needed in the new service. The interest then was only half-hearted. . . . When I eventually got back to Edinburgh, the place was seething with young doctors. All the junior training posts were full and, there was obviously no future in clinical medicine in Edinburgh. Then I had a call from Bradford asking me to go there temporarily as Medical Superintendent of St. Luke's hospital. After some months the appointment became substantive and thereafter my career was in medical administration and public health.

Epilogue

The scheme for the future of health services in Scotland was first set out in the Cathcart Report in 1936. The plan was modified in the White Paper of 1944 and again in the National Health Service (Scotland) Act of 1947. The necessary changes were made with the same 'complex of motives that had inspired' reformers in Scotland between the wars.[1] The habit of co-operation that had grown up among the bodies contributing to health services in Scotland was brought forward into the new NHS. The confusion of interests, the acrimony and the often bitter squabbles that accompanied the sudden creation of the NHS for England and Wales – and, in folk memory, make up the history of the foundation of the NHS – did not disturb the consensus in Scotland.

The provisions of the National Health Service (Scotland) Act, delayed until the disputes over the English Bill had been settled, were put in place without friction. The Department of Health made full use of its devolved powers to make special provisions for Scotland. Douglas Haddow toured the United States to study what were then generally recognised as the world's most modern hospital services. Norman Graham travelled to Switzerland to negotiate a contact for the treatment of Scottish tuberculosis patients in the sanatoria that had lain almost empty since the outbreak of war:

> When money was made available for Civil Defence on the outbreak of the Korean War the Ministry of Health spread its share around in penny packets here and there. But since the Clyde was the most likely target area for a nuclear attack we decided to build a new hospital at Vale of Leven and to build it to a higher standard than other hospitals. We meant it to be an experience for everybody of what a hospital should be.[2]

There was no such harmony or sense of common purpose in England and Wales. The NHS had been put together in a 'precipitous and haphazard manner.'[3] A distinguished Professor of Medicine visiting England in 1949[4] saw the NHS as the creation of a country 'in extremity.' At the end of the Second World War there had been 'no economic recourse but to establish

1 Cathcart Report, p. 313.
2 Sir Norman Graham, recorded interview
3 C. Webster, *The Health Services Since the War*, ii (London, 1996), p. 27.
4 J. H. Means, Professor of Medicine, Harvard University.

some sort of national health programme' but he did not expect this hasty creation to last. Its structure had been negotiated in a climate of 'acrimonious controversy'[5] and, under pressure to have the new service in place within the lifetime of the first post-war Labour Government, it had been found necessary to make counter-productive concessions to the teaching hospitals and to the local authorities in England and Wales. The fault lines in the tripartite organisation of the service caused by these concessions were soon revealed when the NHS ran into unforeseen financial difficulties.

In the first nine months the Estimated Gross Expenditure had already been exceeded by 39%.[6] The Treasury had failed to foresee the increase in costs that would come with the change from a limited system of supply-led state medical services to a universal demand-led system of free medical care. The Beveridge Report's section on the 'Social Security Budget' had included the surprising projection that the cost of health care under his scheme would remain stable.[7] In Whitehall the NHS came as a consequence of Government acceptance of the Beveridge Report and it may have seemed reasonable to accept Beveridge's prediction. In retrospect this projection can be seen as wildly improbable. It can only be explained by Beveridge's confidence that the existing health services, in spite of their defects and anomalies, were already efficient and 'unmatched and scarcely rivalled in any other industrialised country.'[8] It may have seemed to Beveridge that it remained only to make the existing unrivalled health services available to everyone. He must also have assumed that by abolishing want, his scheme of social welfare would reduce the total burden of disease to a level that could be easily contained without major outlay on medical services.

Beveridge was mistaken. He might have been forewarned by the twenty-year experience of the Highlands and Islands Medical Service. But he could not have foreseen the rise in the cost of medicines. The revolution in medical care that would come from the discovery and exploitation of new drugs was inconceivable at the time of the Cathcart Report. When Beveridge reported, penicillin had been discovered, and although it had not yet been released for use in civilian practice, it had been used to 'miraculous' effect on war wounds. The therapeutic revolution had begun but the full implications of that revolution were still not obvious to Beveridge, and his failure to recognise the size of the financial burden his assumption of free treatment would place on the state's medical services was not corrected in the White Paper in 1944 or in the National Health Service Acts.

5 J. H. Means, 'Medicine and the State', *Edinburgh Medical Journal*, 1953, clxx, p. 56.
6 C. Webster, *The Health Services Since the War*, i (London, 1988), p. 134.
7 Beveridge Report, p. 33.
8 Ibid., p. 38.

In 1948, both north and south of the border, general practitioners were almost overwhelmed by the demand for their services. In Scotland there were 2,364 doctors on the lists of the Executive Councils in the first years of the service.[9] The average number of patients on a general practitioner's list was only a little over 2,000. In England and Wales there were relatively fewer general practitioners. Lists were correspondingly greater but, on average, still not unacceptably large by present-day standards. But suddenly after July 1948 consulting hours had to be extended, waiting rooms were uncomfortably full and, in many cases, there were queues outside doctors' surgeries. It was not only that both the doctors' services and the medicines were now free that attracted patients. The new medicines were infinitely more effective than anything that had been available before.

Already in 1949, Bevan complained of 'the cascade of medicine which is pouring down British throats.'[10] Thereafter expenditure on medicines continued to increase. By far the greatest part of this expenditure was in general practice. Under the provisions of the contract negotiated with the general practitioners, government was unable to interfere directly with the doctors' right to prescribe freely for their patients. Government had therefore attempted to reduce costs by imposing prescription charges in the National Health Service (Amendment) Act at the end of 1949. The charge of one shilling for each prescription had virtually no effect on the level of demand, either in Scotland or in England and Wales and a Joint Committee of the English and Scottish Health Service Councils was appointed to advise on prescription practices in both countries.[11] It had been hoped that general practitioners could be persuaded to prescribe only the cheapest brands of the new drugs. In the Budget in 1951 further attempts at economy were made by imposing charges on spectacles and false teeth. The annual number of applications for dentures in Scotland immediately dropped from 284,000 to 150,000. The effect on the prescription of glasses was much less; patients continued to use the free eye-testing services but used the results to have spectacles prescribed privately.[12] The responses to the imposed economies in general practice were similar both north and south of the border and the new charges continued to cause complaints and criticism. Nevertheless, in 1953, Iain Macleod, the Minister of Health, reported that the annual drugs bill of £46,000,000 was prejudicing even the most urgently necessary developments of the NHS.[13]

Almost from the beginning it had become clear that there was little

9 *Annual Report of the Department of Health for Scotland*, 1948, Cmd. 7659, p. 13.
10 A. Bevan, quoted by J. Campbell, *Nye Bevan; A Biography* (London, 1987), p. 183.
11 *Annual Reports of the Department of Health for Scotland*.
12 *Annual Report of the Department of Health for Scotland*, 1952, Cmd. 8799, p. 21.
13 *Lancet*, ii, 1953, p. 828.

prospect that the cost of the NHS could be contained by restricting the use of necessary medicines in general practice. The hospital service was the largest element within the NHS and the section over which central Government had most direct control. It was therefore the hospital service that came under the most critical review in the effort to contain costs, and the chosen target for economy was the growing cost of its staff.

The Secretary of State for Scotland, Arthur Woodburn, who had objected vigorously to other restriction on NHS spending in Scotland, did not stand out against the Government proposals to contain expenditure in the hospital service.[14] Sir Norman Graham, then in charge of the Hospital Division of the Department of Health for Scotland, remembers that on this issue he was at an advantage over his opposite number in the Ministry of Health.[15] In 1948, Scotland already had a hospital bed complement 15% greater per head of population than England and Wales and his Division had been quicker to increase capital investment. Since it was Treasury policy that revenue moneys should follow capital investment, Scotland was relatively well placed financially. By 1948 Scotland also had proportionally 30% more nurses and 45% more hospital medical and dental staff manning only 15% more beds and was therefore in a better position to withstand any limitation of recruitment that the Government might impose.

In England and Wales there was active and effective resistance to the Treasury's proposed restrictions. At the Treasury's first call for the control of recruitment of hospital staff in 1949, Bevan insisted that the prescription of staffing levels by the Ministry of Health would be inconsistent with the Ministry's established policy of local autonomy.[16] The Treasury pointed out that, in Scotland, staffing levels were controlled centrally and recommended that the same practice should be followed by the Ministry of Health in England and Wales. The Ministry was not only reluctant, on principle, to adopt the Scottish practice, it also had to confess that it held neither the relevant statistics nor the results of any reviews of staffing levels that might already have been carried out. Under additional pressure from the Public Accounts Committee and the Select Committee on Estimates, the Ministry was persuaded to set up a complex enquiry into establishment levels in each separate section of the hospital service. Boards of Governors and management committees in England and Wales created difficulties and the Treasury very quickly decided that this enquiry was 'a farce set up to appease the Public Accounts Committee but without any real prospect of its recommendations becoming effective.'[17] The medical elite in England and

14 *Ibid.*, p. 148.
15 Sir Norman Graham, recorded interview.
16 Webster, 1988, *op. cit.*, p. 299.
17 *Ibid.*, p. 301.

Wales, the 'voice at court,' operating directly at a personal level and also through the Boards of Governors and medical committees that they dominated, had demonstrated their ability to influence or even obstruct recommendations of Government.[18] For its part, the Ministry of Health continued to exhibit a lingering opposition to any avoidable increase in central administration, which, as one of its senior officers has recorded, was its traditional stance.[19]

In October 1951, a Conservative government came into office. The new Chancellor insisted that the Treasury's recommendations for restrictions on spending on hospital staff must be carried out. From its position of strength 'the Scottish Department of Health acceded readily.'[20] In England and Wales, the Ministry of Health, now under a new Minister, was persuaded to relax its opposition to any increase in central administration and began to force the restrictions required by the Treasury. The consultants and administrators of the London teaching hospitals, now acting in their own sectional interest and not on behalf of the hospital service as a whole, made public their resentment at what they regarded as Ministerial interference with the privileged position that they had been given in the National Health Service Act. But any private assurances that may have been given by Aneurin Bevan over dinner at the Café Royal and elsewhere[21] now counted for nothing. In a letter to the *Times*, Mr. A. H. Burfour, a consultant surgeon, wrote:

> The London Teaching Hospital at which I am now employed has a tradition of independence going back for more than two and a half centuries and is respected world-wide. On the introduction of the National Health Service there were high hopes that that tradition would be respected and its reputation enhanced.[22]

Mr. Burfour was supported in the correspondence columns of the *Times* by consultants and administrators at other London teaching hospitals. All wrote of their surprise and resentment at the unexpected loss of independence by their hospitals. Sir Russell Brain presented their case in the *BMJ*.[23]

The teaching hospitals did not have the sympathy of the general hospital service in England and Wales. London's Medical Officer of Health, Sir Allen Daley, devoted his Croonian Lecture to the Royal College of Physicians of London to pointing out that the great London hospitals were

18 *Ibid.*
19 J. Pater, *The Making of the National Health Service* (London, 1981), p. 26.
20 Webster, 1988, *op. cit.*, p. 302.
21 Campbell, *op. cit.*, p. 171.
22 Leader, 'Frustration in the Hospitals', *BMJ*, ii, 1953, p. 319.
23 Sir Russell Brain, *BMJ*, ii, 1953, Supplement, p. 206.

not pulling their weight. 'The individual hospitals must remember that they are part of a national hospital service with a collective responsibility for the institutional care of the sick.'[24] To what was presumably a hostile audience, Sir Allen argued that the concessions made to the teaching hospitals had been a mistake and that, 'in spite of the practical difficulties,' it would be better 'to go back to the Willink proposals.' This would have effectively put the administration of all NHS hospitals under the control of the local authorities to be managed by joint committees of the county councils and county boroughs. Such restructuring might have found support among the local authorities themselves and possibly some lingering sympathy among the longer serving officers of the Ministry of Health who had originally favoured such a scheme. But the Willink proposals had been vigorously resisted by the medical profession when they were first put forward in 1944[25] and, as Bevan had informed the Cabinet in 1945, 'few local authorities run a good hospital system. The majority are not suited to run a hospital service at all.'[26] In 1953, Sir Allen Daley's proposals came to nothing. Teaching hospitals continued in their privileged position while the former local authority hospitals were thereafter tacitly acknowledged by the Ministry as second-rate.

The local authorities later came under criticism in a different context. In 1953, the Minister of Health, now Ian Macleod, made public his dissatisfaction with the local authorities in the exercise of the powers that they had been given in the administration of general practitioner services in the National Health Service Act for England and Wales.[27] He had it in mind to change the constitution of the Executive Councils as set out in the Act. 'Lay members did not always attend and in that respect the members appointed by the local authorities appear to be by far the worst.'[28] The Minister had been aware that relations between the local authorities and the general practitioners had long been unsatisfactory but he had been somewhat reassured in recent special reports from the local authorities that in 1953 there was 'growing cooperation.'

The general practitioners did not share this view. A survey of general practice found that local authority services and the general practitioners were often in conflict and seemed 'to be treading different paths . . . Maximum benefit for the patient cannot result from a bisected service

24 Sir Allen Daley, 'The Place of the Hospital in a National Health Service', *BMJ*, ii, 1953, p. 249.
25 P. Bartrip, *Themselves Writ Large: The British Medical Association 1932–1966* (London, 1996), p. 240.
26 The Future of the Hospital Services, CP (45) 205, PRO CAB 129/3, quoted by C. Webster, *Aneurin Bevan on the National Health Service* (Oxford, 1991), p. 33.
27 National Health Service Act, para 50.
28 *Lancet*, ii, 1953, p. 828.

... The NHS is crying out for a unified administration'[29] – the unified administration that already existed in Scotland.

After five years, the NHS in England and Wales had not yet become an established as a settled part of the structure of society. Those it served seemed satisfied but only 'sometimes enthusiastic about it.' Its medical personnel had become only 'by and large more reconciled to it.' The observer of 1949 had at last some confidence that in England the 'National Health Service is here to stay and in all probability it will gradually be improved.'[30] But it was not until the mid-50s that the NHS had the support of 'a broad consensus, embracing all social classes, both political parties and all but an eccentric fringe of the medical profession.'[31] However, the differences and tensions that had been perpetuated by the late concession in the National Health Service Act (1946) remained institutionalised in England and Wales for almost 30 years and lingered for over half a century.

The NHS for Scotland had come after years of preparation. There had been no entrenched opposition to overcome and the service had been planned, introduced intact and consolidated in a spirit of co-operation and there had been no last-minute deviations from the concept of a tripartite organisation. From the start, the NHS was welcomed wholeheartedly in Scotland, by the public,[32] the civil service and the medical profession. Even Scotland's leading conservative newspaper, the *Scotsman*, supported the creation of this new state service. The *Scotsman* was also confident that the NHS would work better in Scotland than in England.[33] From the beginning, the NHS in Scotland was accepted as a welcome and permanent addition to the social structure of the country.

29 S. J. Hadfield, 'A Field Study of General Practice', *BMJ*, ii, 1953, p. 706.
30 Means, *op. cit.*, p. 60.
31 Webster, 1988, *op. cit.*, p. 389.
32 *Glasgow Herald*, 5 July 1948.
33 G. McLachlan, *Improving the Common Weal* (Edinburgh, 1987), p. 93.

APPENDIX I

Should the BMA Speak
for the Medical Profession?

Throughout 1912, from its London base, the British Medical Association conducted an aggressive campaign to dictate the terms and conditions under which doctors would take part in the National Health Insurance Scheme. The outcome of the campaign was 'the eventual trouncing of the British Medical Association'[1] and a distortion of the public perception of the medical profession as united in support of the intemperate behaviour of the officers of the BMA, a perception that has been reinforced by frequent repetition. Misconceptions of the authority of the BMA as the single voice of the medical profession persisted, causing misunderstandings during the evolution of the National Health Service. Historians of this period have overestimated the degree to which the officers of the British Medical Association faithfully represented the views of the members and have tended to perpetuate the myth that, in the struggles to launch the NHS, the BMA and the medical profession in Great Britain were synonymous. Eckstein refers to the BMA as the 'nearly monolithic formal organisation'[2] of the profession. Eder equates the BMA leadership with the medical profession without question and goes so far as to say that 'professional solidarity was unshakeable.'[3] Pater[4] refers to the BMA but not to any other section of the profession. Honigsbaum[5] writes of 'the doctors' and the 'BMA' indiscriminately. For Ross the 'BMA' and the 'medical profession' are interchangeable (even in his index).[6]

Jones has noticed that the British Medical Association in 1911 and 1912 'recognised a crucial opportunity to achieve its desires for the profession and to enhance its own position'[7] but makes no reference to the power struggle then taking place within the medical profession which had reached a climax as Lloyd George negotiated the introduction of his scheme for National Health Insurance.

1 V. Berridge, *Health and Medicine*, in F. Thompson (ed.), *The Cambridge Social History of Britain 1750–1950*, iii (Cambridge 1990), p. 183.
2 H. Eckstein, *Pressure Group Politics: The Case of the British Medical Association* (London, 1960), p. 49.
3 N. Eder, *National Health Insurance and the Medical Profession* (London, 1982).
4 J. Pater, *The Making of the National Health Service* (London, 1981).
5 F. Honigsbaum, *Health, Happiness, and Security* (London, 1989).
6 J. Ross, *The National Health Service in Great Britain* (Oxford 1952).
7 P. Jones, *Doctors and the BMA* (Farnborough, 1981), p. 25.

At the turn of the century there was no Ministry of Health, and Government authority over medical matters lay with the Privy Council and the Secretary of its Medical Committee. In turn the Medical Committee of the Privy Council was guided informally by the Royal College of Physicians of London which had 'always been close to the Crown and the establishment.'[8] It had long been the routine practice of the Privy Council to consult the London College on routine matters. In one typical year (1907) the Privy Council referred to the College requests for advice: from the Secretary of State for India on the control of plague; from the Home Office Committee on Ambulance Services; from the Board of Trade (Marine Department) on the medical inspection of seamen; from the Colonial Secretary on the management of beriberi in St Helena; from the Local Government Board on the management of an outbreak of plague in East Anglia.[9] The London College had also been acting as advisor to the Army Medical Department since the Crimean War.

Even on matters on which it had not been formally consulted the College often 'decided to use its influence.'[10] Although it spoke as from the medical profession, the College was by no means a representative body. In 1909, when its position was finally challenged, there were 40,257 medical practitioners on the Medical Register; of these a total of 12,524 were Fellows, Members or Licentiates of the Royal College of Physicians of London. However, only the 339 Fellows were entitled to vote at the Ordinary General meetings that were held only four times a year, and at which as few as 10 fellows constituted a quorum. (In practice, the real business of the College was conducted by a Council of 17 Fellows including the President, the four Censors and the Treasurer.) Nevertheless, as Eckstein has observed, the Fellows of the Royal College of Physicians of London regarded themselves as the high court of British Medicine.[11]

In 1909, the College faced a challenge to its position from the British Medical Association. In the last days of 1908 the British Medical Association had lodged a petition for the Grant of a Royal Charter of Incorporation 'in order to enable the Association to undertake more completely than hitherto all the proper means for promoting the efficiency and welfare of the medical profession and the advancement of the sciences of medicine and surgery.'[12] This political bid by the BMA was a major departure from the original concept of the Association's founder.

In 1828, Charles Hastings, an Edinburgh graduate, founded a medical

8 A. Cooke, *A History of the Royal College of Physicians of London* (Oxford, 1972), p. 1123.
9 Minutes of the Royal College of Physicians of London, 1907.
10 Cooke, *op. cit.*, p. 835.
11 Eckstein, *op. cit.*, p. 50.
12 *BMJ*, i, 1909, p. 3.

journal, the *Midland Medical and Surgical Reporter*, as a vehicle by which provincial practitioners could communicate with each other, sharing their experience and making their contribution to the advance of medical science. In 1832 its promoters formalised themselves as the Provincial Medical and Surgical Association (PMSA). Membership was not restricted to medical practitioners but its aims were confined to 'gathering information from medical practice, increasing knowledge of medical topography, investigating disease, and advancing medico-legal science.'[13] The Association centred on Worcester but wider participation was encouraged by holding the annual meetings in different provincial towns. This was a case of the Mountain going to Mohammed. Few of the foot soldiers of the profession could afford, in time or in money, to travel far from home for 'science, good fellowship and philanthropy.'[14] For each annual meeting a President was selected from the most distinguished of the local practitioners in the area in which the meeting was to be held; the President held nominal office for one year only and took no part in the conduct of the Association's affairs. In time the PMSA evolved to become the British Medical Association and moved its headquarters from Worcester to London. An attempt to amend the constitution in 1896 failed because of the lack of interest shown by the members.[15] The fundamental problem was that the Association had a very high proportion of unattached members (i.e. not affiliated to a Division) whose membership allowed them free subscription to the Association's journal, the *BMJ*, but who had no further interest in the affairs of the Association. In order to encourage greater participation by members, in 1901 the Annual Representative Meeting restructured the Association, creating a constitution later described by Michael Foot as 'a democratic machine seemingly constructed by Dr. Strabismus.'[16] At Annual Representative Meetings, each Division would now be represented by a delegate, able to vote according to the instructions of his Division and exercising a number of votes that reflected the number of members in his Division. Resolutions passed at the Annual Representative Meeting, if secured by the votes of two-thirds of those present, were to be binding on the Council. A quorum was to be half of the number entitled to attend. In order to encourage attendance the Association undertook to pay the delegates' expenses. However, ordinary members could not attend Annual Repre-

13 P. Bartrip, *Themselves Writ Large: The British Medical Association, 1832–1966* (London, 1996), p. 5.
14 *Ibid.*, p. 36.
15 'Of the association's 37 United Kingdom branches, only 18 offered views on the proposed reforms. There was only one question to which all 18 replied. Of the proposals tabled, not one received a ringing endorsement.' Bartrip, *op. cit.*, p. 140.
16 M. Foot, *Aneurin Bevan* (London, 1973), p. 117.

sentative Meetings and there was no postal voting system; the new constitution was intended to increase membership but the Council of the BMA in London was careful to retain its ability to 'tower'[17] over the Annual Representative Meetings. Effective power remained in the hands of 'a small circle of inner council members and permanent officials.'[18] Within this inner circle the most powerful political figure was the Chairman of Council, elected by the Council 'for such time as it determines' but in practice . . . that seems as long as he wants to hold office.'[19] The Chairman of Council and his inner circle were supported by a secretariat of permanent officials, headed by a Secretary with wide powers to supervise the whole organisation. While scientific questions were farmed out to *ad hoc* committees made up of the many experts available within the wide membership, the inner circle retained the monopoly on political issues through appointed medico-political committees of activists. Theoretically, ordinary members could contribute to decision-making through their Divisions but as Alfred Cox, a former Secretary of the Association, recalls in his memoirs,[20] at the turn of the century meetings were infrequent and it was the medico-political committees, convened in London, that produced the reports which formed the substance of all official statements made by the BMA.

At the turn of the century the BMA carried little weight. In 1897 the *Times* declared:

> It would be impossible to point to anything the association has done, either for the benefit of the medical profession or for mankind, at all adequate to the apparent possibilities of the case. Probably no statesman was ever influenced by its views with regard to any matter of legislation, whether purely medical or relating to some one of the many social questions upon which medicine is calculated to throw light.[21]

In 1904 the Annual Representatives Meeting was held at the height of the agitation over the evils of club and contract practice ('mass medicine'). Medical Unions had been formed in various parts of the country, often in mining areas, to secure reform. The campaign had been taken up by the *Lancet* in a series of articles entitled 'The Battle of the Clubs.' It was Cox, who later became its Secretary, who persuaded the BMA in 1900 to take up the cause.[22] But almost nothing was achieved; the ineffectiveness of the

17 Eckstein, *op. cit.*, p. 60.
18 Bartrip, *op. cit*, p. 148.
19 Eckstein, *op. cit.*, p. 60.
20 A. Cox, *Among The Doctors* (London, 1950).
21 *The Times*, 1 September 1897.
22 Eskstein, *op. cit.*, p. 75.

BMA's advocacy on behalf of the profession was becoming more and more obvious. Recruitment was falling as a result. In the period 1890–1895 membership had increased by 15%; from 1895 to 1900 the increase was 14%. Now for the years 1900 to 1905 the increase was only 6%.[23] In the worst year ever, 1907, only 130 new members were recruited[24] while the number in the profession increased by 444.[25]

To a number of those attending the annual meeting in 1904 it seemed that some attempt should be made to increase the authority of the BMA:

> A resolution was passed instructing the Central Council to take steps to effect such changes in the Constitution of the Association as would enable it to carry out its objectives more freely. When this task came to be undertaken the Council was advised by the eminent lawyer consulted that the time had come to consider whether application should not be made for a Royal Charter.[26]

A first draft of the Petition for a Royal Charter was brought before the annual meeting in July 1906 and a revised version in May 1907. The formal application was submitted to the Privy Council by the BMA leadership on 21 December 1908. Over four years, drafts of the proposed Chapter had been debated at successive Representative Meetings[27] but support had remained much less than wholehearted.

The Petition stated that 'greater freedom of action is desirable in order to enable the Association to undertake more completely than hitherto all proper means for the promoting of the efficiency and welfare of the medical profession and the advancement of the sciences of medicine and surgery.'[28] The full intention is clear from the text of the *Draft Charter, Ordinances and Byelaws* presented to the Annual Representative Meeting in 1908 and from the reports of the debates on the drafts at Representative Meetings. Armed with a Charter, the leaders of the Association could expect to be consulted by Government in 'the framing and carrying out of legislation affecting the public health, the Poor Law, the treatment of lunacy and inebriety and other matters as to which the members of the medical profession have special knowledge.'[29] The BMA would become a disciplinary body controlling standards of practice and conduct. It would also act for individual members 'against unjust attacks and accusations;' it would 'establish benevolent funds

---

23 Calculated from figures supplied by the Archivist of the BMA.
24 *BMJ*, i, 1908, p. 290.
25 *Medical Register*, 1908.
26 *BMJ*, i, 1908, p. 1267.
27 Reported in full in *BMJ*, Supplements, ii, 1907; i, 1908; and ii, 1908.
28 The text of the Petition is reproduced in *BMJ*, Supplement, i, 1909.
29 *Ibid.*, p. 3.

for the benefit of members of the medical profession and their families.' Most contentious of all, the ultimate responsibility for the exercise of these wide-ranging powers would be vested in the Representative Meetings.

The petition was submitted to the Privy Council. In accordance with its long-standing practice, the Privy Council consulted the Royal College of Physicians of London. Since a Charter in the terms set out by the BMA would inevitably undermine the position of the Royal College of Physicians, the College at once sought legal advice. Counsel's opinion (Sir Alfred Cripps) reads:

> The Charter would in effect constitute a body of co-ordinate and parallel jurisdiction.
>
> The object of the Association to take any legal proceedings, civil or criminal, on which the honour or interests of the medical profession or any member of the Association in his professional capacity is or are involved, is one which should be opposed. It would constitute the Association a public prosecutor and the power might be exercised against medical men who were not desirous to join the Association.[30]

The College advised the Privy Council that the application for a Royal Charter should be refused.

The Royal College of Physicians of London was not alone in its opposition. Counter-petitions were submitted to the Privy Council by the Royal College of Physicians of Edinburgh, the Royal College of Surgeons of Edinburgh, Edinburgh University, the British Medical Benevolent Fund, and the Society for the Relief of Widows and Orphans of Medical Men. Counter-petitions were also lodged by a number of branches of the BMA itself (including the Edinburgh Branch) and by individual members of the Association.[31] Members of the medical profession, not members of the BMA, wrote in protest to the *BMJ*.

The objections were on two main grounds. There were many, especially in Scotland, who believed that the BMA should not follow this path at all. There would be a conflict of interests with the General Medical Council and '. . . political proposals would be impracticable and would raise internal dissension in the Association. It was very much better that the Association should take no part whatever in political matters.'[32] There was even more objection that the structure and procedures of the BMA made it unsuitable for the exercise of such power. In particular, it was felt that the ultimate authority should not be vested in the Annual Representative Meeting that

30 *Annals of the Royal College of Physicians of London*, lxv, 26 January 1909.
31 *BMJ*, ii, 1909, Supplement, p. 66.
32 *BMJ*, i, 1908, Supplement, p. 111.

could not pretend to be a democratic body. One general practitioner wrote to the *BMJ*:

> No one desires to see a large majority of the Association disenfranchised, or the control of the affairs placed permanently in the hands of an unrepresentative assembly. It is well known that in many Divisions, if not in most, only a handful of members, chiefly residents in the towns where the meetings are always held, attend these meetings which elect and instruct Divisional Representatives. Men in most parts of the Division cannot neglect their patients in order to record their votes. This disability, special to medical men, must not be lost sight of in dealing with their representative government. Therefore the 'Representative Body' as provided for in the Charter is a gravely unrepresentative body and discussions at which it arrives can in no sense be finally taken as the decision of the Association.[33]

Even within the Representative Body there were many who agreed. The Scottish Representatives were particularly strong in their objection. Dr Norman Walker[34] supported an amendment that proposed that Representatives should be elected by postal vote:

> . . . because he knew that in the scattered districts of Scotland members had very rarely an opportunity to attend a meeting and could not do so as it would mean losing an entire day and perhaps more than one day. In the case of any important matter like the election of Representatives, he thought each member should have the opportunity of voting.[35]

The Scottish arguments were not well received by the Council of the BMA.[36] 'In Scotland they live in a sort of heaven of their own and have no interest in common with the English members.'[37] Dr. Walker's proposal for postal voting was not put to a vote and was lost. The leaders of the BMA brushed aside all opposition. When expedient, their methods could be dictatorial; in the preparation of the final draft of the Charter they attempted to overturn legitimate decisions of the Representative Meeting. The Representatives had wished to change the practice by which voting could only be done by show of hands. The Council resisted the change:

> As a result of the Special representative Meeting in May 1907 certain resolutions for the proposed new Charter were passed, but some of

33 W. Gordon, *BMJ*, ii, 1908, p. 1520.
34 Later Sir Norman Walker.
35 *BMJ*, i, 1908, Supplement, p. 117.
36 Described by the *Edinburgh Medical Journal* as the 'reverend seigneurs of the Association.' *Edinburgh Medical Journal*, NS i, 1908, p. 192.
37 *BMJ*, i, 1908, Supplement, p. 111.

them were considered by the Council not to properly represent the wishes of the Association. Consequently an instruction was issued to every Division throughout the Association that a direct vote should be taken on each resolution of the Representative Meeting.[38]

This referendum, unauthorised by the Representative Meeting, was directed to all 220 Divisions. Replies were received from 149 Divisions in the UK and 10 from overseas. The total attendance at these meetings was 1,831 within the UK and 147 outside. The largest number attending any one of these meetings was 46, the smallest two. The meetings clearly demonstrated the general apathy of the members on political matters; even so, those who did attend voted decisively against the Council by majorities of at least 2 to 1.[39]

There was little evidence that the leaders of the BMA could, with confidence, claim the substantial support of the membership. There was even less evidence that the leaders of the BMA were justified in claiming the support of a majority of the medical profession in the United Kingdom, as was implied in the sophistical statement in the Petition: 'The present membership of the Association comprises upwards of 50 per cent of practitioners on the medical register.'[40] In 1908, when the petition for a Royal Charter was submitted to the Privy Council, 12,392 (49%) of the 25,017 medical practitioners registered in England and Wales were voting members of the BMA; in Scotland 1,825 (47%) of 3,829, and in Ireland, 862 (32%) of 2660.[41]

In the Petition to the Privy Council, the Council of the BMA, hoping to establish the Association as a political body, failed to make clear the extent to which the Association depended for its mere existence on its scientific journal. Not only was the *BMJ* responsible for the Association's reputation worldwide, the journal also supported the Association financially. In 1907, for example, it was only the journal's income of £25,259, with a profit of £6,505, which saved the Association from a trading deficit. Very many members opposed any further advance of the Association's political activities that might cause them to overshadow its scientific reputation.

Despite the lack of united support from the membership and what on examination seems an insubstantial case, the leaders of the BMA persisted. At a meeting of the Representatives in July 1908, with only 107 of the 220 Representatives present, the motion to present the Petition for a Royal Charter was carried. The Petition was lodged on 21 December 1908.

The Privy Council, after deliberation, refused to grant a Charter. The

38 *Ibid.*, p. 290.
39 Minutes of the BMA.
40 *BMJ*, i, 1909, Supplement, p. 2.
41 Figures from the *Medical Directory*, 1908 and *BMJ*, i, 1908, Supplement, p. 311.

British Medical Association made no further application. Indeed the *BMJ* makes no further reference to the Charter after 1909. The rebuff was received in silence.

The affair of the Royal Charter can be seen as a test of the right of the British Medical Association to manage and to represent the medical profession in Great Britain. In 1908 the BMA failed to establish that right. The BMA continued to be a limited company registered with the Board of Trade, neither a trade union nor with rights established by Charter. Nevertheless, the BMA went on to assume some of the powers it had been refused in 1908. From the disputes over the National Insurance Act until the difficulties in the creation of the National Health Service the BMA was uninhibited in its pretension to speak for the whole of the medical profession. In this it was so successful that in the end the identification of the BMA with the medical profession, in the eyes of the public, was almost complete.

Forgotten in the rest of the UK, the affair of the Royal Charter had a more lasting effect on the medical profession in Scotland. The facetious comment that 'in Scotland they were in a sort of heaven of their own' had drawn attention to the truth. As had been frequently pointed out by Scottish Representatives, the Scottish Divisions were exceedingly scattered and the Divisional structure that worked in England was unsuitable in Scotland. This had been illustrated by the response to the Referendum on the Charter. At two of the Divisional meetings called to allow members to record their votes no members attended and only one meeting in Scotland attracted more than 16 members. Of all members of the BMA entitled to vote in Scotland, only 12% were able to attend these special and important meetings.

At the final meeting of Representatives of the BMA before the Petition was presented, Dr. Walker of Edinburgh had made a final appeal. He asked that 'the same consideration should be shown to Scottish Divisions as to those in His Majesty's Dominions beyond the seas.' The Chairman ruled that this request could not be put to the meeting.

The *Edinburgh Medical Journal*, in its only reference to the Royal Charter affair, expressed the growing uncertainty about the relevance of the political activities of the BMA to the medical profession in Scotland:

> It is evident that Scotland will gradually have less and less to say in the policy of the Association . . . Sooner or later Scotland will discover that the dominant partner resides south of the Tweed – a good way south.[42]

42 *Edinburgh Medical Journal*, NS I, 1908, p. 193.

APPENDIX II

British Health Statistics, 1889–1948

	1898	1903	1908	1913	1918	1923	1928	1933	1938	1948
Scotland										
Population	4,249	4,579	4,826	4,728	4,886	4,901	4,893	4,912	4,993	5,169
Deaths	78,397	76,002	77,838	73,069	78,372	63,283	65,271	64,848	62,953	60,979
Death Rate	18.4	16.6	16.1	15.5	16	12.9	13.3	13.2	12.6	11.8
Births	130,861	133,525	131,362	120,516	98,554	111,902	96,822	86,546	88,627	100,344
Birth Rate	30.8	29.2	27.2	25.5	20.2	22.8	19.8	17.6	17.8	19.4
Infant Deaths	17,554	15,693	15,900	13,214	9,836	8,825	8,299	7,019	6,163	4,486
Infant Mortality Rate	134.1	117.5	121	109.6	99.8	78.9	85.7	81.1	69.5	44.7
Phthisis Deaths	7090	6130	6079	5103	5217	3996	3318	3810	2581	3415
Phthisis Death Rate	167	134	126	108	107	82	68	78	52	66
Puerperal Sepsis Deaths	227	303	241	160	113	218	234	212	150	30
Puerpeal Deaths	578	709	676	708	688	718	676	512	432	161
MMR	4.4	5.3	5.1	5.9	7	6.4	7	5.9	5	1.6
Sepsis Death Rate	1.7	2.3	1.8	1.3	1.1	1.9	2.4	2.5	2	0.3
England & Wales										
Population	29,002	32,527	35,348	36,919	37,507	38,403	39,482	40,350	41,215	43,502
Deaths	552,141	514,628	520,456	504,975	611,861	526,858	543,664	579,467	489,100	468,700
Death Rate	19	15.8	14.7	13.7	16.3	13.7	13.8	14.4	11.9	10.8
Births	923,265	948,271	940,383	881,890	662,661	758,131	660,267	580,413	621,204	775,306
Birth Rate	31.8	29.2	26.6	23.9	17.7	19.8	16.7	14.4	15.1	17.8
Infant Deaths	148,013	125,136	113,254	95,608	64,386	52,311	42,917	36,566	32,924	29,461

Infant Mortality Rate	160	132	120	108	97	69	65	63	53	38
Phthisis Deaths	41,335	40,132	39,299	37,055	42,247	37,627	34,399	31,860	21,282	18,798
Phthisis Death Rate	143	123	111	100	123	98	79	79	52	42
Puerperal Deaths	4,367	3,857	3,361	3,492	2,509	3,761	3,733	3,263	2,096	809
Puerperal Sepsis Deaths	1,707	1,668	1,395	1,108	845	1,246	1,458	1,949	682	187
Maternal										
Mortality Rate	4.7	4.1	3.6	4	3.8	5	5.7	5.6	3.4	1
Sepsis Death Rate	1.8	1.8	1.5	1.3	1.3	1.6	2.2	3.4	1.1	0.2

Sources: *Annual Reports of the Registrar General for Scotland, Annual Reports of the Registrar General for England Wales, Annual Abstract of Statistics*

Populations in thousands

Scottish Health Statistics, 1860–1945

	1860	1865	1875	1885	1895	1905	1915	1925	1935	1945
Population										
Highlands	381,610	381,610	369,562	370,601	357,466	352,941	295,355	316,209	290,436	274,754
Ayrshire	199,063	199,063	201,168	200,908	229,883	254,468	264,335	306,458	289,442	207,631
Scotland	3,062,294	3,185,439	3,495,214	3,735,573	4,155,654	4,472,103	4,785,598	4,893,032	4,952,500	4,673,900
Deaths										
Highlands	5,698	6,081	7167	5,961	6,210	5,541	5,331	4,406	4,952	4,663
Ayrshire	4,054	4,053	5006	4,171	4,392	3,974	4,049	3,371	4,475	3,341
Scotland	63,539	70,821	81,767	74,607	81,852	74,536	81,631	65,507	65,331	62,655
Death Rate										
Highlands	14.9	15.9	19.4	16.1	17.4	15.7	18	13.9	15.4	12.2
Ayrshire	20.4	20.4	24.9	20.7	19.1	15.6	15.3	11	12.3	11.6
Scotland	20.7	22.2	23.4	19.4	19.7	16.7	17.1	13.4	13.2	13.2
Births										
Highlands	10,607	9,992	9186	9326	8,366	7,297	5,132	4,827	4,302	3,501
Ayrshire	7,464	7,538	8233	7623	7,564	7,824	6,689	5,947	5212	3,624
Scotland	104,418	113,126	123,578	126,100	126,494	131,410	114,181	104,137	87,928	86,932
Infant Deaths										
Highlands	906	935	919	749	704	681	452	284	234	146
Ayrshire	851	760	948	824	850	785	763	560	394	127
Scotland	12,622	14,099	14,950	15,200	16,874	15,275	14,441	9,430	6,754	2,932
Infant Mortality										
Highlands	85	94	100	80	84	93	88	59	54	53

Ayrshire	114	101	124	108	112	100	114	94	76	61
Scotland	121	125	132	121	133	116	127	91	77	60
TB Deaths										
Highlands	541	592	644	518	554	506	390	308	158	146
Ayrshire	586	502	569	476	409	344	260	138	116	127
Scotland	7264	7416	8699	7922	7,688	6374	5292	3722	2823	2,932
TB Rate										
Highlands	142	155	174	140	155	143	132	97	54	53
Ayrshire	294	252	283	237	178	135	98	45	40	61
Scotland	237	231	249	212	185	143	111	76	57	62

Source: *Reports of the Registrar General for Scotland*

The Scottish Board of Health, 1919

Sir George McCrae	Chairman, Local Government Board. Member of Parliament for Edinburgh East.
Sir James Leishman	Chairman, Scottish Insurance Commission. Treasurer, City of Edinburgh.
Sir Leslie Mackenzie	Medical Officer, Local Government Board. Highlands and Islands Medical Service Board.
Dr. John McVail	Deputy Chairman, Scottish Insurance Commission. Medical Officer of Health.
Ewen MacPherson, KC	Legal Secretary to the Lord Advocate. Local Government Board.
Muriel Ritson	Secretary, Women's Friendly Society.

The Consultative Committee on Medical and Allied Services, 1919

O. Chanock Bradley	Principal, Royal (Dick) Veterinary College, Edinburgh
A. J. Campbell	Secretary, Berwick Medical Panel Committee
A. K. Chalmers	Medical Officer of Health, Glasgow
D. Elliot Dickson	Convenor, Fife Colliery Surgeons Committee
J. R. Drever	Scottish Secretary, BMA
Anne Gill	Lady Superintendent of Nurses, Royal Infirmary of Edinburgh
Professor M. Hay	Aberdeen University
J. Rutherford Hill	Secretary, Pharmaceutical Society in Scotland
Sir Donald McAllister	Principal, University of Glasgow
John Mackay	Principal, University College, Dundee
Sir James Mackenzie	Clinical Institute, St Andrews
Sir Robert Philip	University of Edinburgh
J. Maxwell Ross	Medical Officer of Health, Dumfries
Laura Stewart-Sanderson	Controller of Medical Services, Queen Mary's Army Auxiliary Corps
Sir Harold Stiles	University of Edinburgh
F. Tocher	Public Analyst, Aberdeen
Norman Walker	General Medical Council
George Williamson	Chairman, Aberdeen Local Medical Committee
John Young	Vice-President, Odonto-Chirurgical Society

The School Health Service: Medical Examinations, 1919–1928

	1919	1920	1921	1922	1923	1924	1925	1926	1927	1928
School Population	850,000	*	837,923	867,689	866,894	866,894	733,362	823,028	830,060	825,440
Pupils Inspected	*	*	*	*	208,706	215,288	220,467	254,570	237,692	249,142
Proportion Inspected	*	*	*	*	24%	24.80%	30%	30.93%	28.62%	30.18%
Nutrition	*	*	*	*	10.8	9.3	8.6	7.4	7.9	6.6
Head Lice	*	*	*	*	2.4	2.2	2.3	2.2	*	1.8
Other Vermin	*	*	*	*	common	common	common	common	common	common
Hearing Loss	*	*	*	*	*	*	*	*	*	*
Poor Sight (specs)	*	*	*	*	6	6	6.2	6.5	5.4	5.7
Skin Disease	*	*	*	*	common	common	*	*	*	*
Discharging Ears	*	*	*	*	1	1	1	1.2	1	1
Enlarged Adenoids	*	*	*	*	4.7	4.4	4.7	4.9	4	6
Rickets	*	*	*	*	*	*	*	*	1.6	1
Tuberculosis(overt)	*	*	*	*	*	*	*	*	*	*
Heart Disorders	*	*	*	*	*	*	*	1.4	1.7	1.8

Source: *Annual Reports of the Scottish Board of Health.*   *No record   Recorded as percentage of children examined

APPENDIX VI (ii)

The School Health Service: Medical Examinations, 1929–1938

	1929	1930	1931	1932	1933	1934	1935	1936	1937	1938
School Population	762,132	816,004	819,537	831,792	827,311	841,991	823,445	808,110	795,079	782,872
Pupils Inspected	254,044	263,334	248,835	247,272	243,345	247,342	236,923	243,240	231,812	233,306
Proportion Inspected	33.33%	32.27%	30.30%	29.72%	29.41%	29.37%	28.77%	30.09%	29.15%	29.80%
Nutrition	6.1	6	6.2	5.5	5.7	5.5	5.5	5.1	5.5	5.3
Head Lice	1.8	1.7	1.4	1.3	1.2	1	0.9	0.9	1.1	0.8
Other Vermin	0.8	0.7	0.5	0.5	0.3	0.2	0.2	0.1	0.1	0.1
Hearing Loss	1	0.9	1	0.8	0.8	0.8	0.8	0.8	0.8	0.8
Poor Sight (specs)	5.8	5.4	4.9	4.9	4.4	4.3	4.4	4.7	4.7	4.7
Skin Disease	3.7	3	2.8	2.9	3	2.9	2.7	3	2.8	2.9
Discharging Ears	2.4	2	2.1	2.3	0.9	0.9	0.9	0.9	0.9	0.9
Enlarged Adenoids	3.9	3.8	3.8	3.5	3.4	3.3	3.3	3.2	3.1	3.3
Rickets	1.6	1.4	1.3	1.4	1.2	1	1.1	1.1	0.9	0.8
Tuberculosis(overt)	0.1	0.1	0.1	0	0.01	0.02	0.02	0.04	0.03	0.03
Heart Disorders	1.9	1.8	2	2	1.9	2.2	2	2.1	1.9	1.8

Recorded as percentage of children examined

Source: *Annual Reports of the Department of Health for Scotland.*

APPENDIX VII

The School Health Service: Dental Examinations

	1929	1930	1931	1932	1933	1934	1935	1936	1937	1938
School Population	762,132	816,004	819,537	831,792	827,311	841,991	823,445	808,110	795,079	782,872
Number Examined	254,044	263,334	248,835	247,272	243,345	247,342	236,923	243,240	231,812	233,306
Dental Decay-number	187,203	188,547	180,654	178,035	172,531	173,139	165,324	171,484	165,745	165,647
Dental Decay	74%	72%	73%	72%	71%	70%	70%	71%	72%	71%
Number Treated	113,325	125,338	135,490	150,000	146,389	143,819	134601	152,670	146,491	149,920
Proportion Treated	61%	66%	75%	84%	85%	83%	81%	89%	88%	90%

Recorded as percentage of children examined

Source: Annual Reports of the Department of Health for Scotland.

Bibliography

Archival Sources

British Medical Association   Minutes of Branches and Divisions in Scotland
Edinburgh University   Lothian Health Board Papers
Glasgow University   Hetherington Papers
Public Record Office:
PRO CAB 26/1 HAC 3rd: 2   (Proposal of Ministry of Health for Scotland)
PRO CAB 21/2032 (CP (45) 205)   (Presentation of Bevan's nationalisation plan)
PRO CAB 129/5 CP (45) 345   (Separate NHS for Scotland)
PRO MH 80/24   (Morant's plan for medical services)
PRO CAB 24/284 CP 77 (39)   (Forecast of air-raid casualties)
PRO CAB 27/659 EHO 1 (39) 2   (Wartime ambulance services)
PRO CAB 87/13 PR (43) 52   (Secretary of State's plan for Scotland)
Royal College of Physicians of Edinburgh   Notes for a History of the College (1838)
   Physicians Inquiry Papers (1851)
National Archives of Scotland:
NAS HH/65/24   (Highlands and Islands Medical Service)
NAS HH/65/25   (Highlands and Islands Medical Service)
NAS HH 1/469   (Consultative Council for Scotland)
NAS HH 1/526   (Reorganisation of Scottish Office)
NAS HH 1/787   (NHS (Scotland) Act delayed)
NAS HH 1/791   (Letter: Collins to Chancellor)
NAS HH 3/20   (Incapacitating Sickness)
NAS HH 45/61   (Gilmour Committee on Scottish Office)
NAS HH 61/787   (Legislation for Maternity Services)
NAS HH 65/50   (Rejection of Cave Committee)
NAS HH 65/549   (Regionalisation of hospitals)
NAS HH 1/467   (Equality of hospitals)
NAS HH 1/469   (Separate Ministry for Scotland)
NAS HH 1/787   (Collins to PM: 'Scottish nationalism')
NAS HH 1/791   (Collins to Chancellor: 'Scottish share')
NAS HH 101/2   (Presentation of Hetherington Report)

Annual Reports and Minutes

British Medical Association
General Assembly of the Church of Scotland
Royal College of Physicians of Edinburgh
Royal College of Surgeons of Edinburgh
Royal College of Physicians and Surgeons of Glasgow
Royal College of Physicians of London
Minutes of the Scottish Board of Health
Minutes of Evidence, Committee on Scottish Health Services

Diaries and Private Papers in Private Hands

Sir Douglas Haddow, KCB
Ekkeharde von Kuenssberg, CBE
James Williamson, CBE

RECORDED INTERVIEWS   Archive of the Royal College of Physicians of Edinburgh
Dr. I. D. Campbell   Hon. Physician to the Queen Lt. Col. RAMC
   Chief Administrative Medical Officer, Lothian Region
Dr. C. Clayson CBE   Consultant Physician (Tuberculosis)
   Chairman, Scottish Council on Postgraduate Education
Dr. C. D. Falconer   Scottish Secretary, British Medical Association Consultant Surgeon,
   Singapore
J. Ford   Registrar General for Scotland
Prof. J. O. Forfar, OBE MC   Professor of Child Life and Health, Edinburgh
   President, British Paediatric Association.
Dr. Constance Forsyth   Consultant Paediatrician, Dundee
Prof. M. Fraser   Professor of Paediatrics, Baroda Medical College, India
R. B. Fraser, CB   Cabinet Office
   Secretary, Scottish Home and Health Department
Sir Norman Graham   Private Secretary to the Secretary of State for Scotland
   Assistant Secretary, Department of Health for Scotland
Dr. Joyce Grainger   Consultant Physician, Edinburgh
Ekkeharde von Kuenssberg, CBE   General Practitioner
   President Royal College of General Practitioners
Lord Kilpatrick   President, General Medical Council
   President, British Medical Association
   Professor of Medicine, Leicester
Prof. R. M. Lee   Professor of Clinical Pharmacology, Edinburgh
Dr. C. P. Lowther   Consultant Geriatrician, Edinburgh
Dr. A. Macewan   General Practitioner, Dunfermline
Dr. James McHarg   Consultant Psychiatrist, Dundee
Dr. J. C. G. Mercer   General Practitioner, East Lothian
R. Moore, CB   Ombudsman, Scotland
   Secretary, Eastern Regional Hospital Board
Margaret Orr   Senior Nursing Officer,
   Western General Hospital, Edinburgh
R. Passmore   Col., Indian Medical Service
   Reader in Physiology, Edinburgh
A. L. Rennie, CB   Private Secretary to the Secretary of State for Scotland
   Secretary, Scottish Home and Health Department
Elisabeth Shaw   Matron, Edinburgh Royal Infirmary
J. Smith, OBE   Col., RAMC
   Deputy Chief Medical Officer,
   Scottish Home and Health Department
Prof. J. Williamson, CBE   Professor of Geriatric Medicine, Edinburgh
   President, British Geriatric Society

Unpublished Theses and Lectures

H. Jones   *The Administration of National Health Insurance in Scotland*, MA (Hons.) Dissertation,
   Edinburgh, 1988
A. M. Keane   *Mental Health Policy in Scotland 1908–1960*, Thesis (Ph.D.), Edinburgh, 1988

J. W. R. Mitchell   *The Evolution and Consolidation of Scottish Central Administration.* Thesis (D.Phil.), Oxford, 1989

S. Stacy   *The Ministry of Health, 1919–1929*, Thesis (D.Phil.), Oxford, 1985

P. K. Underhill   *Science, Professionalism and the Development of Medical Education in England*, Thesis (Ph.D.) Edinburgh, 1987

J. Burnet   'A Context for Boyd Orr: Glasgow Corporation and the Food of the Poor', International Committee on Research into European Food History, Aberdeen, September 1997

C. Lawrence   'Edward Jenner's Jockey Boots and the Great Tradition in English Medicine', Society for the Social History of Medicine, Glasgow, July 1999

Parliamentary Papers and Official Reports

Report on the Sanitary Conditions of the Labouring Population of Scotland (Edinburgh, 1842)

Report of the Inquiry into the Condition of the Crofters and Cottars of the Highlands and Islands of Scotland, 1884, Cmd. 3980 (the Napier Report)

Royal Commission on Physical Training (Scotland), 1903, Cd. 1507

Report of the Interdepartmental Committee on Physical Deterioration, 1904, Cd. 2175

Report of the Royal Commission on the Poor Laws and Relief of Distress, 1909 Cd. 4499

Report of the Poor Law (Scotland) Commission, 1909, Cd. 4922

Report of the Royal Commission on the Poor Laws and Relief of Distress (Scottish Report), 1909, Cd. 4620

Report of the Board of Education, 1909, Cd. 4566

Report of the Royal Commission on the Poor Laws and Relief of Distress (Evidence Relating to Scotland), 1910, Cd. 4978

Report of the Royal Commission on the Poor Laws and Relief of Distress (Condition of Children in Scotland), 1910, Cd. 5075

Report of the Highlands and Islands Medical Service Committee, 1912, Cd. 6559 (the Dewer Report)

Report of the Royal Commission on the Housing of the Industrial Population of Scotland Rural and Urban, 1917, Cd. 8731

Report of the Committee on Working Classes Cost of Living, 1918, Cmd. 1918

A Scheme of Medical Services for Scotland, 1920, Cmd. 1039 (the MacAlister Report)

The Future Provision of Medical and Allied Services, 1920, Cmd. 693 (the Dawson Report)

Interim Report of the Committee on Smoke and Noxious Vapours Abatement, HMSO, 1920

Report of the Ministry of Health Voluntary Hospital Committee, HMSO, 1921 (the Cave Report)

Report on the Voluntary Hospitals Accommodation in England and Wales, 1925, Cmd. 2486 (the Onslow Report)

Report of the Royal Commission on National Health Insurance, 1926, Cmd. 2596

Report of the Hospital Services (Scotland) Committee, HMSO, 1926 (the Mackenzie Report)

Report of the Joint Committee of the Board of Education and the Board of Control on Mental Deficiency, HMSO, 1929

Report of the Committee on Local Expenditure (Scotland), 1932, Cmd. 4201 (the Lovat Report)

Report of the Committee on Local Expenditure (England and Wales), 1932, Cmd. 4200

Report on Hospital Services, HMSO, 1933 (the Walker Report)

Report of the Inter-Departmental Committee on Food Laws, 1934, Cmd. 4564

Report of the Departmental Committee on Sterilisation, 1934, Cmd. 4485

Report of the Committee on Scottish Health Services (Interim Report), HMSO, 1934

Report on Maternal Mortality and Morbidity in Scotland, HMSO, 1935

Report of the Committee on Scottish Health Services, 1936, Cmd. 5204 (the Cathcart Report)

Report of the Committee on Social Insurance and Allied Services, 1942, Cmd. 6404 (the Beveridge Report)

Report of the Committee on Post-War Hospital Problems in Scotland, 1943, Cmd. 6472 (the Hetherington Report)

Report of the Interdepartmental Committee on Medical Schools, HMSO, 1944
A National Health Service, 1944, Cmd. 6502
Annual Reports of the Highlands and Islands Medical Service Committee
Annual Reports of the Highlands and Islands Medical Service Board
Annual Reports of the Scottish Board of Health
Annual Reports of the Department of Health for Scotland
Annual Reports of the Registrar General for Scotland
Annual Reports of the Registrar General for England and Wales
Annual Reports of the Chief Medical Officer of the Ministry of Health
Health Bulletins of the Chief Medical Officer for Scotland

Other Published Reports

Royal College of Physicians of Edinburgh *Statement Regarding the Existing Deficiency of Medical Practitioners in the Highlands and Islands* (Edinburgh, 1852)
Russell, J. B. *Report on Uncertified Deaths in Glasgow* (Glasgow, 1876)
Paton, N. Dunlop, J. Inglis, E. *A Study of the Diet of the Labouring Classes in Edinburgh* (Edinburgh, 1901)
Chalmers, A. K. *Proceedings of the National Conference on Infant Mortality* (Liverpool, 1912)
Medical Research Council *Some Facts Concerning Nutrition for the Guidance of those Engaged in the Administration of Food to Famine Stricken Districts*, HMSO, 1910
Cathcart, E. P. Boyd Orr, J. *The Energy Requirements of Recruits in Training* (HMSO, 1919)
Leighton, G. McKinlay, P. *Milk Consumption and the Growth of School Children* (HMSO, 1930)
British Medical Association *A General Medical Service for the Nation*, 1930
Cathcart, E. P. Murray, A.M.T. *A Study on Nutrition: An Inquiry into the Diets of 154 Families in St. Andrews* (HMSO, 1931)
Cathcart, E. P. Murray, A.M.T. *A Dietary Survey* (HMSO, 1936)
British Hospitals Association *Report on the Voluntary Hospitals Commission*, 1937
Cathcart, E. P. Murray, A.M.T. *Studies in Nutrition: An Inquiry into the Diet of Families in the Highlands and Islands of Scotland* (HMSO, 1940)
Political and Economic Planning *Report on the British Health Services*, 1941
British Medical Association *Interim Report of the Medical Planning Commission*, 1942
Rowett Research Institute *Family Diet and Health in Pre-War Britain*, 1955
King Edward Hospital Fund for London *Trends and Prospects for Health*, 1989

Periodicals and Newspapers

British Medical Journal
Blackwood's Magazine
Bulletin of the Royal College of Physicians and Surgeons of Glasgow
Dundee Advertiser
The Economic History Review
Edinburgh Medical Journal
Fortnightly Review
Glasgow Herald
Glasgow Medical Journal
Hansard
Health Bulletin
History Workshop Journal
Journal of Physiology
Journal of the Royal Society of Medicine
Journal of Social History

Kölnische Zeitung
Lancet
Maternity and Child Welfare
Medical History
Nature
Past and Present
Population Studies
Practitioner
Proceedings of the Royal College of Physicians of Edinburgh
Quarterly Review
Scotsman
Scottish Economic and Social History
Scottish Historical Review
Sociology Review
Times
Transactions of the Edinburgh Obstetric Society
Transactions of the Gaelic Society of Inverness
Transactions of the Medico-Chirurgical Society of Edinburgh
Vesalius

Articles in Journals

Anderson, M. Morse, D. J. 'High Fertility, High Emigration, Low Nuptialty: Adjustment Processes in Scotland's Demographic Experience', *Population Studies*, xlvii, 1993, pp. 324–343

Blackden, S. 'From Physician's Enquiry to Dewer Report: A Survey of Medical Services in the West Highlands and Islands of Scotland', *Proceedings of the Royal College of Physicians of Edinburgh*, Part I, xxviii, 1998, pp. 51–66; Part II, xxviii, 1998, pp. 207–217

Brown, J. 'Charles Booth and Labour Colonies', *The Economic History Review*, xxi, 1968, pp. 349–360

Brown, J. 'Scottish and English Land Registration', *Scottish Historical Review*, xlvii, 1968, pp. 72–85

Brown, J. 'Social Judgements', *The Economic History Review*, xxiv, 1971, pp. 106–113

Bryden, L. 'The First War: Healthy or Hungry?' *History Workshop Journal*, xxiv, 1987, pp. 139–157

Caldwell, J. 'Paths to Lower Fertility', *BMJ*, cccix, 1999, pp. 985–987

Cameron, E. A. 'Land Raids and Land Raiders in the Scottish Highlands, 1886–1914', *Scottish Economic and Social History*, xvii, 1997, pp. 43–64

Cathcart, E. P. 'Preventive Medicine and Public Health', *Glasgow Medical Journal*, cxix, 1933, pp. 185–191

Chalmers, A. K. 'Our Provision for Treating the Sick', *Glasgow Medical Journal*, cxviii (1932), pp. 1–15

Collings, J. S. 'General Practice in England Today', *Lancet*, i, 1950, pp. 555–585

Craig, R. W. 'Discussion of the Report of the Departmental Committee on Scottish Health Services', *Transactions of the Medico-Chirurgical Society of Edinburgh*, 1936, pp. 1–24

Crofton, J. 'The NHS Revolution: Before and After', *Proceedings of the Royal College of Physicians of Edinburgh*, xxviii, 1998, pp. 576–584

Crosfil, M. 'The Highlands and Islands Medical Service', *Vesalius*, ii, 1996, pp. 118–125

Davidson, A. 'The Contribution of the Emergency Medical Service to Medicine and Surgery in Scotland', *Edinburgh Medical Journal*, xlix, 1942, pp. 553–567

Dupree, M. W. Crowther, A. 'A Profile of the Medical Profession in Scotland', *Bulletin of the History of Medicine*, lxv, 1991, pp. 209–233

Fairbairn, J. S. 'Changes in Thought in Half a Century of Obstetrics', *Transactions of the Edinburgh Obstetrical Society*, xciv, pp. 63–82

Findlay, L.   'The Aetiology of Rickets; A Clinical and Experimental Study', *BMJ*, i, 1908, pp. 13–17

Findlay, L.   'A Review of the Work Done by the Glasgow School on the Aetiology of Rickets', *Lancet*, i, 1922, pp. 825–831

Gillanders, F.   'The West Highland Economy', *Transactions of the Gaelic Society of Inverness*, 1962, p. 250–261

Honigsbaum, F.   'The Evolution of the NHS', *BMJ*, xxxi, 1990, pp. 694–699

Horder, Lord   'Medicine and Old Ethicks', *BMJ*, i, 1924, pp. 485–491

Horder, Lord   'Eugenics and the Doctor', *BMJ*, ii, 1933, pp. 1057–1060

Horder, Lord   'The Approach to Medicine', *Lancet*, i, 1939, pp. 913–918

Holmes, G. I.   'Trial by TB', *Proceedings of the Royal College of Physicians of Edinburgh*, xxvii, 1997, pp. 1–53

Leitch, A. G.   'Two Men and a Bug: A Hundred Years of Tuberculosis in Edinburgh', *Proceedings of the Royal College of Physicians of Edinburgh*, xxvi, 1996, pp. 295–308

MacLennan, W. J. Sellars, W.I.   'Ageing Through the Ages', *Proceedings of the Royal College of Physicians of Edinburgh*, xxix, 1999, pp. 72–75

Mackay, H. M.   'The Etiology of Rickets: Some Experiences based on Work in Vienna', *Maternity and Child Welfare*, viii, 1923, pp. 250–255

Manchester, K.   'Tuberculosis in Antiquity and Interpretation', *Medical History*, xxviii, 1984, pp. 162–173

Mayhew, M.   'The 1930s Nutritional Controversy', *Journal of Contemporary History*, xxiii, 1988, pp. 445–464

Means, J. H.   'Medicine and the State', *Edinburgh Medical Journal*, 1953, clxx, pp. 56–60

Mellanby, E.,   'The Part Played by an Accessory Factor in the Production of Experimental Rickets', *Journal of Physiology*, lii, 1918, pp. xi–xii and lii–liv

Montagu, J. D.   'Length of Life in the Ancient World', *Journal of the Royal Society of Medicine*, dxxxvii, 1994, pp. 25–26

Paton, D. N. Findlay, L. Watson, A.   'Observations on the Cause of Rickets', *BMJ*, ii, 1918, pp. 625–626

Paton, D. N.   'Relationship of Science and Nutrition', *Edinburgh Medical Journal*, xxx, 1919, pp. 1–12

Paton, D. N.   'Physiology: The Institutes of Medicine', *Glasgow Medical Journal*, xii, 1920, pp. 321–329

Simmons, H. G.   'Explaining Social Policy: the English Mental Deficiency Act of 1913', *Journal of Social History*, xi, 1978, pp. 386–403

Smith, D. Nicolson, M.   'Chemical Physiology Versus Biochemistry: The Glaswegian Opposition to Melanby's Theory of Rickets', *Proceedings of the Royal College of Physicians of Edinburgh*, viii, 1989, pp. 51–60

Smith, D. Nicolson, M.   'The Glasgow of Paton, Findlay and Cathcart: Conservative Thought in Chemical Physiology, Nutrition and Public Health', *Social Studies in Science*, xix, 1989, pp. 195–238

Smith, J.   'The Scottish Air Ambulance Service', *The Practitioner*, clxx, 1953, pp. 67–74

Soloway, R.   'The Perfect Contraceptive: Eugenics and Birth Control in Britain and America', *Journal of Contemporary History*, iv, 1995, p. 639

Tredgold, A. F.   'Heredity and Environment in Regard to Social Reform', *Quarterly Review*, cccxix, 1913, pp. 344–383

Tully, A.   'A Study of the Diet and Economic Conditions of Artisan Families in Glasgow', *Glasgow Medical Journal*, ci, 1924, pp. 1–13

Webster, C.   'Hungry or Healthy Thirties?', *History Workshop Journal*, xiii, 1982, pp. 111–129

Webster, C.   'Health, Welfare and Unemployment During the Depression', *Past and Present*, cix, 1985, pp. 204–230

Whatley, C. A.   'Women and the Economic Transformation of Scotland', *Scottish Economic and Social History*, xiv, 1994, pp. 19–40

Wright, J. H. 'Current Topics', *Glasgow Medical Journal*, cxx, 1933, pp. 135–37
Young, J. 'The Universities and the Nation's Health', *Transactions of the Edinburgh Obstetrical Society*, xciv, 1933, pp. 1–19
Young, J. 'The University and the Public Health Services', *Edinburgh Medical Journal*, 1, 1943, pp. 474–490

Memoirs, Biographies and Autobiographies

Aldred, G. *John Maclean* (Glasgow, 1940)
Allen, B. *Sir Robert Morant: A Great Civil Servant* (London, 1934)
Blake, R. Louis, W.R. (eds.) *Churchill* (Oxford, 1996)
Boyd Orr, J. *As I Recall* (London, 1966)
Brivati, B. *Aneurin Bevan, 1897–1960* (London, 1997)
Brown, G. *Maxton* (Edinburgh, 1886)
Campbell, J. *Nye Bevan* (London, 1987)
Clark, R. *J.B.S: The Life and Work of J.B.S. Haldane* (London, 1968)
Coates, T. *Lord Rosebery* (London, 1900)
Coote, C. *A Companion of Honour: the Story of Walter Elliot* (London, 1965)
Cox, A. *Among the Doctors* (London, 1950)
Dugdale, B. *Arthur James Balfour* (London, 1936)
Dunnett, A. *Among Friends* (London, 1984)
Elletson, D. H. *The Chamberlains* (London, 1966)
Foot, M. *Aneurin Bevan* (London, 1973)
Garry, R. C. *Life in Physiology* (Glasgow, 1992)
Girdwood, R. *Travels With A Stethoscope* (Edinburgh, 1991)
Grigg, J. *Lloyd George: The People's Champion* (London, 1978)
Harris, J. *William Beveridge* (London, 1977)
Hill, Lord *On Both Sides of the Hill* (London, 1964)
Horder, M. *The Little Genius* (London, 1966)
James, R. *Rosebery* (London, 1963)
Jenkins, R. *Gladstone* (London, 1995)
Johnston, T. *Memories* (London, 1952)
Laugharne, P. *Aneurin Bevan: A Parliamentary Odyssey* (Liverpool, 1996)
Lee, Jenny *The Great Journey* (London, 1963)
Lovell, R. *Churchill's Doctor: A Biography of Lord Moran* (London, 1992)
Lubbock, D. *The Boyd Orr View from the Old World to the New* (Aberdeen, 1992)
Marquand, D. *Ramsay Macdonald* (London, 1997)
Monkton-How, R. *The Health Service versus the Family Doctor* (London, 1972)
Morgan, K. Morgan, J. *Portrait of a Progressive: The Political Career of Christopher Addison* (Oxford, 1980)
Morgan, K. *Bevan, Architect of the NHS* (Oxford, 1991)
Pottinger, G. *The Secretaries of State for Scotland* (Edinburgh, 1979)
Robertson, E. *Glasgow's Doctor: James Burn Russell* (East Linton, 1998)
Small, H. *Florence Nightingale: Avenging Angel* (London, 1998)
Somerville, A. *The Autobiography of a Working Man* (London, 1848)
Sykes, C. *Nancy: The Life of Lady Astor* (London, 1979)
Walker, G. *Thomas Johnston* (Manchester, 1988)
Watson, F. *Dawson of Penn* (London, 1950)
Williamson, P. *Stanley Baldwin* (Cambridge, 1999)
Zebel, S. *Balfour: A Political Biography* (Cambridge, 1973)

Histories of Institutions

Andrews, J. Smith, I. *Let There Be Light: Gartnavel Royal Hospital* (Edinburgh, 1993)

Bartrip, P. *Themselves Writ Large: The BMA, 1832–1966* (London, 1996)

Cameron, H. C. *Mr. Guy's Hospital* (London, 1954)

Catford, E. *The Royal Infirmary of Edinburgh, 1929–1979* (Edinburgh, 1984)

Clark-Kennedy, A. *The London* (London, 1963)

Cooke, A. *A History of the Royal College of Physicians of London* (Oxford, 1972)

Cope, Z. *The Royal College of Surgeons of England: A History* (London, 1959)

Craig, W. S. *History of the Royal College of Physicians of Edinburgh* (Edinburgh, 1976)

Crawford, D. G. *Roll of the Indian Medical Service* (London, 1930)

Dow, D. *Paisley Hospitals* (Glasgow, 1986)

Dow, D. *The Rotten Row: A History of the Glasgow Royal Maternity Hospital, 1834–1984* (Edinburgh, 1984)

Eastwood, M. Jenkinson, A. *A History of the Western General Hospital* (Edinburgh, 1995)

Gibson, J. *The Thistle and the Crown: A History of the Scottish Office* (Edinburgh, 1985)

Gosden, P. *The Friendly Societies in England, 1815–75* (Manchester, 1961)

Grant, Sir A. *The Story of the University of Edinburgh* (London, 1884)

Gray, J. A. *The Edinburgh City Hospital* (East Linton, 1999)

Grey-Turner, E. Sutherland, F. *History of the British Medical Association* (London, 1982)

Guthrie, D. *The Royal Edinburgh Hospital for Sick Children* (Edinburgh, 1960)

Hull, A. Geyer-Kordesch, J. *The Shaping of the Medical Profession: The History of the Royal College of Physicians and Surgeons of Glasgow, 1858–1999* (London, 1999)

Levitt, I. *The Scottish Office: Depression and Reconstruction, 1919–1959* (Edinburgh, 1992)

Mackenzie, T. C. *The Story of a Scottish Voluntary Hospital* (Inverness, 1946)

Masson, A. H. *History of the Blood Transfusion Service in Edinburgh* (Edinburgh, 1998)

Tait, H. P. *A Doctor and Two Policemen: The History of the Edinburgh Public Health Department* (Edinburgh, 1997)

Other Secondary Sources

Abel-Smith, B. *The Hospitals* (London, 1964)

Abel-Smith, B. *The Philosophy of Welfare* (London, 1987)

Addison, C. *Politics From Within* (London, 1924)

Addison, P. *The Road to 1945* (London, 1994)

Addison, P. *Churchill on the Home Front, 1900–1955* (London, 1995)

Aldcroft, D. *The Inter-war Economy: Britain, 1919–1939* (London, 1970)

Alison, W. P. *Observations on the Management of the Poor in Scotland and its Effects on the Health of the Great Towns* (Edinburgh, 1840)

Alison, W. P. *Remarks on the Report of Her Majesty's Commissioners on the Poor in Scotland Presented to Parliament in 1844* (Edinburgh, 1844)

Allsop, J. *Health Policy and the National Health Service* (London, 1984)

Anderson, M. (ed.) *British Population History* (Cambridge, 1996)

Anderson, R. *Education and Opportunity in Victorian Scotland* (Edinburgh, 1989)

Ashford, D. *The Emergence of the Welfare States* (Oxford, 1986)

Ballantyne, J. *Manual of Ante-natal Pathology and Hygiene* (Edinburgh, 1904)

Begg, T. *Housing Policy in Scotland* (Edinburgh, 1996)

Bevan, A. *In Place of Fear* (London, 1952)

Booth, C. *Life and Labour of the People of London* (London, 1903)

Booth, W. *In Darkest England* (London, 1890)

Bowie, J. A. *The Future of Scotland* (Edinburgh, 1939)

Bowley, A. L. *Wages and Income* (Cambridge, 1977)

Boyd, D. *Amulets to Isotopes: A History of Medicine in Caithness* (Edinburgh, 1998)

Boyd Orr, J. *Food, Health and Income* (London, 1937)
Boyd Orr, J. *Family Diet and Health in Pre-war Britain* (London, 1955)
Braithwaite, W. *Lloyd George's Ambulance Wagon* (London, 1957)
Brendon, V. *The Victorian Age* (London, 1996)
Briggs, A. *Victorian People: A Reassessment of Persons and Themes* (London, 1996)
Brooke, S. *Reform and Reconstruction* (Manchester, 1995)
Brotherston, J. *Observations on the Public Health Movement in Scotland* (London, 1952)
Brown, A. McCrone, D. Paterson, L. *Politics and Society in Scotland* (London, 1996)
Brown, J. *The British Welfare State* (Oxford, 1995)
Brown, S. J. *Thomas Chalmers and the Godly Commonwealth* (Oxford, 1982)
Buchan, W. *Domestic Medicine or the Family Physician* (Edinburgh, 1769)
Burnett, J. *Plenty and Want: A Social History of Diet in England from 1815 to the Present Day* (London, 1966)
Bynum, W. F. Porter, R. (eds.) *William Hunter and the Eighteenth Century Medical World* (Cambridge, 1985)
Cairncross, A. K. (ed.) *The Scottish Economy: A Statistical Account of Scottish Life* (Cambridge, 1954)
Cameron, C. Lush, A. Meara, G. *Disinherited Youth* (Edinburgh, 1943)
Campbell, R. H. *The Rise and Fall of Scottish Industry, 1707–1939* (Edinburgh, 1980)
Carlyle, T. *Chartism* (Boston, 1840)
Carr-Saunders, A. *The Population Problem: A Study in Evolution* (London, 1922)
Cathcart, E. P. *The Human Factor in Industry* (London, 1928)
Cathcart, E. P. Murray, A.M.T. *A Study in Nutrition* (London, 1940)
Cave, R. A. *The Scottish Poor Law, 1745–1845* (Edinburgh, 1981)
Chalmers, A. K. *Public Health Administration in Glasgow* (Glasgow, 1905)
Chalmers, A. K. *The Health of Glasgow, 1818–1925* (Glasgow, 1930)
Checkland, O. *Philanthropy in Victorian Scotland* (Edinburgh, 1980)
Checkland, O. Lamb, M. (eds.) *Health Care as Social History: The Glasgow Case* (Aberdeen, 1982)
Checkland, O. Checkland, S. *Industry and Ethos: Scotland, 1832–1914* (Edinburgh, 1989)
Checkland, S. *British Public Policy, 1776–1939* (Cambridge, 1985)
Cherry, S. *Medical Services and the Hospitals in Britain, 1860–1939* (Cambridge, 1996)
Clarke, J. S. *An Epic of Municipalisation* (Glasgow, 1928)
Clyde, R. *From Rebel To Hero* (Edinburgh, 1995)
Cole, G. D. H. Cole, M. T. *The Condition of Britain* (London, 1937)
Collins, K. *Go and Learn: The International Story of Jews and Medicine in Scotland* (Aberdeen, 1988)
Conant, T. B. *Harvard Case Histories in Experimental Science* (Boston, 1957)
Cowan, R. *Vital Statistics of Glasgow* (Edinburgh, 1838)
Craig, D. *On the Crofter's Trail* (London, 1997)
Craig, W. S. *Child and Adolescent Life in Health and Disease* (Edinburgh, 1946)
Crewe, F. A. E. *Organic Inheritance in Man* (Edinburgh, 1927)
Curry, J. R. *The Mustering of Medical Service in Scotland, 1914–1919* (Edinburgh, 1922)
Daunton, M. *Progress and Poverty* (Oxford, 1995)
Davidson, S. Passmore, R. *Human Disease and Dietetics* (Edinburgh, 1975)
Davis, J. *A History of Britain, 1885–1939* (London, 1999)
Daunton, M. *Progress and Poverty* (Oxford, 1995)
Day, J. *Public Administration in the Highlands and Islands of Scotland* (London, 1918)
Devine, T. M. Mitchison, R. (eds.) *People and Society in Scotland*, i (Edinburgh, 1988)
Devine, T. M. *The Great Highland Famine* (Edinburgh, 1988)
Devine, T. M. (ed.) *Improvement and Enlightenment* (Edinburgh, 1989)
Devine, T. M. (ed.) *Conflict and Stability in Scottish Society* (Edinburgh, 1990)
Devine, T. M. (ed.) *Irish Immigration and Scottish Society in the Nineteenth and Twentieth Centuries* (Edinburgh, 1991)

Devine, T. M. (ed.)   *Scottish Emigration and Scottish Society* (Edinburgh, 1992)

Devine, T. M. (ed.)   *Scottish Elites* (Edinburgh, 1994)

Devine, T. M.   *Clanship to Crofters' War* (Manchester, 1994)

Devine, T. M.   *Exploring the Scottish Past* (Edinburgh, 1995)

Devine, T. M. Finlay, R. (eds.)   *Scotland in the 20th Century* (Edinburgh, 1996)

Devine, T. M. Young, J. R. (eds.)   *Eighteenth Century Scotland* (East Linton, 1999).

Devine, T. M.   *The Scottish Nation* (London, 1999)

Dewey, P.   *War and Progress* (London, 1997)

Dickson, A. Treble, J (eds.)   *People and Society in Scotland*, iii (Edinburgh, 1992)

Digby, A. Bosanquet, N.   *Doctors and Patients in an Era of National Health Insurance and Private Practice, 1913–1938* (London, 1988)

Digby, A.   *Making a Medical Living* (Cambridge, 1994)

Digby, A.   *The Evolution of British General Practice* (Oxford, 1999)

Doig, A. Ferguson, J. P. S. Milne, I. A. M. Passmore, R. (eds.)   *William Cullen and the Eighteenth Century Medical World* (Edinburgh, 1993)

Donaldson, G.   *Scotland: The Shaping of a Nation* (Nairn, 1993)

Donnachie, I. Whatley, C. A.   *The Manufacture of Scottish History* (Edinburgh, 1992)

Donnachie, I. Harvie, C. Wood, I.   *Forward: Labour Politics in Scotland* (Edinburgh, 1989)

Dow, D.   *The Influence of Scottish Medicine* (Edinburgh, 1986)

Dubois, R. Dubois, J.   *The White Plague: Tuberculosis, Man and Society* (London, 1953)

Dyos, H. Wolff, M.   *The Victorian City* (London, 1973)

Eckstein, H.   *The English Health Service* (Harvard, 1958)

Eckstein, H.   *Pressure Group Politics* (London, 1987)

Eder, N.   *National Health Insurance and the Medical Profession* (London, 1982)

Fenton, A.   *The Turra Coo* (Aberdeen, 1989)

Fildes, V. Marks, L. Marland, H.   *Women and Children First* (London, 1992)

Ferguson, T.   *Scottish Social Welfare, 1864–1914* (Edinburgh, 1958)

Finlay, R.   *A Partnership for Good?* (Edinburgh, 1997)

Finlayson, G.   *Citizen, State, and Social Welfare in Britain, 1830–1990* (Oxford, 1994)

Fisher, R. A.   *The Genetic Theory of Natural Selection* (London, 1930)

Flinn, M.   *Scottish Population History* (Cambridge, 1977)

Flinn, M. (ed.)   *Report on the Sanitary Condition of the Population of Great Britain by Edwin Chadwick 1842* (Edinburgh, 1965)

Floud, F.   *The People and the British Economy* (Oxford, 1997)

Fordyce, A.   *The Care of Infants and Children* (Edinburgh, 1911)

Foster, D.   *The Evolution of the British Welfare State* (London, 1984)

Fox, D. M.   *Health Policies and Health Politics: The British and American Experience* (Princeton, 1986)

Fraser, D.   *The Evolution of the British Welfare State* (London, 1984)

Fraser, D.   *Cities, Class and Communication: Essays in Honour of Asa Briggs* (London, 1950)

Fraser, W. H. Morris, R. (eds.)   *People and Society in Scotland, ii, 1830–1914* (Edinburgh, 1990)

Freemantle, F. E.   *The Health of the Nation* (London, 1927)

Fullerton, A. (ed.)   *Gazetteer of Scotland* (Glasgow, 1840)

Gallichan, W. M.   *Sterilisation of the Unfit* (London, 1929)

Geddes, Sir A.   *A Voice from the Grandstand* (Edinburgh, 1937)

Geddes, G.   *Statistics of Puerperal Sepsis and Allied Infectious Diseases* (Bristol, 1912)

Gilbert, B. B.   *The Evolution of National Insurance in Great Britain: The Origins of the Welfare State* (London, 1966)

Gilbert, B. B.   *British Social Policy* (London, 1970)

Godber, G.   *The Health Service: Past, Present and Future* (London, 1975)

Goodman, G.   *The State of the Nation: The Political Legacy of Aneurin Bevan* (London, 1997)

Gosden, P.   *Self-Help* (London, 1973)

Gosney, E. S. Popenoe, P.   *Sterilisation for Human Betterment* (London, 1929)

Green, M. E.   *Health in the Home* (London, 1927)

Guthrie, D. *Janus in the Doorway* (London, 1963)
Ham, C. *Health Policy in Britain* (London, 1992)
Hamilton, D. *The Healers* (Edinburgh, 1981)
Harris, R. *National Health Insurance* (London, 1945)
Harvie, C. *Scotland and Nationalism* (London, 1977)
Harvie, C. *No Gods and Precious Few Heroes* (Edinburgh, 1998)
Harvie, C. *Travelling Scot* (Argyll, 1999)
Henderson, D. *Highland Soldier* (Edinburgh, 1989)
Henrick, H. *Child Welfare: England, 1872–1989* (London, 1994)
Hodgkinson, R. *The Origins of the National Health Service* (London, 1967)
Honigsbaum, F. *Health, Happiness, and Security* (London, 1989)
Honigsbaum, F. *The Struggle for the Ministry of Health* (London, 1970)
Honigsbaum, F. *The Division in British Medicine* (London, 1979)
Horder, Lord *Health and a Day* (London, 1937)
Hunter, J. *The Making of the Crofting Community* (Edinburgh, 1976)
Hunter, J. *The Claim of Crofting* (Edinburgh, 1991)
Hunter, J. *A Dance Called America* (Edinburgh, 1994)
Hunter, J. *The Other Side of Sorrow: Nature and People in the Scottish Highlands* (Edinburgh, 1995)
Hutt, A. *The Condition of the Working Class in Britain* (London, 1933)
Jenkinson, J. *Scottish Medical Societies, 1731–1939* (Edinburgh, 1993)
Jewkes, J. Jewkes, S. *The Genesis of the National Health Service* (Oxford, 1962)
Johnston, T. *Our Scots Noble Families* (Glasgow, 1909)
Johnston, T. *The History of the Working Classes in Scotland* (Glasgow, 1920)
Jones, H. *Health and Society in Twentieth Century Britain* (London, 1994)
Jones, P. *Doctors and the BMA* (Farnborough, 1981)
Joshi, H. (ed.) *The Changing Population of Britain* (London, 1989)
Kamminga, H. Cunningham, A. (eds.) *The Science and Culture of Nutrition, 1840–1940* (London, 1995)
Kinloch J. Butt, J. *The History of the Scottish Co-operative Wholesale Society* (Glasgow, 1981)
Kiple, D. (ed.) *The Cambridge World History of Human Disease* (Cambridge, 1993)
Kitchen, A. H. Passmore, R. *The Scotsman's Food* (Edinburgh, 1949)
Knox, W. W. *Hanging By A Thread: The Scottish Cotton Industry* (Preston, 1995)
Knox, W. W. *Industrial Nation: Work, Culture and Society in Scotland, 1800 – Present* (Edinburgh, 1999)
Krige, J. Pestr, D. (eds.) *Science in the Twentieth Century* (Amsterdam, 1997)
Kuczynski, J., *Hunger and Work* (London, 1938)
Land, A. Lowe, R. Whiteside, R. *The Development of the Welfare State, 1939–1951* (London, 1992)
Langdon-Brown, W. *Thus We Are Men* (London, 1938)
Lawrence, C. *Medicine in the Making of Modern Britain, 1700–1920* (London, 1994)
Leneman, L. (ed.) *Perspectives in Scottish Social History* (Aberdeen, 1988)
Levitt, I. Smout, T. C. *The State of the Scottish Working Class in 1843* (Aberdeen, 1979)
Levitt, I. *Poverty and Welfare in Scotland, 1890–1948* (Edinburgh, 1988)
Levitt, I. *Government and Social Conditions in Scotland, 1845–1919* (Edinburgh, 1988)
Linklater, M. Dennison, R. *The Anatomy of Scotland* (Edinburgh, 1992)
Lowe, R. *The Welfare State in Britain since 1945* (London, 1983)
Lynch, M. (ed.) *Scotland, 1850–1979: Society, Politics and the Union* (London, 1993)
MacDougall, I. *Voices from the Hunger Marches. Personal Recollections by Scottish Hunger Marchers of the 1920s and 1930s* (Edinburgh, 1991)
Macfarlane, A. Mugford, M. *Birth Counts* (London, 1984)
McGonigle, G. M. Kirby, J. *Poverty and Public Health* (London, 1936)
Macgregor, A. *Public Health in Glasgow* (Edinburgh, 1967)
Macintosh, J. *Trends of Opinion about Public Health* (Oxford, 1953)

Mackenzie, W. L.   *The Health of School Children* (London, 1906)

Mackenzie, W. L.   *Health and Disease* (London, 1911)

Mackenzie, W. L.   *Scottish Mothers and Children* (Dunfermline, 1917)

McKibben, R.   *Classes and Cultures, 1918–1951* (Oxford, 1998)

McLachlan, G. (ed.)   *Improving the Common Weal* (Edinburgh, 1987)

Maclehose, A. (ed.)   *The Scotland of Our Sons* (London, 1937)

McNulty, A.   *The History of State Medicine in England* (London, 1948)

Marshall, T.   *The Population Problem* (London, 1938)

May, T.   *An Economic History of Britain, 1790–1990* (London, 1995)

Mazower, M.   *Dark Continent* (London, 1998)

Mellor, D. H.   *Science, Belief and Behaviour: Essays in Honour of R. B. Braithwaite* (Cambridge, 1980)

Meston, M. C. Sellar, W.D.H. Cooper, Lord   *The Scottish Legal Tradition* (Edinburgh, 1991)

Mitchell, B.   *British Historical Statistics* (Cambridge, 1988)

Mitchison, R.   *A History of Scotland* (London, 1982)

Mitchison, R.   *The Old Poor Law in Scotland* (Edinburgh, 2000)

Morgan, K.   *Consensus and Disunity* (Oxford, 1979)

Morgan, K.   *The People's Peace* (Oxford, 1990)

Morgan, K.   *Bevan: Architect of the NHS* (Oxford, 1991)

Mowatt, C.   *Britain Between the Wars* (London, 1968)

Muir, E.   *Scottish Journey* (Edinburgh, 1935)

Newman, C.   *The Evolution of Medical Education in the Nineteenth Century* (London, 1957)

Newman, G.   *The Health of the State* (London, 1907)

Newman, Sir G.   *The Building of a Nation's Health* (London, 1939)

Nicolls, Sir G.   *A History of the Scotch Poor Law* (London, 1856)

Novak, T.   *Poverty and the State; A Historical Sociology* (London, 1988)

O'Malley, C.   *The History of Medical Education* (Berkeley, 1970)

Orwell, G.   *The Road to Wigan Pier* (London, 1937)

Osler, W.   *The Principles and Practice of Medicine* (New York, 1892)

Pater, J.   *The Making of the National Health Service* (London, 1981)

Paterson, L.   *The Autonomy of Modern Scotland* (Edinburgh, 1994)

Perkins, H.   *The Rise of the Professional Society* (London, 1990)

Phillipson, N. T. Mitchison, R. (eds.)   *Scotland in the Age of Enlightenment* (Edinburgh, 1970)

Pope, R.   *War and Society in Britain, 1899–1948* (London, 1991)

Porter, D.   *Doctors, Politics and Society* (Amsterdam, 1993)

Porter, D. (ed.)   *The History of Public Health and the Modern State* (Amsterdam, 1994)

Porter, J. D. H. McAdam, K. P.   *Tuberculosis: Back to the Future* (Chichester, 1994)

Power, Sir D.   *Medicine in the British Isles* (New York, 1930)

Poynter, F. N. L.   *The Evolution in Medical Education in Britain* (London, 1966)

Richards, E. A.   *A History of the Highland Clearances* (London, 1985)

Robbins, K.   *The Eclipse of a Great Power* (London, 1994)

Ross, J.   *The National Health Service in Great Britain* (Oxford, 1952)

Rowntree, B. S.   *Poverty: A Study of Town Life* (London, 1902)

Royle, E.   *Modern Britain* (London, 1987)

Saleeby, C. W.   *Parenthood and Race Cultures* (New York, 1909)

Sanderson, M.   *Medical Services and the Hospitals in Britain, 1860–1939* (Cambridge, 1996)

Saul, S.   *The Myth of the Great Depression, 1873–1896* (London, 1969)

Seaman, L. C. B.   *Post-Victorian Britain, 1902–1951* (London, 1995)

Searle, G. R.   *Quest for National Efficiency* (Oxford, 1971)

Searle, G. R.   *Eugenics and Politics in Britain* (Leiden, 1976)

Searle, G. R.   *Science and History* (Leiden, 1976)

Searle, G. R.   *Country Before Party* (London, 1995)

Searle, G. R.   *Morality and the Market in Victorian Britain* (Oxford, 1998)

Skidelsky, R.   *Politicians and the Slump* (London, 1967).

Smith, F. *The People's Health, 1830–1910* (London, 1990)
Smout, T. C. (ed.) *The Search for Wealth and Stability* (London, 1979)
Smout, T. C. *A History of the Scottish People* (London, 1969)
Smout, T. C. *A Century of the Scottish People* (London, 1986)
Soloway, R. *Demography and Degeneration* (North Carolina, 1990)
Spring Rice, M. *Working Class Wives: Their Health and Condition* (London, 1939)
Stevenson, J. Cook, C. *The Slump* (London, 1974)
Stevenson, J. Cooke, C. *Britain in the Depression: Society and Politics, 1929–1939* (London, 1977)
Stevenson, J. *British Society, 1914–1945* (London, 1984)
Sutherland, I. (ed.) *Health Education* (London, 1979)
Taylor, A. J. P. *English History, 1914–1945* (Oxford, 1965)
Thane, P. *Foundations of the Welfare State* (London, 1996)
Thompson, F. (ed.) *The Cambridge Social History of Britain* (Cambridge, 1993)
Thomson, G. M. *Scotland, That Distressed Country* (Edinburgh, 1935)
Timmins, N. *The Five Giants* (London, 1995)
Titmuss, R. M. *Poverty and Population: A Factual Study of Contemporary Social Waste* (New York, 1985)
Titmuss, R. M. *The Philosophy of Welfare* (London, 1987)
Townsend, P. Davidson, N. (eds.) *The Black Report* (London, 1992)
Tranter, N. L. *British Population in the Twentieth Century* (London, 1996)
Tuchman, A. *Science, Medicine, and the State in Germany* (Oxford, 1993)
Waites, B. *A Class Society at War* (Leamington Spa, 1987)
Watkins, B. *The National Health Service: The First Phase* (London, 1978)
Watt, H. *Thomas Chalmers and the Disruption* (Edinburgh, 1943)
Webster, C. *Biology, Medicine and Society, 1840–1940* (Cambridge, 1981)
Webster, C. *The Health Services Since the War*, i (London, 1988)
Webster, C. *Aneurin Bevan on the National Health Service* (Oxford, 1991)
Webster, C. *The National Health Service: A Political History* (Oxford, 1998)
Webster, C. (ed.) *Caring for Health: History and Diversity* (Milton Keynes, 1993)
Whatley, C. A. *The Industrial Revolution in Scotland* (Cambridge, 1997)
White, A. *Efficiency and Empire* (London, 1901)
Whitehead, M. *The Health Divide* (London, 1992)
Williams, H. *A Century of Public Health in Britain* (London, 1932)
Winter, J. M. *The Great War and the British People* (London, 1985)
Withers, C. *Urban Highlanders* (East Linton, 1998)
Wrigley, W. Schofield, R. *The Population History of England* (Cambridge, 1989)
Wolfe, J. (ed.) *Government and Nationalism in Scotland* (Edinburgh, 1969)
Wordsworth, D. *Recollections of a Tour in Scotland* (Yale, 1997)

Index